The Psychology of

The Psychology of Nursing Care

Second edition

NEIL NIVEN

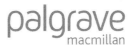

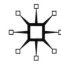

First edition 1994
Second edition 2006 published by
PALGRAVE MACMILLAN
Houndmills, Basingstoke, Hampshire RG21 6XS and
175 Fifth Avenue, New York, N.Y. 10010
Companies and representatives throughout the world

PALGRAVE MACMILLAN is the global academic imprint of the Palgrave
Macmillan division of St. Martin's Press, LLC and of Palgrave Macmillan Ltd.
Macmillan® is a registered trademark in the United States, United Kingdom
and other countries. Palgrave is a registered trademark in the European
Union and other countries.

ISBN–13: 978–1–4039–4217–3
ISBN–10: 1–4039–4217–X

This book is printed on paper suitable for recycling and made from fully
managed and sustained forest sources.

A catalogue record for this book is available from the British Library.

10   9   8   7   6   5   4   3   2   1
15   14   13   12   11   10   09   08   07   06

Printed in China

Neil Niven dedicated this book to Josephine.

This book is dedicated to the memory of its author, our father, Neil Niven, who sadly died in hospital at the end of 2005. Dad's writings on health psychology were an extremely important part of his life, and he continued to proof read and to correct this latest edition right up until the end. Dad always said that he became a health psychologist in order to help people. He was part of a generation who passionately believed that psychological theory should not be confined to academia or to a limited clinical context, but that it had a potential to enlighten and practically improve in all walks of life: that it should be available to everyone. The textbooks he wrote for healthcare professionals were very much a reflection of this. If this book is able to help even one person to better understand their job and their patients then he will have succeeded in a career-long undertaking. We would like to thank Lynda Thompson and all at Palgrave for their help in getting this book published.

Iona and Alex Niven
March 2006

Contents

List of Illustrations

List of Tables

List of Exercises

Acknowledgements

I would like to thank Bob Price for all his work on the conundrums at the beginning and end of each chapter. Jill Robinson for her help with the first edition. Jan Reed for her advice on nursing older people. (She points out that whilst there is a category of Paediatric Nursing there is none for nursing older people.) Sue Milner for information on current developments in the area of health promotion. Carolyn Hicks for comments, advice and most of all support. During my formative years teaching nurses I had invaluable advice from Rosemary Crow as external examiner on the BA Nursing, and of course thanks to my nursing colleagues, in particular Alison Hagel and Senga Bond, with respect to post-registration courses. Finally, thanks to Adrian Swales for the artwork.

Copyright

Preface

Over the last ten years since the first edition there have been quite a few developments in the psychology of nursing care and I hope the changes are reflected in this new edition. The aim of the book remains the same. As Jill Robinson said in her foreword to the first edition: 'What nursing courses and the texts that support them need to provide is an explication of those aspects of psychology which nurses are required to understand and utilise in any given nursing context in order to practise most effectively. *That* is the starting point in this text.'

There are some new chapters on community health psychology and decision making, as well as a reorganisation of the others into blocs that are more representative of the themes of the book. Within each chapter there are whole new sections and the research has been updated to represent recent findings. Another change is the inclusion of a series of 'conundrums' at the beginning and end of each chapter by Bob Price. I felt that scenarios should be presented at the start of the chapter and then be revisited at the end after the reader has, hopefully, taken on board some of the concepts presented in the text. I have not included any references to information available on the internet, the reason being that in five or ten years hence they will be out of date. However, I have set out as many web sources as I can on my site (www.neilniven.co.uk) which I can hopefully update when needed.

I first started lecturing on the BA Nursing course at what is now the University of Northumbria in 1977. At the time I had very little lecturing experience, so I consulted my former research supervisor N. E. Wetherick and asked him what constituted a good lecture. He said I must only try to get across one or, at the most, two main points. Looking at the contents of this book, it seems I have gone way over his limit, but on reflection there is only one central theme running right the way through the book: that the psychology of nursing care is all about the nurse's ability, and motivation, about trying to see things from other people's point of view – patients, clients and colleagues. Of course this is not easy to do but I hope that this book goes some way to making it easier.

Neil Niven

Introduction

If you happen to mention to someone who has never studied psychology that you are taking the subject as part of your nursing studies, you are likely to be met with two responses. The first is 'Psychology, eh? Bet you're analysing me, then,' and then, after you've explained a bit about the subject, the second response is 'Well, that sounds like common sense to me. Surely you don't have to be taught that?' The first response reflects the all too common view of psychology as a form of therapy used to make people better. Whilst some therapies are based on psychological principles, psychology has a much broader remit and can be defined as the 'science of human behaviour'. Psychology is similar to other sciences such as physics, chemistry and biology in that it also is based on a general set of methods, focusing on systematic observation and direct experimentation. We tend to be most familiar with the image of the scientist bending over his microscope and taking notes, yet the scientific method has been used to study other topics such as geography and archaeology as well. Just as the geographer would use a scientific approach to investigate the relationship of climate and natural resources with human culture, the same basic methods of science can be used by the psychologist to study many aspects of human behaviour. Different sciences employ different measuring devices and equipment but the methods they use are similar.

The comment that psychology is just common sense is another misconception. Consider the following well known sayings.

> Opposites attract.
> Haste makes waste.
> Many hands make light work.
> Time and tide wait for no man.
> Out of sight, out of mind.

In commonsense terms they all seem reasonable comments about the human condition. However, consider these other well known sayings.

> Birds of a feather flock together.
> He who hesitates is lost.

> Too many cooks spoil the broth.
> Don't cross your bridges before you come to them.
> Absence makes the heart grow fonder.

The second set of sayings seems to contradict the first, so which is correct? They all are. Sometimes opposites attract, and sometimes birds of a feather flock together – it depends on the circumstances. What psychology tries to do is to identify under what conditions opposites attract and under what conditions 'birds of a feather flock together'. By using the scientific method we can set up a study to investigate these sayings (see Chapter 2).

Exercise 1 *Understanding psychology*

You might like to ask a friend who hasn't studied psychology whether he or she thinks the following statements are true or false.

- Newborn babies do not really feel any pain.
- Women are more conforming and open to influence than men.
- The amount of time nurses spend talking to patients is directly related to the patients' sense of well-being.
- If you toss a coin and it comes up heads five times in a row, chances are that the next time you toss it it will be tails.
- It is always better to tell patients exactly what is going to happen to them.
- Intellectual ability declines in old age.
- Only some people dream every night.
- It usually takes many years to remedy strong irrational fears (for example, fear of needles, or of snakes).
- People who have emotional problems will always benefit from nurses who are willing to talk about their own experiences.

In fact, studies have found all these above statements to be false, and all these statements will be addressed in the text.

In order to investigate what constitutes a scientific approach to human behaviour, let us examine the suggestion that it is a good idea for nurses to reassure anxious patients by gently touching them on the arm whilst speaking to them. It might seem obvious that using touch to reassure patients is a good idea, but how do we go about finding out for sure?

The first step is to obtain a reasonably large sample of patients for our study, for if there are too few, they will not be representative of the general population.

We could just observe nurses touching patients and note their responses, but it would be much better to have two conditions: one where nurses touched patients, and one where they did not. We could then see if there were any differences between the two groups. Thus the next step is to randomly allocate our patients to the two conditions – touch and non-touch.

Having obtained our two conditions, it is necessary to examine how and under what circumstances the touching is going to take place. Let's decide that patients are understandably anxious whilst being given details of a forthcoming operation. Therefore the patients in the touch condition will be touched lightly on the arm while the nurse is giving them information about the operation, and the patients in the non-touch condition will be given the information by the nurse with no contact at all.

How do we measure whether touching is a good idea? We could just look at the patients' faces and see whether they look happy or not, but that would not be a particularly precise measure of 'reassurance'. There are several alternatives:

- We might decide that blood pressure is a good indicator of anxiety and choose to measure it just after the information has been given.
- Alternatively, we could measure the time it takes each patient to recover from surgery and see if there are any differences between the two groups.
- We may decide to ask the patients about their feelings towards the hospital after the operation.
- All three.

It doesn't matter which one we choose, but it will determine the exact outcome of the investigation, for example 'The effects of touch on patients' blood pressure before surgery' or 'The effects of touch on time taken by patients to recover from surgery.'

Finally, it is very important to keep all the variables that we do not want to measure and which could affect the results of the study constant. Thus we would want to have exactly the same instructions given to each patient by the same person the same amount of time before the operation. We would like the patients to be having surgery for exactly the same medical conditions, and to be operated on by the same surgeon. In this way we would hope to control for any extraneous variable that might interfere with our experimental design.

Having constructed a basic design, we might like to examine one or two additional variables, such as gender of nurse and patient. This would now produce the following four conditions.

- Male nurse touches male patients.
- Male nurse touches female patients.
- Female nurse touches male patients.
- Female nurse touches female patients.

By extending our conditions in this way we can investigate the effects of gender as well as touch on patients' responses to information about forthcoming surgery. (An experiment examining this topic is described in Chapter 1, and the findings show that gender does make a difference.).

All this sounds fine until we go back to the beginning and consider what it was that we were really interested in, which was 'is it a good idea to touch patients lightly on the arm to reduce their anxiety while speaking to them?' We can now provide some information concerning the gender of the participants and nature of outcome but by controlling such variables as same hospital, same type of surgery, same amount of time before operation, etc., we have restricted the applicability of our findings and our approach lacks ecological validity in that it doesn't really represent what happens between nurses and patients in a whole host of different circumstances. What then can we do to be more 'realistic' in our method of investigation? Another approach might be to concentrate on observing the responses of patients to nurses touching them in a variety of contexts and maybe use interviews with the patients to see how they felt about it. We may even choose to take part in the study and become 'participant observers'. For instance, the psychologist Marie de Hennezel (1997) worked with doctors and nurses in a hospital for the terminally ill in Paris. She recorded her observations in the form of a diary and notes the use of touch in following extract:

> Sometimes there is no substitute for the touch of a hand. It embodies the sense of true meeting. As I hold Louis's face in my hands and take in all its 'lostness' as his features soften and his skin warms to my touch, the contact between us is profound. Nothing is said, but we are together. When I see nurses keeping there arms straight and stiff while they are taking care of patients, I often tell them that if they curve their arms and make a cradle of them, their movements will be imbued with delicacy and tenderness.

This approach gives a depth of insight into the use of touch that no experimental study could match, yet it is still the observations of one person, in one situation at one period in time.

Whilst both approaches are very different they have one thing in common and that is they were both conducted in 'Western society'. Consider the following observation by Lutz (1999): he talks about a curious custom of the Andaman Islanders of Malaysia and the Maoris of New Zealand.

> In both cultures when two friends or relatives have been separated, they greet each other in an odd way. The two sit down, one in the other's lap, arms around each other's necks, and weep or wail together for several minutes. Relatives who have been separated by as little as a few weeks weep and howl so violently when they see each other again that 'there is no difference observable between their demonstrations of joy on these occasions and those of grief at the death of a close relative'.

Observing this behaviour, one might conclude that the two are weeping 'with tears of joy'. But ask the islanders and they say that they are in fact mourning for the people who had died since their last meeting. Radcliffe-Brown, from a social anthropological perspective, said that because the weeping behaviour occurred even if no one had died and the islanders had only been separated a few weeks, the natives' description of the behaviour as mourning was in fact more of a 'ceremonial act', rather like our handshake or two-cheek kiss, whose origins have been lost long ago. He may be right but if Maori social anthropologists were to observe us crying in a 'weepie' movie in the cinema and interpret it as ritualised ceremony whose origins we had forgotten we would not be pleased. The true meaning of the situation may be accessible only to the participants themselves and require skilled 'hermeneutic' investigation using in-depth interviews with many people.

The above examples illustrate a wide diversity of enquiry, and the 'scientific approach' referred to in this book is one of many. A broad range of approaches are discussed and evaluated, each having its own advantages and disadvantages, each having its own methodological integrity.

Psychology and nursing

There are distinct similarities between the scientific method as embodied in psychological research and as embodied in the nursing process. The nursing process is made up of four elements: *assessment, planning, implementation* and *evaluation*. These elements are similar to the processes involved in psychology: assessing the problem and locating it within a background of research; planning a course of action and experimentation; putting the plan into action; and finally evaluating the results in relation to the goals of the research and background literature.

Also, just as there are different models of nursing, there are different models of psychology. In each case none of the models is either right or wrong; they merely represent different perspectives. Thus Peplau's (1988) model emphasises the importance of the personal process between nurse and patient, both working together to solve problems, whereas Altschul (1978) prefers to use a systems approach (that is, analysing human behaviour as an individual system, a social system and a community/environmental system) to nursing. Similarly, Orem's (1980) self-care model is concerned with human needs whereas Roy's (1980) model chooses to see patients as adapting to an ever-changing environment. Each perspective is valuable in its own right.

Likewise, psychology has a number of different perspectives. Social psychologists may investigate the effect on human behaviour of being a member of a group, whereas personality theorists prefer to explore the individual differences between people; developmental psychologists not surprisingly think it important to examine human behaviour as it changes throughout the life span whilst behavioural psychologists tend to see behaviour purely in terms of what can be overtly observed. One might suggest that it would be particularly narrow to view both the discipline of psychology and the discipline of nursing from just one perspective.

The psychology of nursing care

Given that there are a number of different models in nursing and that the position is the same in psychology, it may seem an impossible task to 'marry' the two together. Attempts to decide 'what goes with what' often end up as a mish-mash of unrelated items with no coherent structure. Therefore, efforts to integrate the two disciplines have tended to concentrate on one to give a lead in providing a structural framework for integration. Early texts used psychology as the framework to examine the relationship between psychology and nursing. Books and articles followed the standard psychological format, with sections on learning; memory, perception, motivation, personality, physiological psychology, cognition, language, social behaviour, and so on. The basic principles of each area would be introduced, followed by some suggestions on how they might be used in a nursing context. The problems with this approach were that often much of the psychological content was not particularly relevant to nursing and because the relevant items were couched in a psychological framework it was difficult for nurses to relate the content to nursing practice.

This book attempts to use nursing as an organising framework, hence the title. There are a number of themes in the book which attempt to use both the nursing process and models of nursing care as their base, and these include the following.

- *The process of nursing care.* Interpersonal skills, a knowledge of 'self' and an understanding of how others view the world are central features in interacting well with people. Thus it is necessary to examine the dynamics of human interaction within different nursing contexts.
- *The systems approach.* This theme involves analysing human behaviour as an individual system, a social system and a community/environmental system. We are unique individuals with different abilities and perspectives on life, yet we are part of a wide range of social, community and cultural groups. Therefore, behaviour should be seen as much a function of context as it is a product of the individual.
- *A developmental approach.* Here behaviour is viewed in the context of the changes that occur throughout the life span. Children have always had a special place in nursing, hence the speciality of paediatric nursing, but just as important are the people approaching or in late adulthood who do not as yet warrant such a specialism. Thus it is important to look at the psychology of nursing care throughout the life span because people differ as much as a function of their psychological and social development as of their 'individual differences'.

- *Adaptation and competence.* The final theme addresses the nurse's role as an agent of health promotion and education as well as treatment. It investigates the process of helping people adapt to their situation and investigates ways that they may develop the competence to deal with other new situations.

One of the problems of psychology, and perhaps of nursing too, is that there is a tendency to concentrate on people as isolated entities rather than viewing them in a wider social context. I hope the themes addressed in this book illustrate the psychology of nursing care in a much broader perspective. In order to interact well with people we have to know about ourselves as well as others, we have to see people not only as individuals but as members of groups, families and communities. Finally, we need to view care in the context of the development of competences as well as just treatment.

1

Interpersonal Skills

A practice conundrum

Nurses are encouraged to individualise care, ensuring that it supports the needs of patients and respects their dignity and privacy. Nurse theorists refer to 'person-centred care' and emphasise that nurses have a key role in ensuring that the experience of disease, illness, treatment and care is appreciated with due respect for the perceptions and aspirations of the patient.

Imagine that you are encountering a new patient for the first time. This person is a relative stranger to you, although you have probably received a brief summary about her circumstances at the start of your shift. For the sake of illustration we will call the patient Ruth and start with the premise that she has been suffering from a chronic illness. Now please choose a chronic illness that is relevant to your area of practice. Suddenly, there has been a complication and some additional tests are necessary. There will be modifications in Ruth's treatment and care and her situation will alter as a result. What Ruth once thought as familiar will become strange and threatening.

Given that you need to understand Ruth's situation, perceptions and needs in order to individualise her care, how will you proceed? What personal resources will you use in order to establish and sustain a rapport with the patient? Most artful of all, how will you know how to manage the care relationship as Ruth's situation changes day by day?

What makes a good nurse? If a representative sample of the population were asked to answer the question, one of the most common responses would be something like 'Well, a nurse has to be able to care for his or her patients.' 'Caring' is a term often used to describe a general attitude towards people involving concern, empathy and expertise. Generally, most people agree that caring is important, but, when asked to determine how it can be developed, usually resort to the response that you are either born with the ability to care or you are not. Caring is not seen as something that can be taught.

This chapter will demonstrate that elements of caring *can* be taught and, perhaps more important, will look at the ways in which a knowledge of interpersonal skills can improve the quality of patient care. Ryden *et al.* (1991) found that the helping skills of nursing students who had taken a course on interpersonal relations resembled those of experienced psychotherapists and crisis interveners. Also, McCabe (2004) says that, far from not being very good at communicating with patients, as some research suggests, nurses can communicate very well if they use a person-centred as opposed to a task-centred approach.

However, a fundamental feature of communicating well with other people is an understanding of ourselves as well as an understanding of those with whom we wish to communicate.

Self-esteem: the affective component of self

Self-esteem may be defined as the feelings, or evaluations, that people have regarding their self-worth. It is important to try to develop one's own self-esteem as well as that of others, for low self-esteem can lead to a number of problems, including the following:

- People with low self-esteem sometimes set themselves unrealistically high or low goals. They feel that if they set goals which are too high they can't be blamed if they do not reach them. Similarly, setting goals which are too low enables them always to succeed. Both sets of behaviour lead to an overall fear of failure.
- Low self-esteem can lead to a tendency to be overcritical of a person's own behaviour and may result in a desire for perfectionism.
- Inevitably, low self-esteem produces a sense of undervaluation which is particularly apparent in social situations where comparisons with others are made.
- A need for approval or to be liked stems in part from having low self-esteem.
- People with low self-esteem run the risk of becoming over-conformist. They may feel that their opinions must be wrong if they are not the same as everybody else's.

On the other hand, people who have high self-esteem tend to believe that they have the resources to confront demanding situations. They feel that they have the strengths to meet the pressures of everyday life, and thus stressful events are perceived more as a challenge than as a threat. Positive regard for the self is an important ingredient in developing one's 'quality of life'.

Moretti and Higgins (1990) say that an important constituent of self-esteem is the degree to which a person's perceived characteristics match his or her concept of an ideal self. In effect, self-esteem asks the question 'Do you like yourself?' However, the most destructive feature of low self-esteem is the tendency to overgeneralise on the basis of one's failures. Kernis *et al.* (1989) studied a group of undergraduate students who had done either relatively well or relatively badly in their first exam. Those students who had been rated low in self-esteem and who had done badly in their exam experienced more negative emotions than those who had done badly but had been rated high in self-esteem. Individuals with low self-esteem overgeneralised the meaning of the poor result in the exam and tended to feel stupid, inadequate, hopeless and discouraged. This led to self-doubt about their ability which manifested itself in low motivation in subsequent exams. Individuals with high self-esteem accurately assessed the meaning of the poor result and were ashamed, scared, angry and disappointed. They attributed the result to lack of effort rather than lack of ability, and maintained high motivation to do better in subsequent exams. Randle (2003) found that, over a three-year period, nursing students on a pre-registration training programme experienced a reduction in self-esteem over the training period. Whilst professional self-esteem was maintained, overall self-esteem declined dramatically. Thus attention should be given in such training programmes to developing strategies to confront the reasons for the decline.

Self-esteem can be increased by giving people rewards for the things that they have done well. Giving a verbal 'pat on the back' and a small present for a task that has been completed correctly serve to boost a person's self-concept. To increase your own self-esteem, it is a good idea to try to worry less about what other people think about you, or your ability, and try to make the same allowances for yourself as you do for other people. Determine to learn from mistakes rather than awarding self-blame and punishment. It is often the case that we think we hold a more prominent position in other people's lives than is actually true.

Self-actualisation

Rogers (1971) believed that each person has an innate drive towards psychological growth. This drive leads ultimately to self-actualisation which Rogers defined as 'the fulfilment of all of an individual's capabilities and the achievement of all of a person's potential'. But how does one determine whether a person is self-actualised or not?

Maslow (1962) studied forty-nine people whom he admired and who he thought might be representative of 'the self-actualised person'. Included in the group were two of his professors and such historical figures as Eleanor Roosevelt, Albert Einstein and Baruch Spinoza. He gathered his data by obtaining biographical information and, wherever possible, interviewing friends, relations and, in some cases, the individuals themselves. On the basis of his data he proposed that self-actualised people share sixteen characteristics:

- the ability to perceive reality accurately;
- the ability to accept reality readily;
- are natural and spontaneous;

- can focus on problems rather than on self;
- have a need for privacy;
- are self-sufficient and independent;
- are capable of fresh, spontaneous, non-stereotyped appreciation of objects, events and people encountered in life;
- have peak experiences (spiritual or ecstatic experiences);
- identify with humankind, and experience shared social bonds with other people;
- have few or many friends, but will have deep relationships with at least some of these friends;
- have a democratic, egalitarian attitude;
- have strongly held values and do not confuse means with ends;
- have a broad, tolerant sense of humour;
- are inventive and creative, and able to see things in new ways;
- resist the pressures of conformity to society;
- are able to transcend dichotomies, bringing together opposites.

Maslow (1972) suggested that some of the behaviours likely to lead to self-actualisation include:

- taking responsibility for events;
- experimenting with new ideas instead of doing the same old things;
- trying to experience life as a child does, using concentration and absorption;
- avoiding being pretentious and trying to be honest;
- trying to identify one's 'defences' and attempting to come to terms with them;
- listening to one's own feelings;
- being prepared to be unpopular if the situation requires.

Exercise 1.1 *Characteristics of a self-actualised individual*   © David Fontana from *Social Skills at Work*, Blackwell Publishing, 1990

To find out how self-actualised you are, work through the sixteen characteristics and see how many of them you possess It should be noted that most of us do not possess them and indeed Maslow proposed that very few people are totally self-actualised

From studying self-actualisation Maslow developed a theory of the self based on a *hierarchy of needs*. On the first level of the hierarchy, Maslow placed physiological needs such as food and water. On the next level he placed safety from such dangers as crime, fire,

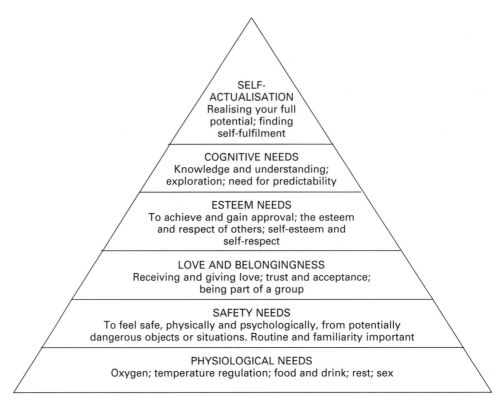

Figure 1.1 Maslow's hierarchy of needs. *After Maslow (1954)*

heat, cold, wild animals and financial disasters. The third level is concerned with love, affection and belonging. Next come self-esteem and a stable, correct evaluation of self-concept, including the need for achievement and self-respect. Finally, when all the other needs have been attained, a person reaches a stage of self-fulfilment or self-actualisation.

There are two main criticisms of Maslow's model of self.

- Satisfaction of a particular need does not necessarily reduce the need's importance as Maslow suggests. Indeed, the greater the level of satisfaction a person has obtained for a particular need, the more important the need seems to become.
- The hierarchy should be much more flexible than the model supposes; people have starved to death for political reasons. Thus the hierarchy cannot be inflexible, and has to take into account deliberate non-fulfilment of certain needs.

Self-examination

In order to be able to relate to other people, it is necessary to identify important facets of ourselves. Fontana (1990) says:

Other people's behaviour doesn't happen in a vacuum. When they relate to us, they are relating to *us*, to the people we are. Their behaviour towards us is a response, in no small measure, to our behaviour towards them. If I want to know why people are intimidated or confused or irritated by me, I need to accept that this says something about me as well as something about them.

He also provides the following exercise to help you examine your social self.

Exercise 1.2 *Self-examination*   (from Fontana, 1990)

Imagine that two people are discussing you. In the course of their conversation they use a number of words which they feel describe you accurately. Study the following list of words and choose those words you think they may have used. Remember, be honest.

friendly	likable	witty
helpful	sensitive	sarcastic
hasty	erratic	warm
communicative	happy	spiteful
cold	talkative	calm
open	devious	anxious
honest	unpredictable	well balanced
reliable	cavalier	quick-tempered
secretive	selfish	forceful
humorous	punctual	unforgiving
depressed	well mannered	kind
creative	thoughtful	remote
slow	able	understanding
formal	mean	empathic

Now select all the words that you think they would *not* have used to describe you. You should now have an outline of the characteristics that you think represent yourself. It remains for you to decide whether you are happy with these qualities. Select the qualities that you dislike in yourself and try to identify the situations that bring them out.

Then select the characteristics that you think you do not possess but would like to. Try to think of situations where you might profitably use them. What is it that stops you from being like this all the time?

Self-disclosure

To what extent should we disclose aspects of our 'self' to other people? On one hand there is the belief that it is important for nurses to maintain a certain professional distance from their patients; they should take care to protect their sense of 'self' and not get too involved. On the other hand, some people think that disclosing aspects of oneself or one's experiences can help a sense of empathy between nurse and patient to develop. The answer is that self-disclosure is correct in some circumstances but not in others. Before exploring when self-disclosure may be appropriate, it is necessary to explore how the 'self' may be displayed to other people.

Luft and Ingham (1955) proposed that there are four aspects of self:

- *the open or public self* – what we know about ourselves and what others know about us as well;
- *the blind self* – aspects of the self that are unknown to us but known to others;
- *the hidden or private self* – what is known to me but hidden from others;
- *the unknown self* – what is unknown to us and unknown to others.

These four 'selves' are represented as 'windows' and have come to be known as *Johari windows,* derived from the christian names of Joe Luft and Harry Ingham. In any given situation one of the windows will take precedence over the other three. In the case of self-disclosure, the open window increases in size and the other three are diminished. Thus self-disclosure gives information about ourselves to others and also, since we are party to information in this window, gives us valuable insights into our own thoughts and feelings.

Functions of self-disclosure

There are several functions of self-disclosure. One is to develop a sense of empathy between nurse and patient. Used correctly, self-disclosure can make a nurse appear more 'human'. It may also be used to direct the focus of attention. Consider the following statement from a patient: 'I just found it impossible to cope with the pain, and you know, nobody seemed to care at all, they just thought I was play-acting.' How would you respond to that statement? One response might be, 'Oh, I'm sure they weren't.' But by using self-disclosure you can empathise and direct the focus of the conversation. This type of response first conveys concern and then directs attention towards the individual, encouraging him or her to disclose more fully: 'I can see that being taken for a play-actor must have made the pain very difficult to cope with.' The next response takes the focus away from the patient and back to the nurse: 'That happened to me too, and it was awful.' Both responses are equally correct but have different functions with respect to the direction and focus of the conversation.

Levels of self-disclosure

As well as fulfilling different functions, self-disclosures can be made on a number of different levels. Usually if two people do not know each other particularly well they rarely divulge details of their innermost feelings. Therefore, talking to someone about one's deep emotions early on in a relationship can be embarrassing. As people get to know each other better they become more relaxed about disclosing intimate information. Even if a patient has an overwhelming desire to divulge sensitive information to a nurse, he or she may not do so because it is too risky and may place him or her in what he or she thinks is a vulnerable position. There are exceptions to the rule, such as what is known as the 'stranger on the plane' phenomenon. Sometimes if two people realise that there is little chance of ever seeing each other again (for example, people sitting next to each other on a plane) they are often tempted to disclose extremely personal thoughts and feelings. Also, people who have recently been bereaved often find it easier to talk to a stranger than to a member of the family. This notwithstanding, it is normal to employ initial self-disclosure carefully in order to avoid embarrassment and patient discomfort.

There are three levels of self-disclosure.

- *Sharing opinions.* This is the best level to start with, as it has the least affective value: 'I think you were quite right to object. What a nerve the man's got.'
- *Sharing experiences.* Slightly deeper than sharing opinions, sharing experiences can help to provide patients with a new perspective on their situation. But it is important that patients have the power to accept or reject the relevance of the experiences.
- *Sharing feelings.* Sometimes it is correct to share feelings with patients, both verbally and physically. Wright (1993) says that although many nurses are worried about the fact that they may cry, on the occasions when he has seen it happen it has increased feelings of caring and understanding.

Nelson-Jones (2002) summarises the positive and negative features of self-disclosure by saying that as some patients may have had little opportunity to practise self-disclosure, owing to lack of knowledge or apprehension about its use, nurses should be able to signal to patients when and where it is appropriate to use such behaviour and how it can be expressed. Also, the correct use of self-disclosure indicates genuineness and the desire to share experiences. An advantage of sharing experiences with patients is that it can provide them with a different perspective on their situation, which may bring about a new approach to dealing with the problem.

There are, however, unfavourable consequences to inappropriate self-disclosures, which we must be aware of.

- *Overloading the patient.* Too much self-disclosure can result in burdening the patient. Patients have problems of their own and do not want to be overloaded with other people's difficulties.

- *Appearing weak.* Too much self-disclosure can make nurses appear 'weak' in the eyes of the patient. Patients like to have health professionals who present themselves as strong and competent. If there is any doubt about the use of self-disclosure, the best approach is to start with 'sharing opinion' disclosures. Then, if communication is proceeding effectively, patients will often pick up the concern and empathy and you can proceed to deeper levels of self-disclosure if necessary.
- *Appearing dominating.* It might seem a contradiction that self-disclosure can make one seem weak *and* dominating, but statements of the nature 'You think you've got problems, well I can tell you . . .' can be perceived as overpowering by patients.
- *Self-serving self-disclosure.* Psychoanalysts call this *countertransference.* It refers to the use of self-disclosure purely for the good of the nurse and not the patient. Sometimes nurses may wish to use self-disclosure to satisfy their own need for approval and affection. Danger signs include going well out of one's way for a particular patient and becoming emotionally involved rather than professionally concerned.

Despite these dangers, self-disclosure can be an essential part of nursing care. Pennebaker (1997) concludes his report on confiding traumatic experiences by saying:

The disclosure of traumas is cognitively beneficial because it promotes the assimilation of the events, it translates the images of the events into language and provides a sense of detachment from the experiences. Socially, the actual or symbolic disclosure of personal experiences to others usually strengthens human relationships and assimilates people's self-definitions with those individuals or institutions in whom they confide.

Social construction: the distributed self

So far the self has been construed as largely self-contained and relatively constant. However, the social construction hypothesis sees the self as being continually 'constructed' according to our experiences throughout life. This is not to say that there isn't some consistent aspect of being that is with us all the time. Rather, our self is largely constructed by way we interact with the world. Who we are is as much part of our childhood experiences and cultural background as it is of our temperament. Thus as our experience of the world continues to change so does our self. One of the first attempts to examine the social construction approach came from Berger and Luckmann (1976) in their book *The Social Construction of Reality.* Since that time the SC perspective has become one of the main themes in psychological epistemology with its emphasis on exploring the meaning of behaviour (hermeneutics). One view of the self is to establish just what remains when all external influences are either discounted or controlled. The social constructionist view is to place the social world at the heart of psychological enquiry. This means where and how a person grew up is important as is the current patterning of social development. Bruner (1990) sees the self as distributed across the cultural and social domain. He uses the analogy of a snooker or pool game where the self is not encapsulated in one ball but is represented by the game as a whole, with the balls continually spreading, grouping and regrouping across the table. This fluency is also manifest in his more recent views (Bruner, 2002) of the narrative creation of self. Here he rejects the idea of the self as 'one that just sits there ready to be portrayed in words'; rather 'we constantly construct and reconstruct ourselves to meet the needs of the situations we encounter, and we do so with the guidance of our memories of the past and our hopes and fears of the future'. For him narrative serves a central role in this process. 'Telling oneself about oneself is like making up a story about who and what we are, what's happened, and why we are doing what we are doing.'

In relation to interpersonal skills, emotions can also be socially constructed. Rosaldo (1984) takes the view that thoughts are inextricably linked to our emotions. This has some substance since the work of Schacter and Singer (1962) found that the experience of an emotion was influenced by the social context in which it occurred (see p. 222). The same physiological change induced by adrenalin was experienced as different emotional states according to the participants' perceptions, or thoughts, about what they should be feeling. For instance Rosaldo (1984) studied the Ilongot people, who believed that anger could be 'forgotten' whereby an angry person could have their anger 'paid for' and then it would vanish. This seems totally alien to our understanding of anger that has its roots in some form of frustration and has to be either vented or repressed – the idea that one can somehow make it disappear seems nonsense. An explanation lies in the fact that their anger is not our anger. Rosaldo (1984) notes that the Ilongot have an emotion they call *liget*. This is similar to what we might call energy/passion. Gergen (1991) explains it thus:

Liget is a distinct possession of the male, and we in Western culture could scarcely imagine its expression among us. A young Ilongot possessed by liget might weep or sing or sulk. He might stop eating certain foods, slash baskets, yet spill water, or demonstrate irritation and distraction. And, when liget has reached its peak, he will be moved to slice the head from a neighbouring tribesman. Having taken a head, he feels his liget transformed and transforming. His resources of energy are increased, he feels passion for the opposite sex, and he acquires a deeper sense of knowledge.

Angry doesn't seem an adequate description of this man's emotional state; more like passionate revenge, perhaps. The central point is that thought, feeling and culture are all bound together such that it may be impossible for a person from one culture to truly appreciate the emotional state of a person from another. If this is the case the question may be asked how far this construction may apply to different groups within cultures. This 'emic' approach (interpretation of meaning) may be contrasted with the somewhat 'etic' approach (observational interpretation) in the next section.

Many people think that non-verbal communication is incidental to conversation, but in fact it is there to supplement speech. Birdwhistell (1970) estimated that about 65–70 per cent of the social meaning of conversation is related in a non-verbal manner. At this point it is necessary to distinguish between verbal and vocal constituents of communication.

- Everyday speech has a verbal (language) component and is vocal (can be heard). It is therefore *verbal/vocal*.
- Morse code or sign language has a verbal component (language) but is nonvocal. It is *verbal/nonvocal*.
- The volume, tone and pitch of a person's voice has a vocal component (it can be heard) but no verbal or language factor. It is *non-verbal/vocal*.
- Gestures, eye contact, proximity and posture are all examples of *non-verbal/non-vocal* communication.

Exercise 1.3 *A group exercise in communication*

This exercise should be carried out in a group. On some cards write down the following emotions/expressions: HAPPY, SAD, SURPRISE, ANGER, DISGUST/CONTEMPT, FEAR, INTEREST, SHAME, AMUSEMENT, BOREDOM, IMPATIENCE, FATIGUE, PAIN, EMBARRASSMENT, LOVE, DOMINANCE. Distribute the cards randomly amongst the members of the group. Give the following instructions:

Written on the card in front of you is an emotion/expression. You have to stand up in front of the group and communicate this emotion nonverbally; that is, you must not use any words. You may communicate vocally by counting from 1 to 5 and altering the pitch and volume of your voice. Other members of the group should write down the emotion they think is being demonstrated.

This exercise has a number of uses. First, it is very good as an initial exercise to break down barriers. Second, it illustrates the dual nature of non-verbal communication. Ask the group members how many they got right. Then ask the members of the group if they can give *any* explanations as to why they did not recognise all the emotions expressions. You will probably find that there are two main reasons.

- The emotions expressed are out of context; thus the lack of background contextual clues and cues makes it difficult to identify them.

- The people expressing the emotions are not actually experiencing them at the time. As we do not normally think about how we appear to others when expressing our emotions, it is difficult to portray them out of context. We don't think about what we are doing/experiencing, we just do it.

Given these difficulties, it may be useful to think about how confidence and competence can be communicated to patients when a nurse really feels nervous and unsure, or how interest and concern can be conveyed when you really don't like the person you are nursing. To what extent do our true feelings 'leak' through our disguises? Can patients detect true emotions through a facade?

Facial expressions

The face probably carries the most non-verbal information. Rosenthal and DePaulo (1979) presented participants with 220 two-second segments of videotape of different combinations of face, body and sound. There were eleven samples of twenty emotions produced by a young woman. The most accurate channels for decoding information were found to be: facial expression (first), body (second), and tone of voice (third). Additionally, certain facial expressions are easier to decode than others. Ekman (2004) produced the following hierarchy of accuracy scores:

EASIEST

Happy
Surprise
Fear
Anger
Sad
Disgust/contempt

HARDEST

Ekman and Friesen (1975) found that there was a great deal of agreement throughout the world with respect to which facial expressions represented happiness and sadness. Moreover, there was a universality of meaning; that is, smiles were recognised as a sign of happiness and frowns as a sign of sadness. Some emotions are shown primarily in certain parts of the face – for instance, fear and sadness are decoded predominantly from the eyes and eyelids, whereas surprise involves the brows and forehead plus the eyes and eyelids and the cheeks and mouth.

An interesting experiment by Zuckerman *et al.* (1981) investigated the question 'Can smiling make people happy?' The experimenters divided their participants into three groups. The first group was shown a film of a pleasant episode. The second group was shown a film of a neutral scene and the third group was shown a film of a nasty event. Within each of the three groups, a third of the group members were asked to suppress their facial reactions while watching the film, a third were told to exaggerate them and a third were not told to do anything at all. The participants' physiological arousal was measured during each of the films and participants were required to rate their emotional reactions to the films after they had finished viewing. The participants who were asked to exaggerate their facial expressions showed higher levels of arousal to both the pleasant and the nasty scenes than the participants in the suppressant groups, and reported stronger positive and negative emotional reactions than the participants asked to suppress their facial expressions.

The experimenters concluded that exaggerating facial expressions increased feelings, both positive and negative, and that suppressing facial expressions decreased emotions. It may be that making patients smile more increases their pleasant feelings, and learning to suppress emotions in times of stress and tension may reduce affective experience. This has been referred to as the *facial feedback hypothesis* (McCanne and Anderson, 1987).

The Duchenne smile

Ekman (2004) says that we can distinguish between a forced smile and a true smile. Two muscles are principally involved in smiling: the *zygomaticus major* and the *orbicularis oculi*. Duchenne, in 1862, had observed that, whilst it was relatively easy to contract the former it was impossible to contract the latter. Thus a false smile could be detected by the absence of contraction of the *orbicularis oculi*. Ekman (2004) confirms this finding but adds that approximately 10 per cent of people can contract this muscle. However, he suggests that these people may be actors or skilled at retrieving a memory that generates the emotion. He also says that we can detect the difference – when happily married couples meet after work, they show contraction of the muscle; unhappily married couples do not. The important part of the muscle pulls down the eyebrows and the skin below, whilst pulling up the skin below the eye and the raising the cheeks. This leads to a somewhat narrowing of the eye, so the place to look to see if someone is really enjoying themselves is the eye cover fold just below the eyebrow.

One important implication of these findings is that it is difficult to portray emotions that are not being experienced at the time, and people are often quite good at picking this up.

Gaze

People have always been fascinated with the messages that are conveyed via the eyes, and eyes have been referred to as the windows of the soul. There are a number of terms used to describe the non-verbal use of the eyes in interpersonal communication:

- *Gaze* is used to describe the process of fixing one's eyes on another person.
- *Mutual gaze/eye contact* are terms used when two people are engaged in focusing their eyes on each other.
- *Staring* is a gaze or a look which persists regardless of the behaviour of others.

As a rule, mutual gaze and eye contact signify friendliness and affection. Research has shown that young couples who are most in love have a high proportion of mutual gaze (Rubin, 1970), whereas married couples with marital discord have low levels of mutual gaze (Beier and Sternberg, 1977). It seems that we prefer those people who look at us, and therefore engaging in eye contact usually signifies that a person wishes to appear friendly. Staring has the opposite effect. Most people become anxious when stared at, partly owing to uneasiness about the intentions of the person who is staring. It may also be due to an innate belief that staring is a prelude to attack, since animals are known to stare before they pounce.

A consequence of the connection between eye contact and friendliness is that it is difficult to look someone in the eye whilst lying to them unless you are a practised liar. Often, if someone has something particularly difficult to say, they will disengage from eye contact while they marshal their thoughts. Therefore, lack of gaze or eye contact often signifies that something is wrong. It is no good saying one thing to a patient and contradicting it with your eyes. In the course of interviewing patients, their eye contact, or lack of it, can signify which issues should be examined in further detail.

However, there are individual and cultural differences in the use of gaze. Direct focus on the eyes is common among Arabs, Latin Americans and southern Europeans while Asians and northern Europeans tend to adopt less, or sometimes, no gaze at all (Mayo and Le France, 1973). Thus our own and others' gaze should be seen in the context of the culture that has socialised our individual behaviour. Since nursing takes place in a multicultural setting, this last point is particularly relevant.

Touch

The use of touch in the healing process has been chronicled since the Bible. In the context of nursing care, touch has a more common function. Touching a patient whilst communicating emotional information usually indicates a degree of warmth and concern (McCann and McKenna, 1993). However, the use of touch may differ between cultures. An experiment often mentioned is one by Jourard (1966). He observed couples

Table 1.1 *Types and number of touches used in a survey of airport greetings (Greenbaum and Rosenfeld, 1980)*

No touch at all	41
Kiss on the mouth	41
Touch on the head, arm or back	38
Kiss on cheek	30
Light hug	23
Solid hug	19
Arm round waist or back	15
Holding hands	12
Handshake	10
Extended embrace	10
Extended kiss	3

talking to each other in coffee shops in different parts of the world and counted the number of times the couples touched each other during a one-hour period. In San Juan (Puerto Rico) they touched each other a total of 180 times during the hour. In Paris the number was 110. In London the number of touches was 0. This study was one of the first to indicate that there are considerable cultural differences in the amount of touching that is socially acceptable, and that in the United Kingdom people do not seem to engage in a great deal of contact with each other. Since 1966 there have been changes in the amount of touching deemed socially acceptable; this may be due to greater exposure to other cultures, leading in turn to a decrease in inhibition in the UK.

In the United States, Greenbaum and Rosenfield (1980) observed 103 greetings between people at airports. The different types of touch used and the number of times they were used are shown in Table 1.1. Men tended to shake hands; females were more likely to kiss and embrace, finishing with a hand touching the upper body.

Davitz and Davitz (1985) cite an American patient's perception of British nurses: 'They're efficient, but they're not sympathetic.' This comment may in part be due to a tendency in British culture to be sparing with body contact. However, what one culture sees as adequate contact between nurse and patient may not be acceptable for another. American patients may perceive British nurses as cold and unsympathetic, but British patients may see American nurses as overfamiliar. It is perfectly reasonable for British nurses to tailor their interactive style to the needs of British patients, but they should realise that their patients came from many ethnic groups who may have different interpersonal norms.

There are also status differences implicit in touching behaviour. Whitcher and Fisher (1979) investigated female nurses' use of touch while providing patients with information about their imminent operation. There were two conditions.

- Nurses touched the patient lightly on the hand while giving them information about the operation.
- Nurses gave information about the operation without touching the patient in any way.

Patients were asked what they thought about the operation and the hospital, and their blood pressure was measured after surgery. Female patients touched on the hand by the nurses described the hospital in positive terms, had lower levels of anxiety and lower blood pressure than those patients who were not touched on the hand. However, the results for male patients were different. Male patients who were touched reported greater anxiety, more negative feelings towards the hospital and were found to have higher blood pressure after surgery than males who were not touched. The experimenters suggest that the differences in response may be due to status differences. Men may dislike being touched, as they perceive it to be a threatening gesture, accentuating the nurse's superior status in the hospital setting, whereas women recognise touch as an indication of warmth and caring. Mulaik *et al.* (1991) collected baseline data about seventy-one female and twenty-seven male patients' perceptions of touch. Although 93 per cent of the patients believed that touch meant caring and affection, only 74 per cent agreed that the nurse's touch felt good, and 77 per cent believed touch conveyed control.

Touching patients can also have a significant effect on nurses themselves. In a Swedish study Edvarsson *et al.* (2003) investigated nurses' experiences of the use of touch in a population of the elderly. They found that giving touch in the care of older patients was valuable for the nurses in a personal as well as professional context. It also transformed the way they viewed patients 'Instead of seeing a severely demanding patient suffering from dementia and/or pain, one is able to see the person behind the disease as a human being, like oneself.'

Presence: just being there

This is one of the most difficult aspects of non-verbal behaviour both to teach and to assess. Because there is no step-by-step procedure, nurses are often at a loss as to when and how to implement 'caring presence' despite it being listed as a nursing intervention in the Nursing Interventions Classifications (NIC) (McCloskey and Bulechek, 1996). Engebretson (2004) says

Most nursing textbooks and beginning curricula stress the importance of non-verbal communication, however, students often feel insecure if they do not know what words to say. Words are a comfortable tool as the non-verbal communication often relates to an inner state of being that is not easily taught. Many professionals are often terrified of being with someone in silence.

However, McKivergin and Daubenmire (1994) suggest there are three categories of presence: physical presence, psychological presence and therapeutic presence. *Physical* presence includes touching but also seeing, examining and hugging too. *Psychological* presence is made up of communicating active listening, reflecting, being empathic, non-judgemental and accepting. *Therapeutic* presence is much more difficult to define. McKivergin and Daubenmire (1994) use words such as centring, intentionality and intuitive knowing to describe the experience. Perhaps it is the last that comes closest to describing therapeutic presence it is 'knowing that words are just not necessary'.

This still leaves the problem of when and where to say something or keep silent. It is always useful to pay attention to cultural as well as individual differences. Western culture is often characterised by doing or saying something, 'filling in the gaps', whereas other cultures accept that just being there is highly valued. But there is no answer, except that it isn't a problem – as one nurse put it, 'Just try to connect is all.'

Spatial behaviour

Interpersonal proximity simply means the space between two people. Edward Hall (1969) was an anthropologist interested in the individual and cultural differences of interpersonal distance. He called this *proxemics* and identified four main proximity zones.

- *Intimate* (0–0.45 m). People allow only intimate friends this close to their bodies.
- *Personal* (0.45–1.2 m). This is what people usually mean by 'personal space'. Invasion of this area causes anxiety, especially if the person who has had their space violated cannot escape.
- *Social* (1.2–3.65 m). This distance is used for day-to-day interaction with strangers and formal business purposes.
- *Public* (3.65–7.6+ m). This is the distance kept from important public figures.

These distances are, of course, averages and there are distinct individual differences in the amount of space people like to place between themselves and others while interacting. Most of us have experienced someone who has come a bit too close, making us take a step back to feel more comfortable. Again, there are cultural as well as individual differences in personal space. In some cultures people stand close to their correspondents, while in others people prefer to maintain a considerable distance from each other. This can cause conflict if a person from one culture feels that the interpersonal distance is too small and takes a step back while a person from another culture feels that the distance is too impersonal and takes a step forward to close the gap. Speaking too close to a person may appear intrusive; too far away, cold and impersonal.

Exercise 1.4 *Investigating interpersonal space*

It is reasonably simple to investigate interpersonal space. One way to determine your own personal 'space bubble' is to stand in the middle of a room and ask a friend to approach you until they get to a distance that feels uncomfortable. Adjust this distance to the point where you are able to accept their proximity and you have one point on the circumference of your 'bubble'. Get your friend to repeat the procedure from different angles and you will end up with your own personal 'space bubble'

Another good exercise is to sit on a chair in the middle of a room with nothing else in it except another chair close to the door. As people come in, ask them to pull up a chair and see how close they place it to you. You can vary the gender of the seated person and their familiarity with you. Measure the different distances and see if there are any interesting findings.

Also watch what goes on in lifts and crowded trains. When people's personal space is invaded by strangers there is a huge reduction in eye contact Eye contact in combination with intrusion into one's intimate space produces too much familiarity.

Although nurses are 'allowed' to invade their patients' personal space by the nature of their job, they should be aware that people do not normally permit this behaviour and therefore may appear nervous for no other reason than that their interpersonal space has been invaded. Winkel *et al.* (1988) found that police officers often tended to stand too close to people whilst interviewing them, thus producing a situation in which the person felt threatened and uncomfortable. These responses were then misinterpreted as suspicious. In a similar vein, if nurses invade personal space they may get reactions which could be interpreted as a general state of anxiety rather than a specific response to proximity.

Spatial behaviour also encompasses *orientation*; this refers to the angle at which people sit or stand in relation to each other. Pietroni (1976) found that when general practitioners sat at a 90° angle to their patients the interaction increased six times as much as when they faced them square on across the table. Co-operation, competition and conversation increase or decrease according to orientation. Cook (1970) found that people who like each other generally sit side by side. People who dislike each other sit opposite. The exception to this rule is that people prefer to eat facing each other.

Body movements

Postures

The way a person stands, sits or even walks conveys non-verbal information about them. Standing erect with the head held high and the hands placed on the hips is a dominant posture. A nurse who adopts this posture whilst asking a patient if he or she wants a bed bath may be seen as aggressive and dominant, giving the patient no room to decline the request. A patient who adopts a hunched posture with eyes lowered and who says that everything is fine and that he or she is not worried in the slightest may be hiding the truth. Depression is often indicated by a slouching, listless posture; anxiety by a tense, stiff, rigid posture. Status may also be conveyed non-verbally through posture. High rank or prestige is denoted by a relatively relaxed sitting posture; low status people tend to sit more upright and rigid in their seats. Interest is indicated by sitting forward in one's seat, whilst leaning backwards in the chair signifies the opposite.

There is evidence that the way nurses walk on the hospital ward influences patients' perception of their personality. Montepare and Zebrowitz-McArthur (1988) showed participants videotapes of people of different ages walking back and forth at what was for them a comfortable pace. The experimenters found that gait affected the participants' ratings of the walkers. Those with a youthful gait were rated as more powerful and happier than those with an older gait. Thus a nurse's style of walking may be an important determinant of the impression she makes on patients.

Gestures

Gestures are used to replace and augment speech and it is very difficult to speak to someone without gesticulating in some way. The majority of people who see themselves on a video-tape are surprised by the type, and amount, of gestures they use. Since nurses are generally unaware of the gestures they employ, it is necessary to provide some form of feedback, as they may be unaware of the messages they are transmitting unwittingly. One specific example of a gesture used in a therapeutic context is the head nod. Not only does it communicate to the speaker that the listener is attending to the conversation, but it also encourages them to keep talking.

Exercise 1.5 *Gestures and emotions*

Try to think of a situation or an incident that made you very, very angry. Keep thinking about the event for a minute or so. Now try to remember an event or incident that made you feel very, very sad and think about that for a minute. Think about your behaviour, your expression, gesture and posture. Did you move your hands, arms, legs as your thoughts moved from the first event to the second? The next time you observe someone making a phone call look at their gestures. Chances are that they will use a whole series of gestures to accompany their conversation even though the person they are talking to cannot possibly see them.

The voice

The quality of vocal expression produces a wide range of messages. Changes in volume can represent the following meanings:

- soft = sadness/affection;
- moderate = pleasantness/happiness;
- loud = dominance/confidence.

Changes in resonance or tone can represent the following meanings:

- sharp voice = complaining/helpless;
- flat voice = sickly/depressed;
- breathy voice = anxious;
- thin voice = submissiveness.

The pitch of a person's voice often varies with the volume of their voice thus:

- high pitch/low volume = submissiveness/grief;
- high pitch/high volume = activity/anger;
- low pitch/low volume = boredom/sadness;
  low pitch/high volume = dominance.

Clarity of speech is often associated with class differences. Hence clipped speech is frequently associated with 'upper-class' people and can convey anger and impatience. Less clearly enunciated speech is often associated with 'lower-class' people and can denote sadness and boredom.

The pace at which people speak varies. Speaking too fast is sometimes linked with anger, surprise, nervousness and occasionally expertise, while speaking too slowly may mean sadness, boredom or sometimes disgust.

Finally, pause fillers such as 'ers' and 'ahs', stutterings, repetitions and omissions all have meanings. They can indicate nervousness, boredom, anger or other emotions.

Conversational sequence

Sacks (2001) illustrates the importance of rules governing conversational sequence with reference to an example from callers to a psychiatric hospital who were reluctant to give their names. The hospital was concerned about whether anything could be done about it. He analysed telephone conversations between staff and patients and found that if staff answered the phone by saying 'This is Mr Smith, can I help you?' patients were much more likely to respond with something like 'Yes, this is Mr

Brown' than if the phone was answered with a simple 'Hello' or 'Hello, emergency psychiatric centre.' He says that if a patient responded with 'I can't hear you' or 'I don't know' then you would have a lot of difficulty getting a name, if you got one at all. The reason, he says, is that there is a procedural rule whereby the person who speaks first can choose their form of address and therefore the form of the other's response. He says that a 'slot' is produced where the patient can provide their name without the member of staff having to explicitly ask for it later. 'Asking for a name tends to generate accounts and counters. By providing a slot for a name, those activities do not arise.'

One good reason for working on one's interpersonal skills is that Faulkner (1984) found that as nurses' communication skills improved so did their empathic and warm responses to patients. She also suggests that if communication with patients is to be effective, the interpretation of conflicting messages should not be left to chance.

Exercise 1.6 *Changing non-verbal behaviour*

This is a popular exercise obtained from Carolyn Kagan. Divide a group of students into threes. Designate one person as A, another as B and the third as the observer. Tell A and B to think about their own non-verbal behaviour in the context of the issues discussed in this chapter. For instance A might like to concentrate on eye contact whereas B might concentrate on posture. Remind them of the components of non-verbal behaviour if necessary. Having thought about their behaviour, ask both A and B to change any *two* aspects of it without telling anybody what the two changes are.

A and B should then have a conversation about what they like and dislike about where they live, concentrating all the time on changing the two aspects of their behaviour they have selected. The observer takes notes on the interaction of A and B, recording all items of interest. Throughout the conversation between A and B the observer should keep reminding them to concentrate on changing their non-verbal behaviour. After about five minutes, stop the conversation and get A and B to reveal their behavioural changes. The observer should then relate his or her observations to A and B.

Ask the groups of three to consider whether it is easy or difficult to change behaviour and whether the changes are easily discernible. Discuss the changes in the context of relating to patients and highlight the problems associated with changing well learned habits.

Questioning and listening

The most important feature of questioning is listening. Liehr (1992) found that nurses who listened to their patients produced lower levels of blood pressure and heart rate in the patients than when they talked to them. Bearing this in mind, consider the following conversation.

'Hello, it's good to see you. How have you been?'

'Absolutely awful. It's my mother, she just won't leave me alone. She rings up at all hours during the night.'

'Mums. They're awful, aren't they? Just like children sometimes. I know mine is, she always wants attention.'

'I mean, I just can't get any sleep and it's ruining all our lives. Not just mine but the whole family's.'

'Yes, I know, they need just as much attention as children. No, I actually think they need more.'

There is not much listening going on in this dialogue. The other person's conversation is being treated as an interruption to one's own dialogue. Therefore a fundamental requirement of asking questions is wanting to hear answers. However, there are different types of questions which serve specific functions in different contexts.

Closed questions

Closed questions, such as 'Do you take sugar in your tea?' or 'Are you a diabetic?' do not allow the respondent any leeway for elaboration. They usually require a fixed or limited number of responses. Closed questions are used to gain factual information about a person or an event, and often form the basis of questionnaires. Closed questions have limited value in allowing patients to explore important concerns, since they return the conversation to the questioner. Try asking a friend a series of closed questions for as long as you can and you will find that you soon dry up. Once your friend has answered your question, you have to think of a new question without much time to do so. As a nurse, if you use a lot of closed questions you will find yourself having to ask more and more to fill the silence. In the end you will be concentrating more on thinking about what you are going to say next than on what the patient is saying. So give yourself some space and use a few open questions.

Open questions

Using open questions gives patients the opportunity to reply in any way they like. It enables them to answer in their own terms and in their own way. There is usually no correct answer and people have the freedom to explore their concerns. The use of this type of question enables the nurse to take stock of the situation and concentrate on how the patient's response may guide the next sequence of questions. A disadvantage of this mode of questioning is that there is no control over the length and relevance of the patient's response. However, closed questions can always be used to bring a wandering conversation back to the relevant issues at hand.

It is important to use both open and closed questions when interviewing patients. Jesudason (1976) illustrated what can happen if only one form of questioning is used. A sample of 1,151 Indian women were asked the open question 'What foods are prohibited during lactation?' Approximately 53 per cent replied that no foods were. Those who said no foods were prohibited were then given a closed question in the form of a list of twelve foods. They were asked if any of the foods on the list were forbidden. About 32 per cent selected five foods or more. Thus, if an open question were used on its own, one would reach a totally incorrect conclusion that 53 per cent of Indian women think that no foods are prohibited during lactation. A better way to elicit correct information would have been to provide the women with a list of foods and ask an open question at the end concerning any foods that were not on the list. When interviewing and constructing questionnaires it is vital to bear these points in mind. Mitcheson and Cowley (2003) found that the use of health needs assessment tools, whilst providing a clear and structured format, did not identify the needs that were specific

Whilst it is a good idea to use both forms of question in conjunction with each other, it is necessary to give some direction to the dialogue and not swap backwards and forwards from one type of question to another. Usually it is a good idea to start off with broad, open questions and then gradually become more focused. Neglecting to provide some sort of sequence can disorientate and confuse patients.

Probing questions

The use of probes or prompts is a verbal strategy designed to help patients talk about themselves and define their condition and concerns more clearly. Probes need not be questions – they can be statements. Furthermore, they can involve just a few words or even a non-verbal response. Here are some examples:

> *Patient*: Look, this is ridiculous; why do I have to see her?
> *A statement prompt*: I can see that you get angry when your wife comes to see you, but I'm not quite sure why.

> *Patient*: Since I was admitted to this hospital I've been treated fairly well; even so I'm not entirely satisfied.
> *An echo prompt*: Not entirely satisfied . . . ?

Patient: Look, after I get home from work, cook the tea and put the kids to bed I'm absolutely exhausted.

Minimal echo prompt: Exhausted?

Patient: Do you know, there are a lot of people who need sorting out?

Non-verbal prompt: Uh-huh?

The use of prompts helps patients to use their own initiative in exploring their situation, but they should not be overused, as dialogue can then turn into interrogation. Once a probe has been used, let the patient talk for a while before responding. Take the opportunity to listen carefully to what the patient has to say, as it will probably indicate the next feature which should be explored.

Leading questions

In most circumstances it is better to avoid leading questions; however, in some circumstances they can be useful. There are three different types of leading question.

- *Conversational leads.* These are not really leading questions at all, since they merely reflect common opinions. An example might be 'She's looking a lot better, isn't she?' Conversational leads can be used to convey interest and friendliness, but only if they accurately reflect other people's thoughts and feelings. The danger lies in misinterpreting what other people are thinking; for example, 'Well, Mrs Appleby, I'm sure you will be really glad to get back home.' Mrs Appleby may not want to go home at all but is unable to say so because the question leads her to respond in the affirmative. In this instance the nurse may not be conscious of leading the patient.
- *Pressurised agreement.* This type of leading question puts pressure on the patient to respond in a prescribed way. An example is 'You do, of course, take your tablets every day?' or 'Hello, John, I bet you could do with a bath, eh?' There is no attempt to ask a question or give the patient any choice. The first example is designed to make the patient feel guilty for not taking his or her tablets, the second is in effect communicating that the patient is going to have a bath and that is it! In very few circumstances, leading questions can serve a useful function. Blatantly incorrect leading questions can stimulate a response in an otherwise uncommunicative person. A question phrased thus: 'Of course, nurses get paid far too much for the job they do, don't they?' will usually precipitate a reply.
- *Subtle leads.* Disturbingly, many people use leading questions without knowing that they are doing so. Subtle leading questions can be found in conversation and in questionnaires. Loftus (1975) interviewed forty people about their headaches and the products they used to alleviate the pain. They were asked either 'Do you get headaches frequently, and if so, how often?' or 'Do you get headaches occasionally, and if so, how often?' Both questions were identical except for the terms 'frequently'

and 'occasionally'. The participants in the 'frequently' condition reported an average of 2.2 headaches a week; the participants in the 'occasionally' condition reported an average of 0.7 headaches a week. Next the participants were asked how many products they had tried for their headaches. Half the participants were given a choice of 1, 2, or 3; the other half were given 1, 5, or 10. Those that were given the choice of 1, 2, or 3 reported an average of 3.3. Those that were given the choice of 1, 5, or 10 reported an average of 5.2. These results indicate that one has to be extremely careful when selecting questions for use in questionnaires. Not only can changing just one word lead to different results, but the degree of choice affects the results as well.

Affective questions

This type of question attempts to address the feelings or emotions of patients. An example of an affective question would be 'How do you feel about your operation?' As well as indicating concern for the patient's emotions, affective questions also offer patients the opportunity to consider how they feel. In many cases, being able to label and define emotions reduces their affective content. It is as if providing some sort of term for feelings objectifies the situation and protects the patient from becoming overwhelmed by emotion. Not all emotions expressed by patients indicate their true feelings. A patient who seems to be angry may in fact be hiding fear. Similarly, a patient who laughs and jokes a lot may be concealing guilt. It is important to allocate time to listen to patients if affective questions are to be used. There is nothing worse than someone asking how you feel and then rushing off. In some contexts, as in the case of a greeting, a matter-of-fact reply to an affective question is appropriate. When a person says 'How are you?' a normal response is 'Fine, and you?' If someone started to say 'Do you know, I feel absolutely terrible, I haven't slept for days. Not only that but I've got this terrible pain in my back . . .' it would cause quite a degree of discomfort to the person, who was just trying to be polite. The nurse should make it clear whether her affective question is a mere greeting or a genuine enquiry about the patient's feelings.

There are other types of question such as multiple questions. Multiple questions should not be used as they can be confusing – patients don't know which one to answer first and often forget what was being asked in the first place. Finally, questions should be used sparingly, since listening to what the patient is saying is more important than concentrating on what to ask next. You should also consider that if you have to ask too many questions, perhaps you are not asking the correct ones to begin with.

Listening

Listening should not be seen as a passive process. It is not time to sit back and have a break from speaking, nor is it an interlude between talking. Active listening involves communicating to the patient that you are interested in what they have to say. There are many ways of indicating concern and consideration, such as:

- *Non-verbal signals.* These have been discussed earlier in the chapter and comprise adopting an interested posture, using nods of the head, 'uh-huhs' and so on, and maintaining suitable eye contact.
- *Reflecting back.* This technique selects the last few words of a person's conversation and repeats, or reflects, them back to the patient. This illustrates that you have been listening to what was being said, and signals to the speaker to continue. For example, a patient's statement such as 'I just couldn't stand the pain. Nobody told me what to expect and when I told him I needed something for the pain I suspect he didn't believe me' could be reflected by saying 'You needed something for the pain and you thought he didn't believe you.' This technique should be used sparingly or you run the risk of sounding like a parrot.
- *Paraphrasing.* This is more difficult to do but has the advantage over reflecting back that it does not make you sound like a parrot and actually conveys understanding as well as listening. An example of a paraphrase response would be:

> *Patient*: I know I keep asking you for help and I don't want to appear difficult but I feel everybody is looking at me all the time.
> *Nurse*: I see, so you think people are looking at you and you don't like asking for help because you think it makes you seem difficult?

Exercise 1.7 *Paraphrasing*

Have a go at paraphrasing some of these statements:

- 'I don't think I can cope any more. It's not just the children, it's my mother as well. My husband is at work all day and I'm at my wits' end.'

  . . . .

  . . . .

- It's the not knowing. I've never had an operation before. I know you've told me everything, but it's just that I think I'm a bit scared.'

  . . . .

  . . . .

- 'It was difficult at first. I just didn't know how I was going to get through the day. But now it's OK, I think.'

  . . . .

  . . . .

● 'I hate hospitals – the smell, the noise, the people, everything. Look, I want out as quickly as possible. I'm not staying here one minute longer than I have to.'

. . . .

. . . .

● 'Every time I say something you parrot it back to me as if I was an idiot. What do you think you're playing at? I'm not stupid, you know.

. . . .

. . . .

The important thing to remember about using active listening techniques is to use them sparingly. If you have any doubts about using paraphrasing, it is probably better not to use it. But sometimes if you don't know what to say and feel that you have to say something, paraphrasing can prove a useful strategy.

Assertiveness

Self-assertion can be a problem for nurses in both their professional and their personal lives. However, assertiveness should not be confused with aggression or arrogance. It is not about getting one's own way but about the freedom to express one's own needs, to stand up for one's own rights whilst respecting the rights and needs of other people. Kagan *et al.* (1986) propose that there are three components to the skill of assertion.

● *Being specific.* The skill in this is in deciding what the point is and stating it succinctly without the unnecessary verbiage that often accompanies statements made when one is uncomfortable and anxious. It is important to know what you actually want to say and then to state it clearly and directly. Example:

> I know it's difficult, and I'm sorry to get you over here again, but do you think that I might have some more water, please? That is, if you're not too busy. Thanks.

Specific question:

> Could I have some more water please? Thanks.

● *Sticking to it.* Not being distracted and being persistent in your requests or instructions produces results, whereas being sidetracked by irrelevant and manipulative comments can divert you from the point you are trying to make. Example:

Nurse: You have to try and stop smoking if you want your breathing to improve.

Patient: Listen, I'm seventy-eight years old and smoking is one of the few pleasures I have left. Surely I deserve *some* enjoyment?

Nurse: But if you stopped smoking you'd feel a lot better and that would be very enjoyable.

Patient: You don't understand, do you?

Nurse: I know it's hard and difficult to give up but if you did manage it for a while you would appreciate the benefits.

● *Fielding responses.* This refers to 'the ability to indicate we have heard what another person has said without getting 'hooked' by what he/ she has said' (Kagan *et al.,* 1986). Example:

> One of your colleagues has asked you to cover for her tonight, but you have made arrangements to go out for a meal with a friend. You do not do this often and know that you deserve a break. You say to your colleague that you had intended to go out for a meal tonight. She says could you please cover for her, as after all she has covered for you in the past. The *easiest* response is to say 'Oh all right. I'll do it'. An *assertive* response is to say, 'No, I'm sorry, I can't work tonight. I appreciate the fact that you've covered for me in the past, and I will help you out as soon as I can, but I'm afraid I just can't work late tonight.' Your colleague may not like this response but you have communicated your willingness to help and at the same time concentrated on your own needs as well as those of others.

It is important to decide on those tasks which you can do, those you might do if possible and those you cannot possibly do. To the first, the response is 'yes'; to the second, 'yes' or 'no' depending on the circumstances, and to the last 'no'. If a 'no' response is selected, it is a good idea to start the reply by saying 'no' as in the reply above. Use a categorical tone of voice and never, never back down. If you do, people will work on you until you agree to help them or do what they ask of you. Most of all, do not feel guilty about saying 'no' if the request falls into the 'cannot possibly do' category. Problems can arise when requests are neither easy nor impossible to comply with. Under these circumstances it is useful to consider your needs in comparison with those of the other person, and if your needs are greater you should decline the request for help (Slater, 1990).

Handling criticism and compliments can be difficult in professional situations. Criticism is never pleasurable but it is made worse if it is perceived as unjust. The assertive nurse will acknowledge justified criticism and confront unreasonable criticism. The way in which unjustified criticism is challenged is important. Often, it is helpful to challenge the basis of the criticism by asking for clarification so that the critics have to examine their own judgements. Example:

Critic: Late again, and scruffy with it.
Response: I'm sorry I'm late, but in what ways am I scruffy?

Some people find dealing with compliments more difficult than dealing with criticism. Genuine compliments should be accepted and rewarded. There is a tendency to concentrate on finding faults in people rather than commenting on how well a person has handled a situation. Therefore one should always respond to praise by thanking the person who has paid the compliment. Example:

Doctor: You handled that patient really well, Nurse.
Nurse: Thank you. I tried to do what I've been taught.

Sarcastic compliments are not compliments at all, but insults, and should be dealt with as such. If in doubt about whether a compliment is genuine or not, ask for clarification. If there was a suspicion that the statement above was meant sarcastically, a warranted response might be:

Nurse: (with a lot of eye contact): Oh, do you think so? In what ways did I handle her well?

Fontana (1990) says:

Self-assertion is essentially having the courage to accept and be the person we are, with all our strengths and weaknesses and individualities. It's the courage to believe in ourselves, and the confidence to convey this belief to others. It has nothing to do with exploiting others, or with always putting our own interests first.

Handling difficult emotions

At times, nurses will encounter the expression of strong emotions in patients, relatives and colleagues. The appropriate use of interpersonal skills at the correct juncture enables nurses to deal with strong emotions in a way that minimises the psychological consequences for all concerned. The following are the most difficult emotions to manage.

Anger and aggression

Aggression in the form of physical assault, threatening behaviour and verbal aggression has become an increasing problem for nurses in general hospitals as well as psychiatric settings. Winstanley and Whittington (2004) investigated aggression in a hospital in the north-west of England by distributing 1,141 questionnaires to members of staff. Their sample of participants was made up of senior nurses (sisters, nurse managers, nurse specialists/practitioners and senior staff nurses), middle-grade nurses (staff nurses and enrolled nurses), basic grade nurses (health care assistants, auxiliary nurses and nursery nurses), professions allied to medicine (physiotherapists, radiographers and occupational therapists) and doctors. Of the 314 who replied to the section on physical violence, ninety-five (30.2 per cent) reported experiencing physical assault once or more than once during the past year, with the staff and enrolled nurses reporting approximately twice as much as the other groups. Although if you compare the ninety-five respondents with the total contacted, including those who did not reply, despite two reminders, the percentage drops to 8.2 per cent. They also found that some staff were repeatedly victimised whilst others experienced no aggression.

Whatever the figures, there really shouldn't be any physical aggression at all, but of course there is, and nurses unfortunately have to deal with it. Thus the management of aggression should feature early on in the nurse's training. Although it is not difficult to identify anger and aggression, dealing with it is a different matter The first stage is to find out the cause of the emotion and whether it is justified or inappropriate. Then the aim is to defuse the hostility and make the situation more manageable. It is no good pointing out to angry people that life is unfair and they have been dealt a 'poor hand'. Usually logic has a limited influence in such circumstances and is unlikely to have an immediate affect. Nurses cannot take away the injustice of life, nor can they restore previous conditions. Therefore, the aim should be to legitimise anger and attempt to disarm it. In similar terms, aggression needs to be managed in a careful way. Coid (1991) says that colleagues who have got into difficulties with aggressive patients recount the following warning signs:

- *Frozen fearfulness.* This represents increasing anxiety in the nurse towards the situation, combined with an awareness that things might be getting out of control. It is necessary to be versatile and intuitive when talking to aggressive patients, and therefore help should be summoned before clarity of thought is lost.
- *Dehumanisation.* Look for indications that the patient is trying to dehumanise the nurse in some way. It is much easier to attack someone who can be made out to be unnatural, uncaring and unlikable, lacking human qualities. Therefore the nurse should pay attention to outbursts such as: 'Nurses are all toerags, they're trash and deserve everything they get.' Sometimes it can help to try to personalise the situation by giving details of oneself to lessen the appearance of being a characterless professional. However, if conditions have got to that stage, it is probably better to get help.
- *Failure to follow a patient's train of thought.* This indicates that a patient may be rapidly losing control. Often it becomes increasingly apparent that the patient has lost touch with reality and may be deliberately withholding information to 'play' the nurse.

● *Point of no return.* A point may be reached where there is no possibility of returning to the rules of a normal nurse–patient relationship. Suggestive speech, sexual innuendoes, invasion of personal space and touching herald a breakdown. Get help.

Ekman (2004) says that one of the first signs of anger is that the red margin of the lips becomes narrower and the lips thinner. This often happens before the person is aware of becoming angry.

Beech (2001) says that health care workers are four times more likely to encounter aggression than the general public, with student nurses being at greatest risk

Guilt

If the focus of aggression or anger changes and shifts from the nurse to the patient him or herself or to a relative, then a feeling of guilt can occur. It is usually very difficult to shift people's guilt feelings away from themselves, but by allowing them to talk about their feelings it is possible to place their guilt in a more appropriate perspective. If feelings of guilt are not examined, they may persist and become a source of psychological problems. The role of the nurse is to appreciate the emotional problems of patients and to accept the reality of their guilt. Although nurses cannot take away people's guilt, they *can* get them to look at it from a different perspective which does not entail individual blame.

Denial

The problem with patients experiencing denial is that it becomes impossible to talk about their true situation. However, there are times when patients may accept some level of reality and provide a 'window' of opportunity for talking about their position. Therefore the nurse should look for an opening and, if one occurs, exploit it. In some cases a patient's denial is complete and they refuse to accept any reality. In that case the nurse must accept the predicament but should not cater to it. For example, a patient who says, 'This time next year I'll be on holiday in the Bahamas,' but very probably will not be alive to do so is clearly using denial. The nurse who responds by saying, 'Yes, it will be wonderful. All that lovely sun', is catering to and feeding the denial. A better way is to accommodate the situation, but not give it substance, by saying, 'Well, I hope things will turn out just as you hope they might.' Thus if the patient does recover, or accepts reality, they will not feel misled by the nurse's responses, and trust can be maintained.

Patients with a terminal illness may never accept reality and die still believing that they are going to get better. Whilst this is unfortunate, and it might have been better if they had accepted their imminent death (see Chapter 6), the situation is ended. This is not necessarily the case for the relatives of patients. Relatives who continue to deny what is happening may suffer a number of psychological problems, and it is necessary to provide much more intervention in such circumstances. (See Chapter 6 for a discussion of how this may be achieved.)

In the majority of cases where strong emotions are apparent, it is a good idea to allow patients and their relatives to vent their feelings before looking for ways forward. People should not be denied the opportunity to express emotion, and moving in too fast with solutions and suggestions may lead to emotional repression and may also lead to issues which have not as yet been expressed being overlooked.

Embarrassment

Edelmann (2004) defines embarrassment as 'a common and often dramatic experience ... a highly uncomfortable psychological state which can have a severely disruptive effect on social interaction'. In a nursing context the phenomenon can have very specific and noticeable consequences. First, embarrassment may be viewed as a feature of a situation involving both nurse and patient and as such it can be viewed from both perspectives. Lawler (1994) suggested that in order for the nurse to help patients manage embarrassment they must first learn to deal with their own. Given that experience by way of greater skill, confidence and knowledge is an important factor in managing embarrassment, there also needs to be what Lawler (1994) calls a sense of purpose. By this she means a sense of purpose associated with having to perform specific nursing procedures. Embarrassment tends to be more of a problem in the initial stages of nurse training, where novel situations allied to inexperience lead to difficulties in managing emotion. Techniques used to combat embarrassment include speeding up nurse–patient interactions, seeking out colleagues in the hope that they have also come across similar circumstances, and perhaps adopting an almost fatalistic view that the situation is absolutely unavoidable and 'I will just have to get on with it'. It may be true that a nurse's embarrassment will disappear with time and experience but this is often little solace to the person, or people, involved.

Patients' embarrassment is often indicated by lack of eye contact, going red, fidgeting, changes in speech patterns and using humour. In most situations patients' embarrassment is relatively easy to spot and, it should be said, perfectly normal, given that patients in the hospital context find themselves in unnatural and abnormal circumstances. Patients can be subjected to invasions of privacy that they would not normally tolerate and it is necessary for the nurse to help redefine the 'rules' such that what was abnormal and uncomfortable is now perfectly acceptable. Also, bodily functions such as vomiting and defecation that are conducted in private can be acceptably performed in a nursing context. Where patients find themselves in a situation where they now are not sure of the rules, it is the task of the nurse to establish an appropriate social order.

Humour

Making people laugh has often been associated with reducing tension and promoting an atmosphere of well-being, But there is little research into when humour can be used to good effect and when an all too well intentioned quip can come seriously unstuck. Furthermore, what is funny for one person is not for another. Sheldon (1996) in a study of the use of humour in the context of children's nursing concluded that 'Although nurses subconsciously use humour in their support of parents it needs to become a conscious activity and incorporated into each individual plan of care'. Although deciding to use exactly what sort of humour in what sort of situation is difficult and certainly lacks spontaneity. Also, one of the reasons for a relative lack of research in this area is hat it is particularly difficult to investigate. One approach used the content analysis of diaries that had been kept over a one-week period (Astedt-Kurki and Isola, 2001) Nurses from two different parts of Finland (Tampere and Oulu) were asked to record incidents at the workplace that involved humour and these were to be written down immediately after work had ceased. Two contexts emerged: that of nurse–patient and that of nurse–nurse humour. The first point to make is that the nurses found the task particularly difficult, as 'it wasn't funny any more' when they came to write the incidents down. However, a number of themes, or categories of humour, emerged:

- Survival oriented humour. Jokes about things going wrong.
- Creative goal-oriented humour. This consists of 'facetious threats' or playfulness on the nurses' part.
- Consensus-oriented humour. Here the nurse is usually the one who laughs at communication problems.
- Patients' observation-based humour. This includes self-irony, cheekiness and witticisms on the patients' part.
- Unintentional contextual humour. This consists largely of patients' mishaps and forgetfulness. Sometime they are not even aware of it.

Humour among staff is categorised as follows:

- Post-mortem-oriented humour. Imagining 'horror' stories related to care, maybe where the patients' safety might have been at risk.
- Skill-oriented humour. This manifested itself in 'black humour' of care styles and forgetfulness.
- Change-oriented humour. Leisure time mishaps experienced by staff and their families outside work

Astedt-Kurki and Isola (2001) give some example of these categories of humour, for instance an example of patients' observation-based humour is:

'Stop rubbing your eyes,' I said.

'Why? I'm not rubbing the other one' – and went on rubbing and giggled.

This may seem not particularly funny. As the nurses in the study said, 'events often didn't seem that funny afterwards', also, what is funny in Finland may not be funny in other countries, and indeed, what is funny in the north of Finland differs from what is funny in the south. The humour was two-way in that it could be initiated by either nurse or patient and thus enabled both to cope with unpleasant procedures and embarrassment. Beck (1997) suggests that humour should be used as a positive nursing strategy to relieve tension and give patients and staff an outlet for their feelings. In this regard it may be seen to facilitate interaction and improve the quality of the working environment.

There remains the issue of when it is appropriate to use the different forms of humour. Unfortunately, there seem to be no clear-cut guidelines but sensitivity to others' perspectives and needs is a prerequisite for avoiding embarrassment and knowing that what worked in one situation for one person or group of people may not work in others.

Summary

This chapter has identified a range of interpersonal skills that can be learnt and developed to improve caring responses to patients. In order to develop these skills it is important to understand and utilise a range of concepts relating to 'self'. These include self-esteem, self-actualisation, self-examination, self-disclosure and the constructed self.

Effective communication skills are an essential element of empathic and sensitive nursing practice. The way in which non-verbal communication complements speech has been examined, and components such as facial expression, gaze, touch, posture and gestures have been explored in relation to cultural, individual and status differences. Verbal communication has been discussed in terms of a range of questioning and listening skills which nurses might use to make their communication with patients, relatives and colleagues more effective.

This chapter concludes with an account of the skills associated with self-assertion and some practical guidance on handling the expression of difficult emotions such as anger, guilt, embarrassment and denial.

Conundrum revisited

The content of this chapter highlights a number of issues and skills important in the care of patients who face uncertainty. Well developed interpersonal skills are central to person-centred care. Before we can claim that Ruth's care is appropriately person- centred, the nurse must gain an appreciation of Ruth as a person and the ways in which she deals with chronic illness and change. Ruth's situation has become unstable. Changes in her illness and new care and treatment prompt her to reappraise what this means for herself (who am I now?) and her future (who will I become?). Adjustments may prove extremely difficult, dependent upon her past experience, support, attitudes, values and beliefs.

Health changes can seriously dent a patient's self-esteem. Previously Ruth felt that she was coping competently with her illness and perhaps even that she had a certain expertise regarding the problem. Now change has reminded her that she needs the assistance of others, and with that may come a loss of confidence. During her health care assessment and rehabilitation Ruth perceived that the locus of control shifted towards the nurses and doctors. She felt angry at a perceived loss of independence and blamed herself for not coping beforehand.

At this point it is tempting to assume that Ruth will simply 'self actualise' by taking charge of her new treatment and regaining independence once more. The nursing goal is certainly to facilitate patient independence, but that still begs the question how we might assist Ruth to 'take charge'? Consideration needs to be given to how she will be helped to compare past, present and imagined future, previous self-care and new self-care. Ruth may for instance perceive controlling her illness once more as simply 'catching up' to her previous (and now less impressive) level of competence. It is important to discuss with Ruth just what meanings she attributes to these events and to anticipate with her what her changed circumstances may represent when she returns home.

Care at this point is quintessentially psychological. The nurse needs to enter into Ruth's world and to appreciate what she defines as problematic and what may represent a solution. To deliver this sort of care it is necessary to facilitate a degree of self disclosure. We need to establish private conditions under which Ruth feels able to rehearse aloud her experiences, thoughts, feelings, values and attitudes concerning her health. Self disclosure involving very intimate matters, those considered closest to the individual's self-identity, is extremely difficult. The nurse must use interpersonal skills to facilitate discussion in these areas and have the confidence to engage in a level of self disclosure too. Whilst nurses are professionally bound not to discuss other patients it may be possible to refer to 'common experiences' – an important reference point that may assist Ruth to take stock of what is happening.

As you thought about your own Ruth conundrum we wonder whether you listed verbal and non-verbal interpersonal skills as key resources? Would you use touch, silence and time discussions to influence Ruth's experience of care? How would you treat the subject of personal space, judging when and how far to intrude into Ruth's thoughts? Patients have varying capacity for and comfort concerning self-disclosure. It is necessary to read the patient's body language in order to judge when to rest a topic of conversation or to suggest a new way of supporting the patient. As you read about the voice and its capacity to represent emotions, the use of different forms of question and listening, you may have identified valuable resources to help you make sensitive decisions regarding a patient such as Ruth.

? Questions for further consideration

1 In what ways is self-actualisation a necessary feature of individual development?
2 Is it possible to hide strong emotions from patients?
3 What is meant by 'active listening'? Describe its use in the nursing context.
4 Define the qualities of the assertive nurse.
5 What are the strengths and weaknesses of open and closed questions?

References

Astedt-Kurki, P and Isola, A (2001) Humour between nurse and patient, and among staff: analysis of nurses' diaries. *Journal of Advanced Nursing* 35 (3), 452–458.

Beck C.T. (1997) Humor in nursing practice: a phenomenological study. *Nursing Studies* 34, 346–352.

Beech B. (2001) Sign of the times or the shape of things to come? A three-day unit of instruction on 'aggression and violence in health settings' for all students during pre-registration nurse training. *Accid. Emerg. Nurs.* 9 (3), 204–11

Beier, E. G. and Sternberg, D. P. (1977). Marital communication. *Journal of Communication, 27,* 92–97.

Berger, P.L. and Luckman, T. (1976) *The Social Construction of Reality.* London: Penguin.

Birdwhistell, R. (1970). *Kinesis and Context.* Philadelphia: University of Pennsylvania Press.

Bruner, J. (1990). *Acts of Meaning.* Cambridge MA: Harvard University Press.

Bruner, J. (2002) *Making Stories: Law, Literature and Life.* Cambridge MA: Harvard University Press.

Coid, J. (1991). Interviewing the aggressive patient. In Corney, R. (ed.) *Developing Communication and Counselling Skills in Medicine.* London: Routledge.

Cook, M. (1970). Experiments on orientation and proxemics. *Human Relations, 23,* 61–76.

Davitz, L. L. and Davitz, J. R. (1985). Culture and nurses' inferences of suffering. In Copp, L. A. (ed.) *Perspectives on Pain.* Edinburgh: Churchill Livingstone.

Edelmann, R. (2004) *Coping with Blushing.* London: Sheldon Press.

Edvarsson, J. D., Sandman, P. and Rasmussen, B. (2003) Meanings of giving touch in the care of elderly patients: becoming a valuable person and professional. *Journal of Clinical Nursing, 12,* 601–609.

Ekman, P. (2004). *Emotions revealed: Understanding Faces and Feelings.* London: Orion.

Ekman, P. and Friesen, W. V. (1975). *Unmasking the Face.* Englewood Cliffs NJ: Prentice Hall.

Engebretson, J. (2004). Caring presence: a case study. In Robb, M., Barrett, S., Komaromy, C. and Rogers, A. (eds) *Communication, Relationships and Care: A Reader.* London: Routledge.

Fontana, D. (1990). *Social Skills at Work.* Leicester and London: BPS Books (The British Psychological Society) and Routledge.

Gergen, K. (1991). *The Saturated Self.* New York, Basic Books.

Greenbaum, P. F. and Rosenfeld, H. M. (1980). Variation of touching in greeting: sequential structure and sex-related differences. *Journal of Nonverbal Behavior, 5,* 13–25.

Hall, E. T. (1969). *The Hidden Dimension.* New York: Doubleday.

Jesudason, S. V. (1976). Open-ended and closed-ended questions: are they complementary? *Journal of Family Welfare, 25, 66–68.*

Jourard, S. M. (1966). An exploratory study of body accessibility. *British Journal of Social and Clinical Psychology, 5,* 221–231.

Kagan, C., Evans, J. and Kay, B. (1986). *A Manual of Interpersonal Skills for Nurses: an experiential approach.* London: Harper and Row.

Kernis, M. H., Grannemann, R. D. and Barclay, I. C. (1989). Stability and level of self-esteem as predictors of anger, arousal and hostility. *Journal of Personality and Social Psychology, 56,* 1013–1022.

Lawler, J. (1994) *Behind the Scenes: Nursing, Somology and the Problem of the Body.* Edinburgh, Churchill Livingstone.

Liehr, P. (1992). Uncovering a hidden language: the effects of listening and talking on blood pressure and heart rate. *Archives of Psychiatric Nursing, 6,* 306–311.

Loftus, E. F. (1975). Leading questions and the eye witness report. *Cognitive Psychology, 17,* 560–572.

Luft, J. (1984). *Group Processes: an introduction to group dynamics.* 3rd edn. Palo Alto CA: Mayfield.

Luft, J. and Ingham, H. (1955). *The Johari Window: a graphic model for interpersonal relationships.* University of California: West Training Laboratory in Group Development.

Maslow, A. (1962). *Towards a Psychology of Being.* London: Van Nostrand.

Maslow, A. (1972). *The Farther Reaches of Human Nature.* New York: Viking Press.

Mayo, C. and Le France, M. (1973). Gaze Direction in Interracial Dyadic Communication. Paper presented to the Eastern Psychology Association Conference, Washington DC.

McCabe, C. (2004). Nurse–patient communication: an exploration of patients' experiences. *Journal of Clinical Nursing, 13,* 41–49.

McCann, K. and McKenna, H. P. (1993). An examination of touch between nurses and elderly patients in a continuing care setting in Northern Ireland. *Journal of Advanced Nursing, 18,* 38–46.

McCanne, T. R. and Anderson, J. A. (1987). Emotional responding following experimental manipulation of facial electromyographic activity. *Journal of Personality and Social Psychology, 52,* 759–768.

McCloskey, A. C. and Bulechek, G. M. (1996) Nursing Interventions Classification. 2nd edn. St Louis MO: Mosby.

McKivergin, M. and Daubenmire, J. (1994) The essence of therapeutic presence. *Journal of Holistic Nursing* 12: 65–81.

Mitcheson, J. and Cowley, S. (2003) Empowerment or control? An analysis of the extent to which client participation is enabled during health visitor/client interactions using a structured health needs assessment tool. *International Journal of Nursing Studies, 40,* 413–426

Montepare, J. M. and Zebrowitz-McArthur, L. (1988). Impressions of people created by age-related qualities of their gaits. *Journal of Personality and Social Psychology, 54, 547–556.*

Moretti, M. M. and Higgins, E. T. (1990). Relating self-discrepancy to self-esteem: the contribution of discrepancy beyond actual-self ratings. *Journal of Experimental Social Psychology, 26,* 108–123.

Mulaik, J. S., Megenity, J. S., Cannon, R. B. and Chance, K. S. (1991). Patients' perceptions of nurses' use of touch. *Western Journal of Nursing Research, 13,* 306–319.

Myles, A. (1993). Psychology and health care. In Hinchliff, S. M., Norman, S. E. and Schober, J. E. (eds) *Nursing Practice and Health Care.* 2nd edn. London: Arnold.

Nelson-Jones, R. (2002). *Basic Counselling Skills: A Helpers' Manual.* London: Sage.

Pennebaker, J. W. (1997). *Opening Up: the healing power of expressing emotions.* New York: Guilford Press

Pietroni, P. (1976). Non-verbal communication in the GP surgery. In Tanner, B. (ed.) *Language and Communication in General Practice,* London: Hodder and Stoughton.

Randle, J. (2003). Changes in self-esteem during a three-year training pre-registration Diploma in Higher Education (Nursing) programme. *Journal of Clinical Nursing, 12,* 142–143.

Rogers, C. R. (1971). *Encounter Groups.* London: Allen Lane.

Rosaldo, M. (1984). 'Toward an anthropology of self and feeling'. In Schweder, R. A. and Levine, R. (eds) *Culture Theory: Essays on Mind, Self and Emotion.* Cambridge, Cambridge University Press.

Rosenthal, R. and DePaulo, B. (1979). Sex differences in eavesdropping on non-verbal cues. *Journal of Personality and Social Psychology, 37,* 273–285.

Rubin, Z. (1970). Measurement of romantic love. *Journal of Personality and Social Psychology, 16,* 265–273.

Ryden, M. B., McCarthy, P. R., Lewis, M. L. and Sherman, C. (1991). A behavioural comparison of the helping styles of nursing students, psychotherapists, crisis interveners, and untrained individuals. *Archives of Psychiatric Nursing, 5,* 185–188.

Sacks, H. (2001) Lecture 1: Rules of conversational sequence. In Wetherell, M., Taylor, S. and Yates, S. (eds) *Discourse Theory and Practice.* London: Sage

Schacter, S. and Singer, J. E. (1962) Cognitive, social and physiological determinants of emotional states. *Psychological Review, 69,* 379–399.

Sheldon L. M. (1996) An analysis of the concept of humour and its application to one aspect of children's nursing. *Journal of Advanced Nursing, 24,* 1175–1183.

Slater, J. (1990). Effecting personal effectiveness: assertiveness training for nurses. *Journal of Advanced Nursing, 15,* 337–356.

Whitcher, S. J. and Fisher, J. D. (1979). Multidimensional reaction to therapeutic touch in the hospital setting. *Journal of Personality and Social Psychology, 39,* 87–96.

Winkel, F. W., Kopelaar, I. and Vrij, A. (1988). Creating suspects in police–citizen encounters: two studies on personal space and being suspect. *Journal of Social Behavior, 3,* 307–318.

Winstanley, S. and Whittington, R. (2004). Aggression towards health care staff in a UK general hospital: variation among professionals. *Journal of Clinical Nursing, 13,* 3–30.

Wright, B. (1993). *Caring in Crisis.* 2nd edn. Edinburgh: Churchill Livingstone.

Zuckerman, M., Klorman, R., Larrance, D. T. and Spiegel, N. H. (1981). Facial, autonomic, and subjective components of emotion: the facial feedback hypothesis versus the externalizer-internalizer distinction. *Journal of Personality and Social Psychology, 41,* 929–944.

Further reading

Ekman, Paul (2003) Emotions Revealed. London: Orion. A classic 'etic' perspective on the meaning of faces and feelings.

Robb, Martin, Barrett, S. and Komaromy, C. (2004) *Communication, Relationships and Care.* London: Routledge. A multidisciplinary selection of readings with a good proportion related to nursing care.

Stevens, Richard (2000) *Understanding the Self.* London: Sage. A very readable discussion of five perspectives on the self (biological, cognitive/experimental, psychodynamic, social construction and experientialist).

Making Judgements about Others

A practice conundrum

The following excerpt comes from a conversation that two nurses held at a conference on practice development. These very experienced nurses were discussing just how complicated practice had become and what might be done to make it more straightforward. Each of the nurses had very different explanations for the current situation and different recommendations for what might be done next.

Nurse A: My friend showed me a textbook on surgical nursing that she had trained with back in the early 1970s. It was amazingly straightforward and gave you a very clear picture of what care consisted of. You could almost feel envious of the situation back then.

Nurse B: But it was a medical model, wasn't it? A list of the problems, operations and associated care procedures. There was nothing about patients as people or what the nurse could initiate for herself. These days you can't start with any assumptions. You have to investigate everything.

Nurse A: True! But I still think that care has got too complicated and we're not willing to trust common sense any longer. A lot of what the textbooks dress up in fancy terms is still common sense, isn't it? Besides, care will grind to a halt if you don't work with at least some assumptions.

Nurse B: Maybe . . . but you have to ask, whose common sense? If you base care on common sense life gets simpler, but you make bigger mistakes, don't you?

The nurses express views about care that are at opposite ends of the spectrum. At one extreme the nurse investigates and analyses everything. At the other extreme a body of knowledge and ideas is considered sound enough to be accepted as a 'given' in care. Where do your sympathies lie, more towards nurse A or towards nurse B? What might the practice consequences be of operating more at one or the other extreme?

Imagine that it is the first day of term of a new course. The course tutor comes into the room and spends a few minutes making some introductory remarks and then leaves. Later that day, over a cup of coffee, a friend asks what you thought of your new tutor. You immediately launch into a description of your reactions, maybe even making predictions about whether you are going to like the course or not. In just a few minutes you have formed a clear first impression of your new tutor. But is your impression correct?

A patient discharges herself after major surgery, against medical advice, only to be readmitted with serious complications at the site of the operation. The nurse on duty may have judged the patient unco-operative and ungrateful for the treatment she received and a source of potential trouble during her future stay in hospital. In reality the patient may have been responding to concern about her children, whom she felt might have inadequate care and support in her absence.

Attribution: understanding the causes of behaviour

If you have known a person a long time you are often able to understand the causes of his or her behaviour. Of course some events may cause unpredictable reactions, but usually you can make reasonable judgements as to why he or she behaved in a particular way. As in the examples given, nurses make, or are asked to make, judgements about people's behaviour with little or no prior knowledge of them. The question arises as to how accurate these judgements can be.

Accurate knowledge of a patient's current mood or feelings is important for the nurse's assessment of the patient's needs and planning of a programme of care. However, a patient's feelings do not always remain the same, and the nurse should be aware that behaviour may change across time and across different situations. The process through which we seek to acquire information about the causes of others' behaviour is called *attribution*.

We draw information from several sources in our attempts to form impressions of the people around us:

- the way they dress, their age and their attractiveness;
- by talking to them;
- by observing their behaviour.

The first two sources of information give clues to the behaviour of others, but they can be misleading. For example, people can dress in a certain way in order to disguise their true personality and may talk in such a way as to camouflage feelings or mood. Many people think that the observation of behaviour provides a much more useful guide, but this too can be fraught with errors. Consider the following example.

A man is standing on a bridge staring down at the water below. Several people observe the man's behaviour. The *artist* sees the scene as a series of colours and shades. The *insurance salesman* thinks the situation represents a bad risk. The *physicist* weighs the force of the man in conjunction with the matter of the bridge.

Each individual's different observation has been influenced by his or her background. The scene is constant, but the observations are different.

There are several questions that need to be asked when considering why people behave as they do:

● How do nurses decide whether a patient's behaviour represents 'true' personality characteristics or whether it is a specific reaction to a specific situation?
● Is a person's behaviour a result of personality and therefore within their control, or is it due to external circumstances beyond their control?
● Do we judge ourselves differently from the way we judge others?
● Do we attribute the cause of our successes and failures correctly to our own behaviour?

Attribution theories

Jones and Davis (1965) proposed a theory called *correspondent inference.* They suggested that attempts to understand the causes of behaviour should focus on a number of different factors.

● Attention is given to acts that are freely chosen by, as opposed to those that are forced on, the individual. If a person is forced to do something, it is difficult to conclude that this behaviour forms a stable dimension of their personality.
● Attention is given to behaviour that gives rise to unique or non-common results. An example would be a friend who says that he wants to get married because his girlfriend is attractive, has a great personality and has just inherited a lot of money. All these three facts seem equally good reasons for wanting to get married. But let us say that the person he proposes to marry is unattractive, complains and moans a lot and has just inherited a large amount of money. You might think the last factor would be more indicative of the real reason for the proposed marriage.
● Greater attention is paid to actions that are not approved or encouraged by society than to those that are. Consider the nurse in his interaction with patients; he might smile at patients when he talks to them, express concern for their anxieties or discomfort and often be seen talking to and reassuring relatives. Such behaviour would seem perfectly normal. But the nurse who scowls at patients when they talk to him, laughs when they say they are frightened and locks himself in the office when relatives are on the ward would seem rather odd. It is much more likely that firm inferences about behaviour will be assigned to the latter nurse, because his actions are both unusual and socially undesirable.

● Finally, we tend to pay more attention to actions that have a direct impact on us than to those that do not. If it is our child that is kissed, or our hand that is shaken by a politician, we will pay more attention than if it is someone else's child or hand.

The main feature of this theory is that not all behaviour is observed; individuals are selective about what they pay attention to. It is important to note just how selective people are in order to gain a better idea of stable personality characteristics.

Another attribution theory, the *co-variation model,* was proposed by Harold Kelley (1972). He was concerned with determining why in some instances a person's behaviour is said to be a result of their personality while in others it is said to be a result of the situation they are in. He gives the following example.

It is lunchtime and the patients on the ward are eating when suddenly Mrs H shouts, 'Take this horrible food away, it's disgusting! I wouldn't give it to my dog.' Is her behaviour due to the quality of the food, or is she just a fussy eater? Kelley says that the answer can be obtained from three kinds of causal information:

● *Consensus.* Do other patients in the ward react in the same way?
● *Consistency.* Has this person reacted to this situation in a similar manner on other occasions?
● *Distinctiveness.* Does this person react to other, different situations in the same way?

If other patients do not react in the same way (low consensus), if Mrs H has done it often before (high consistency) and has also reacted in a similar fashion to other situations (low distinctiveness), then one can assume that her behaviour stems from internal causes such as her personality. If other patients react similarly (high consensus), if Mrs H has reacted to this situation in a similar manner before (high consistency) and she has not reacted to different situations in this way (high distinctiveness), then the food is at fault.

There is empirical support for this theory (Harvey and Weary, 1989), but there are some problems with the extent to which people are willing to spend the time and effort to go through the whole process. Indeed, Fiske and Taylor (1984) say we are *cognitive misers* – 'unwilling to expend the energy necessary' to attribute the cause correctly. Furthermore, people are most 'miserly' when circumstances are against them, for example when events occur unexpectedly and when events are extremely unpleasant.

Kelley has put forward a theory that describes an ideal attribution process, but, as individuals do not always have the time or are unable to make the effort, mistakes are made. Suppose you were in charge of the busy ward where Mrs H is having lunch. Can you imagine having time to work through consensus, consistency and distinctiveness questions before making a judgement about her behaviour?

First impressions

One view of impression formation is that a limited amount of information about a new person influences our overall impression of them. This view was illustrated by a famous study conducted with two groups of people by Asch (1946).

The first group was given a list of adjectives describing a fictitious person – intelligent, skilful, warm, determined, practical, and cautious. The second group was given the same list but the word 'cold' was substituted for the word 'warm'. Both groups were then presented with another list of eighteen words and asked to underline those they thought described this fictitious person.

Whilst some words, such as reliable, good-looking, restrained and honest were chosen by both groups, the 'warm' group viewed the person as generous, humorous, sociable and popular, whereas the 'cold' group viewed the person as having opposite personality characteristics. Merely changing the word 'warm' to 'cold' caused the participants in the experiment to view the fictitious person in a different way.

Would all pairs of opposites have the same effect as 'warm' and 'cold'? Asch said they would not. When he used the words 'polite' and 'blunt' instead of 'warm' and 'cold', he found that participants in both groups underlined almost identical words. He concluded that there were certain words like 'warm' and 'cold' that represented a central or dominant trait and which were influential in determining first impressions, whilst there were others that did not have the same effect, and which represented a peripheral trait or dimension largely unimportant in impression formation. There is still debate about what words represent a central trait, but more important perhaps to consider is whether people respond to a real person in the same way as they do to a fictitious one.

Nisbet and Wilson (1977) conducted a similar experiment to Asch's, but using a real person. They showed one group of students a film in which an instructor behaved in a warm, considerate and friendly way. A second group of students saw a film in which the same person behaved in the opposite manner: cold, aloof and distant. In both films the instructor spoke with a French accent. After viewing the films the students were asked how much they liked the instructor and what they thought of his appearance and French accent. The students assigned to the 'warm' group liked the appearance of the instructor and thought that his French accent had contributed in a positive way to the delivery of his lecture. Those students assigned to the 'cold' group did not like him and thought that his accent hindered the delivery of the lecture.

Although the students in the 'warm' group said that they had developed a liking for the instructor, they felt that this had not influenced their judgement in any way. When a first impression influences the perception of other personality characteristics it is called the *halo effect*. This effect can also lead to making judgements beyond the information given. A person who presents herself as smart and well dressed may also be thought of as punctual, intelligent and hard-working, even when there is absolutely no evidence to support these attributions.

In a study of nurses' initial assessment of patients Price (1987) concluded that current nurse education conceives assessment as relating to the physical status of patients and their abilities to care for themselves. He says:

> This research would suggest that we must quickly review the reality of nursing assessment criteria, skills and protocols. It would indicate that we should take much more account of the psychosocial areas of assessment and the nurses' own feelings of insecurity, control or reward in such interviews.

Consider this example. A nurse admits to the ward a patient who cannot speak clearly and is hard to understand. Much of his speech is slurred. He has difficulty in controlling the movements of his mouth and has a tendency to dribble. The nurse may assume that he is unintelligent, highly dependent and unable to understand anything she says to him. Alternatively she might assume that he is drunk, irresponsible, potentially aggressive and likely to be a nuisance. In reality he may well be none of these things, but consider what the impact of being treated in such a fashion would be.

In a study of what factors lead to a patient being seen as unpopular, Stockwell (1993) proposed that the reasons were mostly related to personality, physical defects such as deafness, nationality and length of stay in hospital being longer than three months. However, Kelly and May (1982) criticised this and other studies on methodological grounds. They suggested that inconsistencies in the research findings stemmed from the use of a variety of research instruments and that there was a failure to define concepts adequately. Furthermore, patients come to be defined as good or bad not because of anything inherent in them, but as a consequence of their interaction with nurses.

The primacy effect

Exercise 2.1 *Forming impressions*

Divide a group of students into two. Split both groups into pairs – one person the experimenter, the other the participant. The participants are then asked to leave the room. The experimenters should take six cards and write the following words on them: *intelligent, industrious, impulsive, critical, stubborn, envious.* Half the experimenters will present the words to the participants in the above order and half present them in reverse, so that half the participants will see the words in the order *intelligent* to *envious* and half will see *envious* to *intelligent.* Cards should be presented to participants at one- second intervals. Participants are asked to form an impression of an imaginary person based on the words shown and then write a brief sketch of the imaginary person's personality. Try and get the participants to use each of the words presented to them as a basis for their sketch. Are there any differences between the impressions of the imaginary people formed by the two groups?

Asch (1946) conducted a similar experiment, giving participants identical lists of personality characteristics but presented in a different order. The first list moved from positive to negative and the second from negative to positive. Asch contended that impressions formed of others are more strongly affected by information received first (*primacy*). Thus subjects given the first list would rate the fictitious person more positively than those given the second list. He found that those participants given the list with 'intelligence' first rated the imaginary person as more sociable, happy and humorous than those given the list beginning with 'envious'.

The explanation given by Asch for this primacy effect was that the adjectives read first changed the meaning of the ones read later. Learning that someone was intelligent caused the participants in the experiment to interpret being stubborn as an intelligent person merely sticking to their intelligent point of view.

Fiske and Taylor (1984) offered another explanation based on their idea that we are cognitive misers (see p. 50); once we have initial information about people, we simply do not bother to pay attention to any additional details.

It is important for nurses to make a good first impression in order to establish the right conditions for the development of mutual trust. However, nurses should be aware that positive first impressions can sometimes inhibit the willingness of the patient to be assertive and necessarily critical when their needs are not being met. Not only may a patient attribute to the nurse positive personality/ability characteristics that are not there, but they may even discount or reinterpret any negative ones that appear subsequently.

Errors and bias

One might predict that psychologists should be less likely to make attribution and first impression errors because of their greater knowledge of human behaviour. Certainly an understanding of the processes involved makes one less susceptible to bias, but greater knowledge can sometimes lead to a concentration on the finer details at the expense of the obvious. There are, however, some attribution errors that we all tend to make.

The fundamental attribution error

The second example at the beginning of the chapter (p. 48) illustrates that, in many circumstances where information is unavailable as to whether a person's behaviour stems from their personality or the situation, it is usually internally attributed to the person's disposition. This is called the *fundamental attribution error* or 'blaming the patient'. Maslach and Jackson (1982) say that it occurs frequently among nurses. Placing the blame on the patient becomes more probable when medical records highlight personal problems at the expense of important background detail. The individual has to be seen within the context of his or her social and economic situation if accurate and useful assessments are to be made.

Case study

Mrs D is 71 and lives in a single room in a hostel. Since her husband died she has been found to be consuming increasing amounts of alcohol, and it was thought that the bereavement had led to dependence on drink. Initially, it was decided to try to change her behaviour by concentrating on improving her attitude and resistance to the temptation to drink. These attempts failed. It was then noticed that the death of Mrs D's husband had resulted in a change in her social arrangements: she had started to socialise with a group of people who drank a lot. Attention was switched from changing Mrs D's attitude to finding her company that did not drink so much alcohol. Subsequently she was observed to cut down her consumption of drink substantially.

Thus attribution errors can be reduced by attention to circumstantial or background details. The likelihood of error is increased if the behaviour is serious and personal; for example, a person spilling coffee over an expensive table increases the likelihood of you making an attribution error that he is clumsy, and the likelihood will be heightened even more if it is your coffee table.

The actor–observer bias

Exercise 2.2 *Personality characteristics and the actor–observer bias*

You can try this exercise on your own or in a group. Think of someone you know very well. Rate this person on the following personality characteristics using the following scale:

+2 Definitely describes
+1 Usually describes
 0 Sometimes describes, sometimes does not
–1 Usually does not describe
–2 Definitely does not describe

Once you have done this, rating someone you know, cover up your responses and rate *yourself* on these personality characteristics.

Personality characteristic	Other person	You
Aggressive	. . . . .	. . . . .
Introverted	. . . . .	. . . . .
Thoughtful	. . . . .	. . . . .
Warm	. . . . .	. . . . .
Outgoing	. . . . .	. . . . .
Hard-working	. . . . .	. . . . .
Ambitious	. . . . .	. . . . .
Friendly		

Add up the score for your friend and then add up your own score. Ignore the plus and minus signs. If the score for your friend is greater than your own score, then you have fallen prey to the actor–observer bias. If both the scores are the same, or you scored higher than your friend – well done!

One day while you are walking along the road you notice a person opposite stumble and fall. You think to yourself 'How clumsy!' or 'They've had too much to drink.' This internal attribution of causality corresponds to the fundamental attribution error. However, while watching the person opposite, you yourself trip up and stumble. You do not think for a moment that you are clumsy, but that the pavements in your town are in need of repair. In short, if you are the observer, you make internal attributions. If you are the actor, you make external attributions, and this is known as the *actor–observer bias* (Jones and Nisbet, 1971).

Janis and Rodin (1979) contend that the actor–observer effect can present particular problems for nurses. If a patient does not take his or her medicine he or she may be perceived by the nurse (the observer) as stubborn and unco-operative. The patient (the actor) will attribute his or her reaction to environmental factors; that is, he or she has stopped taking the medicine because it makes him or her feel sick and thinks that it is not doing him or her any good. The nurse and the patient see the same event from two different perspectives and are reacting to two different cues. Effective care becomes hampered by a conflicting set of perspectives which can lead to severe communication difficulties.

The self-serving bias

Imagine that you are faced with a two-part physiology exam. The first part is much more difficult than the second, but you feel quietly confident because you spent a considerable amount of time revising and feel you know most of the areas reasonably well. After taking the first part of the exam your results confirm your optimism, and your performance ranks with the best in the group. Not surprisingly, you feel quite proud and feel that all your revising was worth while. The second part of the exam approaches and you feel more confident than you did before. After taking the exam you relax in expectation of similar results. It comes as quite a shock when you find that you have not done very well at all and have barely achieved average results. This time you start to blame the irrelevant questions, not having had enough time, or even the heat in the exam room, for your poor performance.

When individuals do well, they attribute the cause of success to internal factors, and when they do badly they attribute it to external factors. This is called the *self-serving bias* (Miller and Ross, 1975) and is an important mechanism for protecting self-esteem in adverse circumstances.

Unfortunately this type of bias can have disastrous consequences for relations between team-workers. If you are working well with a partner and everything is going to plan, attributing the cause of the success to your ability, although this may be incorrect, will not necessarily affect the relationship with your partner. When things start to go badly you may blame external factors, including your partner, and he or she will do the same to protect his or her self-esteem. The ensuing conflict can lead to a great deal of interpersonal friction (Greenberg *et al.*, 1982). This error can be particularly detrimental in the context of primary nursing where nurses work in close relationship with individual patients to plan and implement programmes of care. If a programme of care is not working as planned, the relationship may be impaired by the nurse attributing its failure to characteristics of the patient, such as low motivation. Think back to the last time things went wrong at home or at work; who did you blame first?

Research on attribution and impression formation suggests that we are all susceptible to errors which can distort our perceptions of social reality (Gilbert and Jones, 1986). However, a knowledge of the psychological processes of attribution can lead to fewer errors and hopefully limit the negative consequences.

Prejudice

A father and his son were driving along a road when the father suddenly lost control of the car and crashed into a telegraph pole. The father was killed instantly and the son was badly injured. The boy was rushed to the local hospital, where it was found that he was suffering from serious internal injuries. A prominent surgeon was immediately summoned. When the surgeon arrived and went into the operating theatre to examine the boy, there was a gasp from the surgeon. 'I can't operate on this boy,' the surgeon said. 'He's my son.' How could the boy be the surgeon's son?

Some of you will know the answer to the riddle, but how many were unable to work it out when they first heard it? A clue is to substitute the word mother for father and read the story again.

The importance of this riddle is to emphasise that prejudice is not just about conscious discrimination against race or class; there are many biases of which we are unaware. If you did not know the answer to the riddle then you are prejudiced. You might have thought up all sorts of weird and wonderful solutions but the simple fact that the surgeon was a woman eluded you. Indeed, McDonald and Bridge (1991) found that the female nurses who were given a vignette that differed in terms of patient gender planned significantly more ambulation, analgesic administration and emotional support time for male patients as opposed to female patients.

Prejudice may be defined as a negative attitude to someone who is a member of a specific group, based upon the fact that they are a member of that group. Prejudice occurs in all sorts of groups and takes many forms. There are three main components of prejudice: thoughts (*cognitive*), feelings (*affective*). actions (*behavioural*).

Thoughts

Stereotypes

One form of prejudicial thought is a *stereotype.* This is a cognitive framework that describes a person's thoughts and beliefs about specific social groups.

If you asked someone to describe the typical Italian male, French farmer or British banker, they would not have too much trouble doing so even if they had never met a person from any of these groups. Not all stereotypes involve negative characteristics, and sometimes there can be a grain of truth in them (Allport, 1954). However, the main problem arises when people hold negative, incorrect stereotypes. Davidio *et al.* (1986) suggest that the stereotype accepts only information that is consistent with its cognitive framework and rejects information that is contradictory. If one searches hard enough or waits long enough, one can usually find examples of a person's behaviour that will support the stereotype; this is usually accomplished at the expense of ignoring all behaviour which disconfirms it. In other words we confirm a cognitive schema or stereotype (Richards and Hewstone, 2001).

Davitz and Davitz (1985) assert that we do not like to believe that we operate on the basis of stereotypes, and that we like to think we can see through them. To investigate stereotypes held by American nurses Davitz and Davitz gave nurses the following brief description of an adult patient:

Name: Gino Giselli
Age: 34
Background: Italian

Mr Giselli was hit by a car when going home from work. He was admitted to hospital and found to have a fractured femur and extensive facial injuries. At the moment he is in traction, and will have to remain in hospital for an indefinite period.

Davitz and Davitz varied the cultural background of the patient each time they read the story. The patient's physical condition, gender, and age remained consistent, but different cultural backgrounds were assigned to them. The six cultures were: Oriental, Mediterranean, Black, Spanish, Anglo-Saxon/Germanic and Jewish. The other factor varied was the severity of the individual's condition: mild, moderate and severe. They measured the nurses' average ratings of physical pain and psychological distress for each cultural group and for each level of illness severity.

It was found that most physical pain and psychological distress was perceived to be suffered by the Jewish and Spanish patients and the least pain and distress was experienced by the Oriental and Anglo-Saxon/Germanic patients. The experimenters summarised their results by saying that the results of their research clearly indicated that one aspect of the American nurse's belief systems about suffering involves the ethnic or religious background of their patients.

Do nurses from other countries have similar stereotypes? Davitz and Davitz also looked at attitudes to pain held by 1,400 nurses from thirteen countries using the same technique and found wide variations. The British nurses, for instance, rated the Italian patient in the story as suffering the least pain and were generally inclined to say that patients from other cultures overreacted. This latter point led to the British nurses working in the United States acquiring the stereotype of being efficient but unsympathetic.

In hospitals and communities where there are a wide range of cultures and ethnic groups, it is important to recognise the existence of stereotypes. It is easy to fall into the trap of selectively abstracting behaviour in order to support the stereotype whilst ignoring import-ant disconfirming details.

Labelling

Another form of stereotyping is *labelling*. Because personality is difficult to define, people often resort to labels to simplify categorisation. If individuals are aware of their label, this can lead to a self-fulfilling prophecy; a person with red hair may acquire the label 'quick to anger' and eventually end up behaving that way because he or she is expected to do so.

Rosenhan (1973) illustrated the powerful effect of labelling in a famous experiment called 'On being sane in insane places'. He arranged for 'normal' people, such as a psychologist, a housewife, a paediatrician and a painter-decorator to present themselves at the admissions offices of eight different psychiatric hospitals in the United States, complaining that they were hearing voices saying 'empty', 'hollow' and 'thud'. All were admitted and diagnosed as schizophrenic or manic depressive. The amount of time spent by the 'patients' in each institution ranged from three–fifty-two days, even though they acted completely normally once they were admitted. The only people to become suspicious of these 'patients' were the other inmates. When the 'patients' were discharged they were labelled 'schizophrenic in remission', which implied that they were still schizophrenic but there was no evidence of it on discharge.

In a follow-up experiment, the staff at the teaching hospital were told about the results from the first study and were told to expect a number of 'pseudo-patients' presenting themselves for admission over the following three weeks. The staff were required to rate 193 patients who had been admitted over this three-week period on a ten-point scale according to whether they thought the patient was a 'plant'. Forty-one patients were confidently alleged to be impostors by at least one member of staff and twenty-three were highly suspected by at least one psychiatrist. In fact, no pseudo-patients had been sent to the hospital. Although the study has been criticised on methodological grounds (Spitzer, 1976), this clearly demonstrates the power of giving people labels.

Further evidence for the labelling effect has been provided by Rosenthal and Jacobson (1968). Pupils in a primary school were tested on a range of verbal and reasoning ability tests. The teachers were told that the purpose of the tests was to detect those pupils who were about to go through an intellectual growth spurt. The teachers were told in confidence the names of these 'intellectual bloomers'. The performance of the children was monitored and after just eight months the tests were repeated. The intellectual bloomers produced significantly higher scores on the tests than the other pupils. These results may not seem too surprising apart from the fact that the bloomers had been selected and given the label 'likely to succeed' entirely at random. In just eighteen months the label had produced significant differences in performance. If this can happen in a positive direction, it can also happen to those labelled 'not likely to succeed'. If this then becomes a self-fulfilling prophecy, the challenge of reacting to such a system becomes practically impossible.

Health professionals have a tendency to categorise patients in terms of illness. This is not surprising, as medical practice tends to do the same; however, Wattley and Müller (1984) have illustrated how illness can affect nurses' perceptions of patients. Two groups of nurses were given a written description of a patient and asked to make an assessment. The descriptions of the patient were similar, except that in one the patient was being treated for cirrhosis of the liver and in the other for a hernia. The experimenters predicted that, as cirrhosis is associated with drinking, the nurses would be more inclined to blame the patient for his condition. The nurses were asked to rate the patient on a list of personality traits and it was found that the man with cirrhosis was rated as less cheerful, more unhelpful, more ungrateful, slightly more unco-operative, more difficult to talk to, more willing to accept treatment and less likely to exaggerate the extent of the illness than the same patient would be if suffering from a hernia.

Implications

- Descriptions/diagnoses/assessments should be made with great caution and awareness of potentially stigmatising effects.
- Labels are powerful and very resistant to change. They affect the way people are treated for a long time.

- It is important to reflect on your reactions to patients and on assumptions you might have made as a result of a label.
- Treat all labels as potentially erroneous, even if they appear as facts or rules.

Feelings

Another component of prejudice is the presence of negative feelings towards individuals on the basis of their membership of a specific group. Many of these feelings are deep-seated and thus difficult to change (Stephan and Stephan, 1988). The first step on the way to dealing with negative feelings is to recognise them.

Exercise 2.3 *Identifying negative feelings*

- Read the following descriptions of people.
- Imagine that they are patients in your care.
- Write down your immediate feelings about them.
- Try to identify how these feelings might interfere with nursing these patients.
- Try to think of the characteristics that would describe the person you would find it most difficult to deal with and state why.
- Examine the stereotypes implicit in the five descriptions:

    1 Arthur is a 44-year-old man who obviously doesn't care about his physical well-being. He swears a lot and makes sexist jokes. He has not had a job for years and does not intend to get one.
    2 Cathy is 18, currently experiencing a lot of problems at home and feels that her boyfriend does not understand her. She does not seem to get on with anyone but sees you as a potential ally. In talking to her you notice she seems to blame everyone but herself.
    3 Joan is 36 and could be classed as 'upper middle-class'. She has a very 'correct' attitude and very traditional views. For instance, she believes that a woman's place is in the home and men should be in charge because they are better than women. She is continually asking you to do things for her.
    4 Ken is only 27 years old and has been trying to commit suicide for the last two years. He says that although he has failed this time, he will succeed eventually. He does not want to listen to you, or indeed have anything to do with you, and continually rejects your attempts to interact with him.
    5 Mary is a young lesbian who has recently been rejected by her partner and feels very depressed. She sees you as a new friend and potential confidant.

Actions

Discrimination

The behavioural component of prejudice involves some sort of action. In many instances prejudicial views do not result in active discrimination; laws, social pressure and fear of retaliation can deter people. However, not all discrimination is obvious. Bigoted people usually prefer if possible to harm the targets of their prejudice without raising suspicion by using subtle forms of discrimination such as *tokenism*.

Tokenism involves the use of small, positive acts towards the target individual or group in order to deflect criticism of more overt discriminatory treatment (Rosenfield *et al.,* 1982). 'What do you mean, I don't like gay people? I bought Jeff a drink last week.' Or, perhaps more subtly, 'Listen, I have nothing against disabled people living here. My goodness, didn't I say so at the meeting? It's just that I think their interests would be better represented . . .'

The majority of people are not bigoted, but the majority of people are prejudiced in some way or another. It is easy to spot the bigots by their overt actions, but it is not so easy to measure prejudices that are less transparent. One method of assessing discriminatory tendencies is by using a *Social Distance Scale*.

Exercise 2.4 *Measuring prejudice*

This measure provides an indication of how distant or dose you like to be to members of specific groups.

First, you would select a group – ethnic, homosexual, mentally ill/disabled, AIDS sufferers, or a group within the nursing profession.

Next, you would produce a scale (see the example) by starting with a statement that involves a large degree of distance between you and a member of that group, such as 'I would find it tolerable for this person to come to my country as a visitor.' End with a statement that represents a close relationship, such as 'I would find it tolerable for this person to marry into my family.'

This person is from . . . . . . group.

I would find it tolerable for this person to:

Tick/Cross

- come to my country as a visitor ☐
- live in my country ☐
- work in the same job as myself ☐
- live in the same city ☐
- live in the same street ☐

- have a meal with me
- be neighbours
- be close friends
- many or become involved with my family

Tick/Cross

☐
☐
☐
☐

If you cannot tick all the statements for individuals representing all groups then you are prejudiced. You might like to discuss whether not wanting someone to marry into your family is prejudice or whether it represents a logical concern for the well-being of your kin.

Of course the Social Distance Scale does not measure actual discriminatory acts, nor does it work for discrimination between men and women. However, if people are truthful whilst completing it, they can gain a useful insight into their behavioural intentions to different social groups.

Origins of prejudice

Several theories have been put forward to try to explain the development of prejudice. Some of the main theories are: inter-group competition; social identity; authoritarian personality; social learning.

Inter-group competition

One theory of prejudice suggests that it is caused by competition and that the greatest prejudices occur during times of economic hardship (Hepworth and West, 1988). However, the roots of inter-group conflict have a much broader foundation. Sherif and his colleagues (Sherif, 1981) conducted an interesting experiment into the nature of the relationship between conflict and prejudice. This is known as the *robbers' cave experiment.*

The participants in the experiment were a group of 11-year-old boys at a summer camp in the United States. On arrival they were divided into two groups and assigned to different cabins. For about a week the boys played, worked and slept together in their respective groups, building up strong attachments to each other. They chose names for their groups – the Rattlers and the Eagles – and each group constructed a flag with their symbol on it.

In the second part of the experiment, the boys competed for a trophy and prizes in a games tournament involving baseball, touch-football, a tug-of-war and a treasure hunt. This situation produced intense competition between the two groups. The games started off in good spirit but quickly turned nasty. The boys started to call each other names and, in one instance, burnt one of the flags. The researchers had to intervene as the experiment was getting out of hand. Clearly, in just a few weeks strong prejudices had build up between the two groups.

To try to reduce the conflict, the groups were brought together for social events such as going to the movies, eating in the same dining room and so on. But far from reducing the conflict it seemed to have the opposite effect, actually increasing the acrimony between the two groups. Eventually Sherif and his colleagues found a solution. They constructed conditions where both groups had to work together to reach mutually desirable goals. For instance, they had to restore the camp's water supply, pool their funds to rent a film, and together mend a truck that had broken down. After a few days of co-operative activities the inter-group rivalry had been eliminated and many cross-group friendships had been made.

There are limitations to the conclusions that can be drawn from this experiment, since it took place over a limited period of time, the summer camp does not necessarily represent everyday life and the boys were all from one social group (Tyerman and Spencer, 1983). Despite these restrictions, the results suggest that competition is a powerful factor in the development of conflict and prejudice.

Social identity

Tajfel (1982) contends that there are two main stages in the development of prejudice: social categorisation and social competition.

Social categorisation

People feel a need to categorise themselves into groups to satisfy a need to belong and receive attention and affection. Also, it is often difficult to achieve certain goals as individuals whereas groups may be more successful. Group membership creates and maintains a sense of social identity, an important constituent of self-esteem. However, this act of categorisation causes people to distort their perception of the social groups. An experiment by Tajfel and Wilkes (1963) illustrates this point very well.

Participants were presented with a series of straight lines and asked to estimate their lengths. There were three conditions.

- Participants were presented with lines of different lengths at random.
- Participants were presented with the same lines but this time they were labelled A or B. The presentation was random and the label was unrelated to the length of the line.
- Participants were presented with four short lines accompanied by the letter A and four long lines accompanied by the letter B.

There were a number of differences in the ways the subjects estimated the lengths of the lines. In the third condition, where there was categorisation, the participants exaggerated the differences in length between the four short lines and the four long ones. The longer lines were seen as more alike than they really were.

We could substitute people for lines and see that we tend to categorise people into groups; exaggerate the differences between groups; and see members of groups as more alike than they really are. Further, membership of a group will enhance an individual's self-esteem only as long as the group status is maintained. Thus groups will not only compare themselves with others but actively seek to reinforce all their own positive characteristics, such as individuality, intelligence, and so on, at the expense of other groups' negative characteristics. This theory has been called the *'us' versus 'them'* or the *social identity theory* (SIT). For example, I may think that psychologists are all reasonably intelligent, know a lot about human behaviour and are generally open to new ideas whereas psychiatrists have little idea of human behaviour (as they have done a medical degree), tend to prescribe drugs for all conditions and are very narrow in their thinking! Hornsey and Hogg (2000) provided further evidence for social identity theory but also found that reducing prejudice between groups by breaking the distinction between 'us and them' would work only if both groups were allowed to maintain their sense of uniqueness, even superiority. It appears that we need to form ourselves into groups because they can provide a 'self-esteem boost' and if this is overlooked then mixing groups together or emphasising similarities between groups will prove counterproductive.

Exercise 2.5 *'Us' versus 'them'*

Think about the following groups in relation to the 'us' versus 'them' theory. Can you identify any ways in which one group might reinforce its status at the expense of the other? (Some sample answers are given at the end of the chapter.)

- Nurses   versus   Doctors
- Students   versus   Teachers
- General nurses   versus   Mental health nurses
- Patients   versus   Nurses
- Student nurses   versus   Qualified nurses

Social competition

Skevington (1981) has examined the applicability of Tajfel's theory to nursing students. She presented sixty-four nursing students with a questionnaire designed to measure status and desired social mobility. The students were prospective registered or enrolled nurses and selected from among first and second-years. Some of the findings supported

Tajfel's theory; the registered nurses were deemed to have a higher status, had more positive subjective characteristics, and a positive social identity. The enrolled nurses had more attributed disadvantages and a less positive social identity.

It was found that the two groups of nurses actually *decreased* the perceived differences between themselves. Skevington notes that since the nurses worked closely with each other on the hospital wards, stereotypes were reduced. Also, the enrolled nursing students were trying to become more similar to the registered nursing students' group by adopting similar interests and seeing themselves as equally competent, as a means of achieving equivalent social identity.

Placing groups together can reduce prejudice but this is insufficient on its own; one needs to take into consideration Sherif's findings that the groups must share mutual goals and have to work together to achieve them.

The authoritarian personality

After the atrocities of World War II a number of psychologists, such as Adorno, Frenkel-Brunswick, Levinson and Sandford, decided to investigate what personality characteristics could be said to constitute fascist behaviour. Their aims were to discover how to raise children in such a way that they would never become fascists, and to devise ways to alter the leanings of those already possessing such tendencies. Their measure of the authoritarian personality was called the *F scale* (F for Fascism; Adorno *et al.,* 1950). Individuals who scored high on the F scale were hostile to people of 'inferior' status, servile to those of 'higher' status and rigidly intolerant of others' views. They were filled with as much fear as hate, hence their frequent association with right-wing, militaristic groups.

Bigoted people have often experienced harsh, punitive parenting leading to low self-esteem (Buri *et al.,* 1988). Typically the child cannot respond to the parents' aggression and thus displaces his frustration on to another individual over whom he has power. This aggression has to be justified along such lines as 'Well, he deserved it. They all do, don't they? Shouldn't be here . . .' There is evidence that prejudiced reactions are associated with authoritarian personality characteristics (Cherry and Byrne, 1976) (Table 2.1).

Thus some, but not all, prejudice is perpetrated by people who score high on the F scale. Little can be done to change their personality, but they are responsive to authoritarian demands.

Social learning

Parents can exert a huge influence over the views of their children. Not surprisingly if parents are prejudiced against certain people their children will tend to hold similar views. Tamara Towles-Schwen and Russell Fazio (2001) explored the developmental

Table 2.1 *Characteristics of the authoritarian personality*

Submission. Obedience and respect for authority are paramount virtues.

Aggression. Gays and blacks should be locked up and the key thrown away.

Cynicism. The old traditions of this country have gone and something must be done about it.

Conventionalism. A person who hasn't got breeding can hardly expect to associate with decent people.

Power. There are two sorts of people: the weak and the strong.

Projectivity. People just do not realise how much our lives are controlled by secret plans.

correlates of racial attitudes by asking undergraduates to complete a questionnaire on their childhood experience of African-American people and their perception of their parents' attitudes towards this group. They found that the students who reported parents as being less prejudiced were less prejudiced themselves; further, the more frequent positive interaction with black people during childhood also correlated with less prejudice.

Reducing prejudice

None of the theories discussed represents a solution to the problem of prejudice, but taken together they do suggest a blueprint for action.

- *Awareness.* Many people do not want to be prejudiced and certainly do not want to transmit prejudiced views and attitudes to their children; however, they are simply not aware of the extent to which their attitudes and behaviour *are* prejudiced. Scales like the Social Distance Scale represent a starting place for discussing prejudiced beliefs.
- *Inter-group contact.* We have seen from the Skevington study that contact can reduce stereotypes. Contact between groups can dispel negative stereotypes through lack of supportive evidence, and both groups may realise that they have more similarities than differences.
- *Co-operation.* Mixing groups together is not good enough on its own (see '*the robbers' cave experiment*' p. 62–3). Stephan (1978) reviewed the research on desegregation of schools in the United States and found that prejudice had increased in as many cases as it had decreased. Contact has to be paired with the pursuit of common goals. As the school environment is quite competitive, conflict can be exaggerated by inter-group contact.

● *Equal status.* Argyle (1991) points out that whilst equal status contact is always difficult to achieve, it has long been regarded as essential if prejudiced and hostile attitudes are not to be reinforced. Without equal status, stereotypes may simply be
reinforced.

Aronson *et al.* (1978) put these points into action by constructing a co-operative classroom structure called *the jigsaw classroom.* Pupils from different cultural backgrounds
were placed into groups of six and each member of the group was given one piece of the
lesson to learn and to relate to the other members of the group. At the end of the lesson
each child was tested on the whole lesson and given an individual score. Each child had
to learn the whole lesson, but could do so only by depending on the others. The status
of the members of each jigsaw group was equivalent, and communication between the
group members improved.

Aronson and his colleagues found that just three forty-five-minute jigsaw sessions per
week produced significant changes in the children's abilities and behaviour. There was an
increase in self-esteem and in liking of other group members, and an improvement in
academic performance. However, although the children from different racial groups who
actually worked together came to like each other better, the reduction in prejudice did
not extend to those ethnic groups as a whole.

Summary

This chapter has focused on the way in which we make judgements about other people
and how this might effect both the way patients are assessed and treated and the way in
which health professionals work together. The process by which causative judgements
are made about the behaviour of others is called attribution. I have explored various
theories of attribution, including those which attempt to account for occasions when
behaviour is inaccurately attributed. This can occur either as a result of inattention to all
the available information or as a result of errors of attribution and biases which distort
perceptions of social reality.

Prejudice is one source of bias and this chapter concludes with a discussion of the
origins, components and measurement of prejudice. The main components of prejudice
are thoughts, feelings and actions. I have looked at the three main theories which
attempt to explain the origins of prejudice; these include the theory of inter-group
competition, social identity theory and the authoritarian personality.

Understanding how errors of judgement can occur and recognising the conditions
under which prejudiced thoughts, feelings and actions are likely to increase can help to
improve the accuracy of nursing assessment and clinical judgement and the way in
which health care professionals work together.

Conundrum revisited

A central problem of nursing practice is that we are faced with making decisions based upon incomplete information, where decisions may have very significant consequences and within a context where there are increasing arguments about what is the *right* way to proceed. Our decisions (to act or not to act) to ascribe something to others or to withhold judgement are conducted within the public arena, with patients, relatives and other health care professionals as stakeholders.

Under these conditions nurses face information overload and information deficit. They are overwhelmed by information about patients, colleagues and situations which is typically fragmented. We have to make sense of what has been seen, heard or discovered. In other aspects of practice, though, there is information deficit. We have too little information with which to interpret situations confidently. Often, therefore, practice has to develop incrementally. We have to respond and react as well as to plan or strategise.

Nurse A approaches this problem by acknowledging the need to simplify complex problems so that distinct actions can be planned. She wishes to plan care that it manifestly helpful. In adopting this approach, she proposes that certain assumptions, about needs, situations and care processes, might be accepted as adequate working models upon which to base care. The models are based upon what she thinks of as common sense. Commonsense care is seen as that which most people would find acceptable, think reasonable or defensible. On the plus side, care may proceed briskly and sometimes to good purpose. Where commonsense care is accurately founded upon what the carers and patients find valuable it is applauded as cost- effective. But nurse A runs the risk of inaccurately attributing meaning to situations that others do not share. She may focus on inappropriate aspects of care, bring prejudices to bear about others (patients, colleagues or situations) and rely too heavily upon certain information (first impressions). This may be compounded where meaning is ascribed not only to the actions of an individual but to whole groups. For example, nurse A might think certain behaviour as 'typical of night staff'.

The consequences of uncritical acceptance of certain information or ways of proceeding as commonsense may be dire. Patients may die, consumers may suffer and conflict may develop between individuals or practice groups. The chances of conflict increase in precisely those areas where we may least assume that others ascribe similar meanings to situations as ourselves. For example, assessing patient histories and the origins of problems, evaluating patients' response to education or discharging patients from hospital might all prove points at which assumptions are erroneous.

Perhaps you favoured the perspective of nurse B, who perhaps proposes a more cautious approach to making practice decisions. Nurse B accepts that there are likely to be multiple interpretations of experience and many different perspectives on what should be done next. Her experience of the mass media and the different interpretation of national and international events emphasise to her just how fraught any form of decision making can be. This nurse is much more concerned with understanding the process of care. She believes that care outcomes will be longer-lasting, more satisfying and equitable if decisions are negotiated *en route* by all the stakeholders.

What nurse B finds stressful about this approach to practice is the shortfall in resources (time, staff and expertise) to enable decisions to be arrived at in a more consensual way. She understands just how harmful biases, prejudices and inaccurate attribution of meaning can be. Nurse B faces compromises, needing to make decisions rapidly in some circumstances and to second-guess how others may respond to her chosen actions. She finds herself becoming increasingly cynical about what health care can achieve because very little of the care that she delivers is what she would describe as 'ideal'. As the years pass nurse B finds practice increasingly difficult and debates whether to move to new work.

In this conundrum the pressure to make decisions and manage limited resources has been described as the context within which inaccurate attributions, prejudices and biases may have negative impact upon practice. The costs of relying naively upon assumptions, though, are balanced by those of making incomplete or unsatisfactory progress because decisions cannot be investigated fully. Perhaps not surprisingly neither extreme (the idealism of nurse B nor the complacency of nurse A) seems likely to enhance practice. Whilst there are no trite solutions to this conundrum you may consider the merits of the following:

- Identifying the more common assumptions and prejudices that impact upon local practice.
- With clients and colleagues, identifying areas of health care where consultation is especially important.
- With clients and colleagues, identifying aspects of health care where there is greater agreement regarding what constitutes acceptable health care (care protocols and principles of good practice).

? Questions for further consideration

1 In an interactive activity such as nursing, can we ever be free from all our prejudices and biases?
2 To what extent are we 'cognitive misers' when forming first impressions?
3 What is meant by the primacy effect in impression formation?
4 How can a knowledge of attribution errors inform the process of nursing care?
5 What theories have been put forward to explain the development of prejudice?

Some sample answers to Exercise 2.5

- *Nurses versus Doctors.* As a nurse I may think that nurses are closer and more caring towards patients than doctors, who are distant and aloof.
- *Students versus Teachers.* As a teacher I might think that teachers are totally committed to learning and education and work hard to deliver a high-quality course, whereas students are only in it for the social life and are generally less committed to work.
- *General nurses versus Mental health nurses.* If I were trained in general nursing I might think that general nurses work hard and are always kept busy, whereas mental health nurses sit in their office and drink coffee all day
- *Patients versus Nurses.* As a nurse I present myself as capable, confident and self-reliant, in contrast to patients, whom I perceive as dependent and demanding.
- *Student nurses versus Qualified nurses.* As a student I might think that I have the most up-to-date knowledge about practices and patient care, whereas I believe qualified staff are resistant to anything new and trained before anyone really knew anything useful.

References

Adorno, T. W., Frenkel-Brunswick, E., Levinson, D. J. and Sanford, R. N. (1950). *The Authoritarian Personality.* New York: Harper and Row.

Allport, G. W. (1954). *The Nature of Prejudice.* Wokingham: Addison Wesley.

Argyle, M. (1991). *Cooperation: The Basis of Sociability.* London: Routledge.

Aronson, E., Stephan, C., Sikes, J., Blayney, N. and Snapp, M. (1978). *The Jigsaw Classroom.* Beverley Hills CA: Sage.

Asch, S. (1946). Forming impressions of personality. *Journal of Abnormal and Social Psychology, 41,* 258–290.

Buri, J. R., Louiselle, P. A., Misukanis, T. M. and Mueller, R. A. (1988). Effects of parental authoritarianism and authoritativeness on self-esteem. *Personality and Social Psychology Bulletin, 14,* 271–282.

Cherry, F. and Byrne, D. (1976). Authoritarianism. In: Blass, T. (ed.) *Personality Variables in Social Behaviour,* Hillsdale NJ: Erlbaum.

Davidio, J. F., Evans, N. and Tyler, R. B. (1986). Racial stereotypes: the contents of their cognitive representations. *Journal of Experimental Social Psychology, 22,* 22–35.

Davitz, L. L. and Davitz, J. R. (1985). Culture and nurses' inferences of suffering. In: Copp, L. (ed.) *Perspectives on Pain.* Edinburgh: Churchill Livingstone.

Fiske, S. T. and Taylor, S. E. (1984). *Social Cognition.* Reading MA: Addison Wesley.

Gilbert, D. and Jones, E. E. (1986). Perceiver-induced constraints: interpretations of self-generated reality. *Journal of Personality and Social Psychology, 50,* 269–280.

Greenberg, J., Pysazaynski, T. and Solomon, S. (1982). The self-serving attribution bias; beyond self-presentation. *Journal of Experimental Social Psychology, 18,* 56–67.

Harvey, J. H. and Weary, G. (1989). *Attribution: Basic Issues and Applications.* New York: Academic Press.

Hepworth, J. T. and West, S. G. (1988). Lynchings and the economy: a time-series reanalysis of Hovland and Sears (1940). *Journal of Personality and Social Psychology, 55,* 239–247.

Hornsey, M. J. and Hogg, M. A. (2000). Intergroup similarity and subgroup relations: some implications for assimilation. *Personality and Social Psychoogy Bulletin, 26,* 948–958.

Janis, I. L. and Rodin, J. (1979). Attribution, control, and decision making: social psychology and health care. In: Stone, G., Cohen, F. and Adler, N. E. (eds) *Health Psychology.* London: Jossey Bass.

Jones, E. E. and Davis, K. E. (1965). From acts to disposition: the attribution process in person perception. In: Berkowitz, L. (ed.) *Advances in Experimental Social Psychology* II, New York: Academic Press.

Jones, E. E. and Nisbet, R. E. (1971). *The Actor and the Observer: Divergent perception of the causes of behavior.* Morristown NJ: Erlbaum.

Kelley, H. H. (1972). Attribution in social interaction. In: Jones, E. E. (ed.) *Attribution: Perceiving the causes of behavior.* Morristown NJ: General Learning Press.

Kelly, M. P. and May, D. (1982). Good and bad patients: a review of the literature and a theoretical critique. *Journal of Advanced Nursing, 7,* 147–156.

Maslach, C. and Jackson, S. E. (1982). Burnout in health professionals. In: Sanders, G. S. and Suls, J. (eds) *The Social Psychology of Health and Illness.* Hillsdale NJ: Erlbaum.

McDonald, D. D. and Bridge, R. G. (1991). Gender stereotyping and nursing care. *Research in Nursing and Health, 14,* 373–378.

Miller, D. J. and Ross, M. (1975). Self-serving biases in the attribution of causality: Fact or fiction? *Psychological Bulletin, 82,* 213–225.

Nisbet, R. E. and Wilson, T. D. (1977). Telling more than we could know: verbal reports on mental processes. *Psychological Review, 84,* 231–259.

Price, B. (1987). First impressions: paradigms for patient assessment. *Journal of Advanced Nursing, 12,* 699–705.

Richards, Z. and Hewstone, M (2001) Subtyping and subgrouping: processes for the prevention and promotion of stereotype change. *Personalty and Social Psychology Review, 5,* 52–73.

Rosenfield, D., Greenberg, J., Folger, R. and Borys, R. (1982). Effect of an encounter with a black panhandler on subsequent helping for blacks: tokenism or conforming to negative stereotype? *Personality and Social Psychology Bulletin, 8,* 664–671.

Rosenhan, D. (1973). On being sane in insane places. *Science, 179,* 250–258.

Rosenthal, R. and Jacobson, L. (1968). *Pygmalion in the Classroom.* New York: Holt Rinehart and Winston.

Sherif, M. (1981). Experiments in group conflict. In: Aronson, E. (ed.) *Readings about the Social Animal.* 3rd edn. San Francisco: Freeman.

Skevington, S. (1981). Intergroup relations and nursing. *European Journal of Social Psychology, 11,* 43–59.

Spitzer, R. L. (1976). More on pseudoscience in science and the case for psychiatric diagnosis. *Archives of General Psychiatry, 33,* 459–470.

Stephan, W. G. (1978). School desegregation: an evaluation of predictions made in Brown versus Board of Education. *Psychological Bulletin, 85,* 217–238.

Stephan, W. G. and Stephan, C. (1988). Emotional reactions to interracial achievement outcomes. *Journal of Applied Social Psychology, 19,* 608–621.

Stockwell, F. (1993). *The Unpopular Patient.* London: Royal College of Nursing.

Tajfel, H. (1982). *Social Identity and Intergroup Relations.* Cambridge: Cambridge University Press.

Tajfel, H. and Wilkes, A. L. (1963). Classification and quantitative judgement. *British Journal of Psychology, 54,* 101–114.

Towles-Schwen, T. and Fazio, R. (2001). On the origin of racial attitudes: correlates of childhood experiences. *Personality and Social Psychology Bulletin, 27,* 162–175.

Tyerman, T. and Spencer, C. (1983). A critical test of the Sherifs' robber cave experiments: intergroup competition and cooperation between groups of well acquainted individuals. *Small Group Behavior, 14,* 515–531.

Wattley, L. A. and Muller, D. J. (1984). *Investigating Psychology: A Practical Approach for Nursing.* London: Harper and Row.

Further reading

Aronson, E. (2003). *Social Animal.* San Francisco: Freeman. There is not much to say about this book except for the fact that it is brilliantly written. It contains a discussion of just about all the main social psychological issues in an interesting and understandable fashion.

Baron, R. A. and Byrne, D. (2003). *Social Psychology.* 10th edn. Boston MA: Allyn and Bacon. There are a number of basic experimental social psychology texts, most of which contain all the standard experiments. However, I think this is one of the best because it is easy to understand and intellectually rigorous at the same time. It is one of the most popular texts and should be easy to get.

The Effect of Groups on Behaviour

A practice conundrum

In this chapter you will read about different groups and their influence upon people, decisions and even contexts. Your practice conundrum starts from a common practice experience where you are a member of several different groups and where as a consequence you have to consider your various allegiances, roles and opportunity to influence outcomes. Begin now by recalling a practice scenario where a decision has to be made about the next steps associated with a patient's care. It should be something that you believe the patient would probably feel emotionally invested in, which is (as you see it) clearly something that nurses know something about and yet, which requires multidisciplinary practice to bring to fruition. Pain management is a good example of a decision that fits these criteria. In this scenario there are three groups in operation:

- The consumer-named nurse group. (This consists of the patient and yourself, but may also consist of a lay carer, partner or other family members as well.)
- The nurse professionals group (yourself and other nurse colleagues contributing care to the patient)
- The multidisciplinary group, including nurses, doctors and therapists.

Now make notes in answer to the following questions. As you read through the chapter identify psychological concepts or research findings that seem to either support or challenge your answers. Our own thoughts on the conundrum appear at the end of the chapter.

1 How does your membership of the above groups (in your chosen scenario) influence your contributions (ideas, actions, arguments)?
2 In practice are you forced to owe more allegiance to one group? If so, is this a constant, or does that pattern change, situation to situation?
3 Given the influence of groups, how do you now think about nursing care?

In the last chapter the focus of attention was upon the individual and his or her behavioural make up. However, individuals do not live in a social vacuum but often interact with others in a variety of contexts. Sometimes our behaviour may be influenced by groups, so it is important to examine the processes by which such influence may be exerted. In order to determine the nature of social influence it is proposed to investigate the psychology of group behaviour and then to concentrate on one specific type of group – the family.

Groups

Paulus (1989) has defined a group as consisting of:

> two or more interacting persons who share common goals, have a stable relationship, are somehow interdependent, and perceive that they are in fact part of a group.

Note that a group is not simply a number of people gathered together at the same time in one place; there needs to be interaction, interdependence, some form of stability and, most important of all, the individuals must perceive themselves as being members of the group.

Robbins (1989) has identified a number of reasons why we like to form ourselves into groups:

- to satisfy a need for belonging and to receive attention and affection;
- to achieve goals that we would have considerable difficulty in attaining as individuals;
- to maintain and develop a sense of social identity. Self-esteem may be enhanced by membership of a group.

Having established why people form themselves into groups, it is necessary to determine how groups exert influence over individual behaviour.

Conformity

Society as a group exerts pressure on individuals to conform in specific ways. There are certain unwritten rules or *social norms* which indicate the ways in which people should behave. Forming a queue at a bus stop, wearing appropriate clothes for a formal or informal function and applauding at a concert are examples of social norms. Some social norms provide a useful function, and thus the pressure to conform has a legitimate justification; others, such as wearing a tie for certain occasions, seem to serve no obvious purpose and demonstrate a different type of conformity.

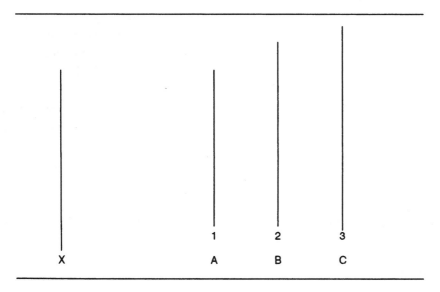

Figure 3.1 How people conform to group pressure. *After Asch (1951)*

An experiment by Asch (1951) illustrated two different features of the ways in which people conform to group pressure. He asked a group of eight people to look at three lines of different lengths and compare them with a line of standard length (see Figure 3.1). The group were asked to estimate which of the three lines was the same length as the standard line. Seven out of the eight people in the group were accomplices of the experimenter, and only one person was the true subject of the experiment. The accomplices gave truthful answers to the first twelve requests to compare the lines, but on the next eight trials were told by Asch to give false responses. Asch then asked each of the group members in turn which of the three lines, A, B or C, was the same length as the standard line X. The first six members of the group all gave a false response and replied that line A was the same length as line X while it was perfectly obvious that the correct answer was line B. Imagine that you were the seventh person in this group – what would you do? Chances are that you would go along with the rest of them and say A, even though you could see that line B was the correct answer. Asch found that 75 per cent of the people tested went along with the rest of the group on at least one occasion, indicating that many people would go along with the group rather than disagree openly with the other members of the group.

Asch put forward two explanations as to why a large proportion of individuals conform to group pressure:

- *Normative social influence.* People do not want to 'rock the boat'. They know the correct answer but feel that they will disadvantage themselves if they disagree with the others.

● *Informational social influence.* If a number of people in front of you have answered in a way that contradicts your opinion, you are likely to doubt your ability to make correct responses. In situations of uncertainty we look to other members of the group for information on how to behave.

These two forms of social influence are not mutually exclusive. Indeed, the subjects in Asch's experiment could very well have experienced both at the same time. A typical mental response of the subjects in the experiment may have been: 'I am pretty sure it is line B, but why is everyone else saying line A? Am I seeing correctly? I think so. Oh well, I might as well go along with everyone else and say line A.'

However, conformity does not occur to the same degree in all situations or among all individuals. Thus it is important to determine the factors that influence the conformity effect.

Cohesiveness

Crandall (1988) has suggested that some groups elicit a greater degree of conformity than others. The more we like others, and wish to gain their approval, the more likely we are to be influenced by them. A group perceived as having high status will generate more conformity than a group perceived as having low status. A nurse who finds him or herself a member of a high-status group, such as consultants, will experience more pressure to conform than when a member of a low-status group. Therefore, when nurses find themselves in the company of people they regard as important or impressive, they should take care not to conform to group pressure, but to respond to the situation with the conformity effect firmly in mind.

Size

Tanford and Penrod (1984) have proposed a *social influence model* (SIM) which says that as group size increases (up to four or five people) conformity increases rapidly. But as further members are added the conformity effect levels off. Therefore, large groups need not necessarily exert more influence than small ones. The implications for team nursing are that working in groups can lead to a higher consistency of approach and a greater common purpose, but they can also maintain an orientation towards old practices which inhibits innovation.

Gender differences

Early studies by Crutchfield (1955) produced evidence that females are more likely to conform than males. However, the tasks used in these studies were more familiar to men than to women, and people tend to conform more in situations of uncertainty. More recent studies (Eagly and Carli, 1981) have found no evidence of gender differences. The differences between the two sets of studies may be resolved by noting that the early studies used male experimenters and male-oriented items, and also, since women may often occupy low-status positions, the apparent *gender* differences are better represented as *status* differences.

Having an ally (social support)

If one member of the group fails to accept the position of the majority, the conformity effect is extinguished. Conformity is reduced even if the ally is viewed as incompetent or does not share the same views. It seems it is the breaking of the group's united front that is important.

Nursing implications

Morris *et al.* (1977) found that the conformity effect is further reduced if someone speaks out at the start of the questioning procedure. These findings are especially important, as, where conformity of approach is required, so too is a forum in which nurses can express nonconformist ideas as a potential source of growth and development. Therefore speaking out in group discussions is an important way of resisting conformity effects which might inhibit the potential for improving practice. Niven (1994) has said:

> Many health professionals find themselves in group meetings to discuss numerous issues. The format of the group may vary, but social influence does not. Sometimes the group may be made up of members of different professions, sometimes the health professional may find him [or her] self in the presence of what he [or she] regards as high-status or influential individuals. In these circumstances conformity to group opinion needs to be avoided.

Social facilitation

Social facilitation is concerned with examining the effect groups have on task performance. Do we accomplish tasks better when in the presence of others or when alone?

Imagine that one of the patients in your clinical area has died. You are familiar with, and competent in, the practices which relate to last offices. Imagine carrying out last offices on your own and then imagine carrying them out with another member of the team. Which would have the best effect on how you practised? Think about the reasons for your answer and how it fits or conflicts with the work described in the following paragraphs.

Zajonc (1965) proposed that the presence of others increases arousal, which leads to better performance on easy or well learned tasks, but worse performance on new, difficult tasks. Further research (Sanna and Shotland, 1990) has indicated that we are also influenced by an audience's evaluation of us and the impression we are making in front of others.

However, an interesting piece of research cast some doubt over the arousal/evaluation explanation of social facilitation. Robert Zajonc and his associates found that they could produce a social facilitation effect in animals (Zajonc *et al.*, 1969). Using cockroaches in mazes, the experimenters found that when a cockroach ran a simple maze observed by four others it did so better than when it was observed running a more complex maze. Clearly, the cockroaches were unlikely to be concerned with 'looking good' or 'making a favourable impression'.

It seems that a supplementary explanation is required. Baron (1986) has put forward a theory based on the distraction caused by the presence of an audience. The presence of others when performing a complex task causes a sort of information overload whereby the individual is unable to concentrate on all the elements of the task requiring attention, thus leading to a poor outcome. Simple tasks, on the other hand, do not suffer from this distraction and focused attention will enhance performance.

Nursing implications

If a nurse is required to perform a new activity in front of others, such as reading out a research report in a seminar, she will not do as well as she did when she tried it out on her own. In order to be successful at new complex activities in front of others, it is necessary to practise and practise until the nurse has a repertoire of strong, well learned, appropriate task responses that will in fact benefit from the presence of others.

Social loafing

One feature of group behaviour is the inequality of an individual's contribution to group goals. Take the following example. A person is having difficulty lifting a heavy object, so a number of people get together to help him. Some people take as much of the load as possible, whilst others are content to appear to help without really doing very much. This is known as *social loafing*. Some people work hard in a group, others employ social loafing and do as little as they can get away with.

A German psychologist called Ringelman was one of the first to investigate the social loafing phenomena, over fifty years ago. He asked people to pull as hard as they could on a rope attached to a meter that measured the amount of force exerted by each individual. He found that one person pulling on their own exerted an average force of 63 kg; when pulling in groups of three the average dropped to 53 kg; and in groups of eight to 31 kg. The greater the number of people, the less effort expended. Further research has indicated that social loafing occurs on all sorts of tasks and in many different cultures (Harkins, 1987).

How can social loafing be reduced?

- Make each person's contribution to the group easily identifiable so that minimal effort cannot be hidden.
- Increase group pressure to succeed. Develop an emphasis on group commitment.
- Provide an opportunity for group members to compare their contributions with members of other groups. People may 'loaf' because they think that their performance cannot be evaluated by others.

Group dynamics and decision making

The following exercise is designed to give you some insights into the group dynamics of decision making.

Exercise 3.1 *Group dynamics and decision making*

Ask for five volunteers from your class or group. Explain to them that they will be required to make some individual decisions and then come together to take part in a group discussion. Take the five volunteers into another room and distribute the Choice Dilemma Sheets (see following). Tell them that they have to make a series of decisions on their own without consulting each other. Example:

> Mrs J likes to go skiing whenever she can. She is quite good at it and seems to get better every time she goes on a skiing holiday. Recently she was involved in a car accident and sustained a serious leg fracture. Although she is now well again, she has been told that a heavy fall could injure her leg permanently, with the possibility that she will walk with a limp.

> Imagine you are advising Mrs J on whether or not to no on a skiing holiday. Use the scale to indicate the lowest probability (the highest risk) of a bad fall which is acceptable if she is to go on holiday.

Please tick

She should not go skiing at all ☐
She should go on the skiing holiday if:

    there is a 10 per cent chance that she will have a bad fall ☐
    there is a 30 per cent chance that she will have a bad fall ☐
    there is a 50 per cent chance that she will have a bad fall ☐
    there is a 70 per cent chance that she will have a bad fall ☐
    there is a 90 per cent chance that she will have a bad fall ☐

Notice that the 'riskier' advice is at the bottom of the list. Work through the following five dilemmas noting your individual response with a tick next to the option you have chosen.

Choice dilemma 1
Ms M is a qualified nurse and has decided to enrol for a psychology course at university. She has been offered a place at two universities. The first has considerable status and a very good reputation for psychology, but quite a large proportion of the students fail to pass the

course. The second university does not have such a good reputation but has a much higher pass rate.

Imagine you are advising Ms M. What is the lowest probability of her passing the course that you thing she should accept to go to the first university?

Please tick

She should go to the second university   ☐
She should go to the first university if:

    there is a 10 per cent chance of failing   ☐
    there is a 30 per cent chance of failing   ☐
    there is a 50 per cent chance of failing   ☐
    there is a 70 per cent chance of failing   ☐
    there is a 90 per cent chance of failing   ☐

Choice dilemma 2

Mr H is a successful programmer in a computing firm. He is well liked by his colleagues and knows that his job is secure, but he has become increasingly disenchanted with it. He feels he needs more excitement and challenge. He has just had an offer from a go-ahead new company which could present an opportunity to develop his talents. He cannot guarantee that the new company or his new job will succeed and he knows he would never get his old job back.

What is the lowest probability that his new job would be successful that you would advise him to accept?

Please tick

He should not risk taking the new job.   ☐
He should take the new job if:

    there is a 10 per cent chance that it will fail   ☐
    there is a 30 per cent chance that it will fail   ☐
    there is a 50 per cent chance that it will fail   ☐
    there is a 70 per cent chance that it will fail   ☐
    there is a 90 per cent chance that it will fail   ☐

Choice dilemma 3

Tony is 41 years old and has developed serious cardiac problems. His life has become increasingly restricted owing to his heart condition. He has great difficulty at work, cannot play any sport, and sex is out of the question. His doctors have estimated that he has about five to ten years to live in this condition. He has been offered the chance of major heart surgery, which, although a dangerous operation, will make him virtually a 'new man'.

Please tick

He should not risk having the operation ☐
He should have the operation if:

there is a 90 per cent chance that it will succeed ☐
there is a 70 per cent chance that it will succeed ☐
there is a 50 per cent chance that it will succeed ☐
there is a 30 per cent chance that it will succeed ☐
there is a 10 per cent chance that it will succeed ☐

Choice dilemma 4

Mary is married with two children aged 10 and 15. She is an infant teacher at a local primary school. Recently Mary has felt that she is in a bit of a rut. She looks upon her marriage as stable but somewhat unfulfilling and in order to make her life more interesting has become involved in community work. As a result of her new interests, Mary has met a man and fallen in love with him. He is single and wants her to leave her unhappy marriage. She would leave but has doubts about whether the new relationship would succeed and be stable enough for herself and her children.

Please tick

Mary should not abandon her marriage ☐
Mary should leave if:

there is a 90 per cent chance that the new relationship
will work ☐
there is a 70 per cent chance that the new relationship
will work ☐
there is a 50 per cent chance that the new relationship
will work ☐
there is a 30 per cent chance that the new relationship
will work ☐
there is a 10 per cent chance that the new relationship
will work ☐

Choice dilemma 5

During a recent case review John, a student in the final year of his nursing course, is asked whether he feels he can manage to participate in the special supervision of a client. The client is on Section 2 of the Mental Health Act and still expresses suicidal intent and a determination to leave the unit. John is worried that the client might be able to leave the unit without him knowing.

John should not become involved with supervising the client   ☐

John should agree to participate if:

there is only a 10 per cent chance that the client will be
able to leave the unit without John's knowledge   ☐
there is a 30 per cent chance that the client will be
able to leave the unit without John's knowledge   ☐
there is a 50 per cent chance that the client will be
able to leave the unit without John's knowledge   ☐
there is a 70 per cent chance that the client will be
able to leave the unit without John's knowledge   ☐
there is a 90 per cent chance that the client will be
able to leave the unit without John's knowledge   ☐

Once the five volunteers have completed the dilemma sheets, return to the main group whose job is to observe the discussion group of the five volunteers in action. Allocate five of them to one group (NVC – non-verbal communication) and divide the others into four groups (Bales A, B, C, D; see following.)

The NVC group

We have already seen that a great deal of communication occurs non-verbally. In order to gain information related to the dynamics of group discussion it is necessary to evaluate the non-verbal signals that take place between the group members. Assign each member of the NVC group to observe one member of the discussion group. For each of the five choice dilemmas they should score the participants using the grid in Table 3.1, according to:

- *Facial expression.* Write down the number of smiles, nods and frowns that occur during each choice dilemma. Also note any other facial expressions that are used.
- *Posture and gesture.* Note the posture of the body. Is the participant leaning forward; tense; relaxed? Also observe any specific gestures used.
- *Voice.* Record the changes in pitch, tone and volume of the voice. Note how fast or slow the person speaks and whether their voice is excited or calm.
- *Holding the floor.* Note the number of interruptions made and the overall time spent speaking on each dilemma. Also write down your overall impressions of the person you are observing.

Table 3.1 *Non-verbal communication grid (adapted from Argyle, 1988)*

Non-verbal category	Dilemma					
	1	2	3	4	5	All total

Holding the floor
Overall time speaking (seconds)
Number of interruptions made

Facial expression
Number of smiles

Posture
Tense versus relaxed.
Open versus closed, etc.

Voice
Speaks fast or slow
High pitch versus low pitch, etc.

Gesture and movement
Type: fidgeting versus still, pointing,
    demonstrating, etc.

Overall impressions
Tense, relaxed, involved, disinterested,
    positive, negative, etc.

Bales A B C D
Bales (1958) developed a system for analysing the verbal content of group interaction, as indicated in Table 3.2.

A 'Dr Feelgood'. For each dilemma write down which people tend to show tension release; joke; laugh; show solidarity; raise others' status; give help; agree; understand; concur.

B 'The Giver'. Note who gives suggestions; direction; opinions; evaluation; expresses feeling or wishes; gives orientation and information; repeats; clarifies, confirms.

C 'The Asker'. Note who asks for information; confirmation; repetition; opinion; analysis; suggestion; direction; possible ways of action.

D 'The Downer'. Note which members of the group disagree, show passive rejection; withhold help: show tension; ask for help; withdraw; show antagonism; deflate others' status.

Table 3.2 *Bales group grid (after Bales, 1958)*

	Participant
Complete only one category	1 2 3 4 5

Socio-emotional area: positive reactions
1 Shows solidarity, raises other's status, gives help, reward
2 Shows tension release, jokes, laughs, shows satisfaction
3 Agrees, shows passive acceptance, understands, concurs, complies

   Total

Task area: attempted answers
4 Gives suggestion, direction, implying, autonomy for others
5 Gives opinion, evaluation, analysis, expresses feeling, wish
6 Gives orientation, information, repeats, clarifies, confirms

   Total

Task area: questions
7 Asks for orientation, information, repetition, confirmation
8 Asks for opinion, evaluation, analysis, expression of feeling
9 Asks for suggestion, direction, possible ways of action

   Total

Socio-emotional area: negative reactions
10 Disagrees, shows passive rejection, formality, withholds help
11 Shows tension, asks for help, withdraws out of field
12 Shows antagonism, deflates other's status, defends or asserts self

   Total

Arrange five chairs in the centre of the room, sufficiently far apart to enable the observers to have a good view of the group. Position the observers around the chairs in the best possible location for them to achieve their objectives. You might chose to video the group discussion and play it back to the observers later. To make sure the observers know what they are doing ask them to give an example of the behaviour they are supposed to be observing. Bring the discussion group into the room and ask them to sit on the chairs. Tell them to go through the five choice dilemmas again, discussing them as a group. They should spend between five and ten minutes on each dilemma.

Results

The individual and group results of the decisions should be collated by noting the number ticked (1–6) on each dilemma by each individual and entering it in Table 3.3.

Table 3.3 *Collating the results*

| | | | *Individual* | | | | |
	1	*2*	*3*	*4*	*5*	*Average*	*Group*
Dilemma							
1							
2							
3							
4							
5							
6							

Place the result of the group decisions in the column marked 'Group'. Take the average of the individual decisions for each dilemma and compare it with the group decision. If the average of the individual scores is less than the group score then the group has arrived at a more 'risky' decision.

The exercise you have just completed is similar to an experiment carried out by Stoner (1961). He found that the decisions made by groups on comparable dilemmas were riskier than those made by the same people on their own. This finding tended to fly in the face of common opinion that groups such as committees and juries would produce

THE PSYCHOLOGY OF NURSING CARE

more cautious, conservative decisions. The phenomenon where group discussion leads to riskier decisions is known as the *risky shift*.

One theory put forward to explain the risky shift was the *diffusion of responsibility*. Simply stated, it proposes that the reason group decisions are more risky is because each member of the group is able to take less personal responsibility for a decision and is able to propose more risk. Undoubtedly diffusion of responsibility does occur in certain situations and people will often behave differently in groups because they do not have to take individual responsibility for their actions.

However, Knox and Stafford (1976) noted that with some dilemmas group discussion actually produced shifts towards caution. Diffusion of responsibility theory would be unable to account for this finding. Further analysis of the risky shift effect has found that there is in fact a shift toward polarisation (Moscovici and Zavalloni, 1969). Group discussion can lead individual members to become more extreme, more risky or more cautious in their decisions. Look at the results obtained in the exercise and see whether group polarisation has occurred in the five dilemmas. If changes have occurred we need to examine the dynamics of the group to find out how and why.

It may be the case that certain individuals exercised more influence in the group discussion than others. Perhaps these individuals converted the other group members towards their more extreme views?

The Bales analysis will provide a guide to the quantity and type of communication made by each member of the group. The non-verbal analysis will give an indication of the influence being exerted via non-verbal channels. Also ask the group participants how they felt about what was going on in the group.

You may be able to identify some of the following characteristics of group behaviour.

Group decision schemes

These schemes are concerned with predicting the final decision of group discussion using simple rules:

- *The 'majority wins' rule.* The group finally adopts the position supported by the majority of its members.
- *The truth wins rule.* The correct solution will ultimately come to the fore as its truthfulness becomes apparent.
- *The two-thirds majority rule.* Used by many juries, if two-thirds of the group favour a decision it is adopted.
- *The first shift rule.* The group adopts a position based on the first shift in opinion shown by any member.

Stasser *et al.* (1989) say that these rules are quite successful at predicting group outcomes, but the nature of the task is important. Thus the 'majority wins' rule is best in situations requiring judgement and opinion, whereas the 'truth wins' rule is best in contexts where there is a correct answer.

The straw poll

This is a procedure used by groups to address the agenda and manage the flow of interaction. Davis *et al.* (1988) found that simply learning about the current distribution of views in the group will influence the final decision. Straw polls do more than simply reflect opinion; they shape it as well.

Groupthink

This term coined by Janis (1982) refers to the process whereby group members are much more concerned with maintaining group consensus than with examining all potential courses of action. McCauley (1989) points out that groupthink is most likely to occur in situations involving an external threat to the group and is thought to have played a role in some of the most disastrous decisions of recent history such as Watergate.

Over-utilising shared information

It was suggested by Stasser *et al.* (1989) that groups are much better at repeating information already shared by most members than at discussing new, unshared information. Furthermore, increasing the number in the group does not increase the chances of bringing original knowledge to the fore; it merely amplifies the utilisation of shared information.

You might also consider how the whole exercise would pan out if the group members could not see each other or had a restricted view by way of a computer conferencing link or even how the exercise would turn out with different forms of on-line communication.

Implications for nursing

It may seem from the preceding discussion that groups are not the best forum for making decisions. Yet, as was stated at the beginning of the chapter, we have a propensity to form ourselves into groups for many reasons. This being the case it is necessary that nurses understand some of the pitfalls inherent in the process of group discourse and are able to employ techniques to reduce the biases. Such techniques are:

- Delay straw polls until there has been considerable deliberation over the matter under discussion.
- Try to promote open enquiry and reservation in group discussion. If necessary, play the devil's advocate and try to find fault with points as they are made.
- Premature group consensus can be avoided by splitting the group into subgroups to consider different aspects of the problem.
- Examine group members' lingering doubts by providing a further opportunity to discuss them.

- Reduce the amount of information dealt with in groups.
- Groups spend much of their time discussing things they already know; therefore try to focus on the expertise of individual members and their unique contributions in order to avoid overusing shared information.

Finally, where there is a choice between using groups or individuals to complete tasks, the following guide proposed by Steiner (1976) may be of help. He proposed that the nature of the task influences group performance and that there are four main types of task.

- *Additive tasks*. Each member pools effort towards the completion of a task.
- *Conjunctive tasks*. The group's final result is determined by the performance of its poorest-performing member. A team of mountaineers cannot proceed at a pace faster than its slowest member.
- *Disjunctive tasks*. Here the final result is produced by the best member of the group. A relevant solution has to be found by one of the group and then he or she has to convince the others of its applicability.
- *Compensatory tasks*. Contributions of all the group members are averaged together to produce the result. A group of experts put all their information together to produce the best possible forecast.

How do groups and individuals compare on these tasks? Put simply, groups outperform even the best individual on both additive and compensatory tasks (with the important exception of social loafing). On conjunctive tasks, groups not surprisingly do not do very well, since they are performing at the level of their worst member. Lastly, on disjunctive tasks groups perform better than most individuals, but are limited to the level of their best member.

The family group

Belsky (2006) noted that one of the limitations of early research on the family was the tendency to view the family merely as consisting of mother–child or father–child interactions. She pointed out that the mere presence of a second parent affects the way the first parent interacts with the child. Belsky argued that the family group should be viewed as a system of social relationships which become more intricate with the addition of each child. Parents do influence the behaviour of their children, but at the same time children play an important role in shaping parental child-rearing practices. Anderson *et al.* (1986) illustrated that children may have nearly as much effect on their parents as parents have on their children. Boys between the ages of 6 and 11 years old were classified either as normal or as having 'conduct disorders'. Conduct disorders were defined as defiant, destructive behaviours often resulting in truancy. The boys' mothers were asked to interact with them for fifteen minutes and then asked to interact with another normal boy, or another boy with conduct disorders, for a similar period of time. The mothers were asked simply to oversee the child's behaviour during the fifteen-minute sessions. Anderson *et al.* found that regardless of whether the mothers were interacting with their own or someone else's son, when they oversaw the conduct of disordered boys they were more coercive and demanding than when paired with a normal boy. The defiant attitude of the conduct-disordered boys brought out the worst in every mother. Furthermore, the mothers of the conduct-disordered boys were found to respond in a calm and positive way when paired with normal boys.

Becoming a family

How do people respond to the birth of a child? Is it a positive event that enriches and enhances the lives of parents or is it a time of stress and disruption of the marital relationship? Dalgas-Pelish (1993) looked at the effects of the first child on the parents' marital happiness and found that marital happiness scales were lower than for a comparative sample of childless couples. She suggests that it is important for nurses to be aware of the implications of these findings. Miller and Sollie (1986) looked at the experiences of 120 couples during their transition to parenthood. The couples were asked to complete and return questionnaires when the woman was in mid-pregnancy; when the baby was about six weeks old; and when the baby was between six and eight months old. The questionnaire was designed to measure personal well-being, personal stress and marital stress.

In general, more stress was reported after the birth of a child than during pregnancy. The mothers' personal stress scores were lower than the fathers' during pregnancy, but considerably higher afterwards. Personal well-being scores declined steadily through the three time intervals. The mother's marital stress increased steadily from pregnancy to eight months after the birth of the child. However, Belsky (1981) had previously found that some couples experience only mildly stressful events when they become parents. Belsky and Isabella (1985) point to two factors that may explain the inconsistency:

- There is less disruption in the family after the birth when the parents are older, conceive after marriage and have been married longer.
- The way both husband and wife were treated by their parents affects how they treat their own children.

Indirect effects

The interactions which take place between members of the family group can have either direct or indirect effects. Direct effects would include findings that teenage mothers who have been rejected by their own parents and who lack social support are somewhat harsh and insensitive parents (Crockenberg, 1987), or research indicating that father–child interaction differs from mother–child interaction both in quantity and in quality (Lamb, 1981).

A view of family groups as a social system implies that parents also have indirect effects on their children's behaviour. Marital disharmony may affect the parents' care-giving routines and thus influence the appropriate interplay of feelings between the children and their parents. Pedersen *et al.* (1977) found that in families that experienced marital strife both mothers and fathers were likely to be unresponsive to their five-month-old infants. Certainly, starting a family in order to shore up personal relationships seems a very bad idea.

Parents can also have positive indirect effects on their children. Fathers play a much more important role in the care of their babies when their partners give them encouragement to find out more and to be more concerned with the behaviour of their children. Similarly, mothers who have a close supportive relationship with their partners are more patient and sensitive to their children's needs (Goldberg and Easterbrooks, 1984). The picture that emerges is one of each family member influencing the behaviour of the others in either a positive or a negative way according to the relationships in the family group itself.

Patterns of parenting

Baumrind (1977) observed 134 children at nursery school and at home. The children were rated on such items as achievement, moodiness, self-reliance, sociability and self-control. She also interviewed and observed parents while they were interacting with their children. The data was collated and three patterns of parenting emerged:

- *Authoritarian.* Adults demand strict obedience from their children. They rarely explain why often harsh and punitive regimes are being employed.
- *Authoritative.* Rules and restrictions are imposed on children with clear rationales and guidelines. Parents are responsive to children's needs, but expect children to abide by the rules and will enforce them.
- *Permissive.* Adults permit their children a wide range of activities and rarely use any method of control. Whilst they do allow children to express their feelings, they pay little attention to them.

Three patterns of child behaviour were also identified: *energetic–friendly*, *conflicted–irritable* and *impulsive–aggressive*. These patterns were related to styles of parenting so that:

- *Authoritative parents* tended to produce energetic–friendly children who were typically curious, co-operative, self-reliant, cheerful/ friendly, self-controlled and purposeful.

- *Authoritarian* parents produced conflicted–irritable children who were moody, aimless, fearful, sulky, vulnerable to stress and passively hostile.
- *Permissive* parents produced impulsive–aggressive children who were rebellious, aggressive, aimless, impulsive, low in self-reliance and self-control, domineering and low in achievement.

These findings suggest that some form of restrictive parenting where rules are important is preferable to a more *laissez-faire* approach. However, it is the way in which the rules are constructed and enforced that distinguishes the energetic–friendly child from the conflicted–irritable one. Clearly Baumrind's findings favour the authoritative pattern of parenting, and when this is combined with a warm, caring family environment an excellent setting for child development can be fashioned.

However, the problem with the study is that the subjects were largely from middle-income Western families. Laosa (1981) makes the point that:

indigenous patterns of child care throughout the world represent largely successful adaptations to conditions of life that have long differed from one people to another. Women are 'good mothers' by the only relevant standards, those of their own culture.

In the socioeconomic context Ogbu (1981) has proposed that the way a family earns its living may affect the strategies that parents use to raise their children. Just as individual behaviour should be seen in the broader context of the family, so too the family should be seen in the broader context of culture and society.

Family dynamics and parenting are not just common sense. Some of the things that were believed to be wrong for children in the 1930s would be considered nonsense today. Duck (1992) has reviewed the research in this area and lists some features of 'problem families'.

- There tends to be an emphasis on punishing poor performance rather than rewarding and praising good performance.
- Parents in the family are not good observers of their children's behaviour. They fail to notice slight improvements in behaviour or effort.
- There is a lack of consistency in the use of punishment. Parents sometimes ignore transgressions whilst at other times will punish the children severely.
- There is an absence of warmth and affection in the family.
- From the children's perspective there is a disproportionate emphasis on power, coercion and force. The model presented to the children is one of aggression.

Brothers and sisters in the family

A survey by Weisner and Gallimore (1977) found that older children were the principal caregivers for infants in 57 per cent of 186 societies studied. This finding suggests that, whether or not siblings have a beneficial role to play in family life, they certainly have an important one. There is also evidence that:

- Children respond differently to siblings than to their parents.
- There are differences in the behaviour of older and younger siblings.

Dunn and Kendrick (1982) found that sibling rivalry tends to occur in families which have just experienced the birth of a second child. When the new baby arrives, older children tend to resent the amount of attention that is directed towards the recent arrival. Happily, most of the older children soon begin to respond in a much less anxious manner and come to play an increasing care-giving role in the family. Parents were found to have a significant effect on the older children by appealing to their maturity and by encouraging them to help with the baby. However, an interesting finding was that showering attention on older girls in the first few weeks after a new baby's birth may not be a good idea. Older girls whose parents went out of their way to give them attention were the ones who played *least* with and were the *most negative* towards their baby brother or sister a year later. It seems that those who played best with their younger siblings had mothers who did not permit them to mope and encouraged them to take a positive view of the baby.

Squabbles among siblings become more frequent as they get older. By the time the younger child is about 2 years old they are able to 'hold their own' and confrontations tend to increase. Not all sibling interactions have a negative effect on family functioning. Stewart and Marvin (1984) found that 4-year olds were able to become an important source of emotional support for infants when the mother was absent. In certain circumstances older siblings were found to be useful role models for their younger brothers and sisters, able to transmit important information from the parents. Norman-Jackson (1982) suggested that siblings can prove productive teachers. A survey showed that young black siblings from low-income families who had older brothers and sisters playing with them at school were less likely to have problems learning to read than a control group.

Relationships between siblings often cause problems in the family. However, older siblings can have a significant and important role to play in the structure and dynamics of the family, and their potential and usefulness should not be overlooked by parents and nurses alike.

Family therapy

Glen and Corland (1993) state that one of the fundamental goals of nursing is to provide family-centred nursing care. They say:

Since the family is a system, no one individual can be effectively cared for if that care does not consider the other members who both affect and are affected by the member seeking nursing care.

One approach that deals with the family as a system is *family therapy*. This technique was developed from the early work of Gregory Bateson and Don Jackson on communication dynamics in groups (Goldenberg and Goldenberg, 1980). It concentrates on understanding the maladaptive communication systems of a group and then restructuring it.

Exercise 3.2 *Role-play*

A problem that often confronts nurse tutors is how to use role-play in teaching students who do not have much experience of the role they are going to play This exercise is more 'acting' than role-play, but hopefully gives some in insights into family therapy.

By far the best way of illustrating the issues involved in treating the whole family is to actually act out a scenario. Indeed, Holmes (1992) sees nursing as a forum for dramatic performance The following scenario is based on an actual case There are five 'actors', Mother, Greg, Jane, Sally and the psychologist The aim of the exercise is to illustrate how a child's problem can be anchored in a network of systems comprising the family and the community

The scene

The family are here because Greg, who is 14 years old, is 'out of control'. His mother does not know what to do with him. He has been playing truant from school and recently broke his leg trying to steal a motor bike. His mother has no complaints about the behaviour of his brothers and sisters, who have come along too. Although the family are here about Greg, the psychologist initially gives the mother an opportunity to talk about herself. She has been married twice. In order to escape from home she married her first husband; in order to escape from her first husband she moved to a new area. She was pregnant with Greg at the time and had no nearby family or friends. Her second husband used to hit her, often in front of the children. We start about fifteen minutes into the session.

> *Mother:* Anyway, we moved again. He was so jealous I couldn't even say 'Hello' to anyone. I tried to stick up for myself and for the children but he just kept hitting me. That's how I got this. (Points to scar under right eye.) He hit me with a lamp.
> *Psychologist:* What you are describing sounds terrible. I don't know how you survived.
> *Mother:* At least my kids won't have to put up with what I did. I used to go to school filthy-dirty because my mum worked and didn't have time to look after us. (Turns to children.) Now, you've heard

all this before. (Turns back.) Every day my father would hit me with this piece of wood. He wanted to have sex with me and beat me every day. Every day I would run away and the neighbours would make me come back. They all wouldn't believe me, said it was rubbish, but my grandmother knew. This went on from 9 to 17 until I finally left home. Now I still think about it. Right now I've got money problems. It always gets to me. But even when I manage not to think about it something just keeps hurting in my head. Today while waiting for my benefit money I just burst out crying. I have to try and live on less than £100 a week with five kids. Christmas is coming up soon and there will be nothing for them. It's like there's this weight and it's suffocating and crushing me.

Discussion

To what extent do you think the woman's social conditions contribute to her vulnerability? What effect has this situation had on the children? She looked to each man that she married for support and seems to have got nothing. You feel it is no wonder that she seems helpless, considering the way she has been treated. What would you do next if you were the psychologist?

Proposal

While the mother was telling her story the psychologist felt that she could not find a way to alleviate the mother's pain. In fact, she felt blocked out in some way by the mother and wondered if her experiences had left her closed to others and unable to trust them. During the initial session she noted that Greg was much more attentive to his mother than the other children were. Perhaps he felt more need to help his mother but was denied the opportunity to help. It was decided to test the hypothesis that the mother would not allow the children to give her support because she had learned not to expect it from anybody. In doing so this would help Greg and the rest of the family.

Psychologist: Do the children know what you are going through at the moment?

Mother: Oh, I tell them, I tell them I don't have any money, but they just make a face, or shout at me. I tried to explain things to them and sometimes they seem to listen but they keep on asking me for things I haven't got. They are upset, get upset and the whole thing just gets out of hand. I say to them that perhaps if they went out and made a bit of money that would help. It seems that I don't have any help.

Psychologist: OK, why don't you ask them for some help here and now? Let's talk about what sort of help you need from them.

Mother: What would really help me is – well, what I hate is when they invite their friends back and they just eat and eat. I don't mind giving hut don't have anything to give and what there is won't even feed them. I tell them not to give food *away* like that and they say, 'Yes, Mum,' but they still go on and do it. It's little things like that. I think they know it upsets me.

Psychologist: Could you speak to them and not to me?

Mother: OK. When I come in and the house is full of kids eating food we can barely afford it's bound to make me upset. All right? It means any food one of you gives to someone else means the rest won't get any, it'll be taken from you and I don't have any money, none unless I go out and beg for it. And sometimes I come in the house and the last thing I want is a lot of noise, because can't hear myself think. I can't think what to do next and there's nobody to talk to. That's my problem . . .

Psychologist: You're asking them for something but they're not answering. The conversation is going one way.

Mother: I've told them this time and time again but . . .

Psychologist: Get an answer. You have a young woman here, Jane, who is 17 years old; and a young man, Greg, who is 14. The others, Sally and John, are listening to you. They can answer you. Go on, get some answers.

Mother: Do you understand what I'm trying to say?

Children: Yes.

Mother: You understand? Well, what do you think about what I've been saying?

Greg: I think about it a lot.

Mother: Do you think we could save money by stopping people coming in? Where else can I get it from? 1 can't even pay the bills, you know. How am I going to get more money? That's what I want to know. I can't get a job . . .

Psychologist: You started to get them to answer you but then you went off on your own. You might find that the only way you're going to find out whether they understand you is to get them to answer you. Find out if they are going to work with you.

Discussion

The mother attempted to get answers from the children but only Greg responded. Discuss how the meeting could progress further. Why did the other children not answer their mother?

Proposal
The role structure in the family is not clearly delineated. The mother addressed all the children as one and did not differentiate between them. The family needs to have precise functional roles that can be allocated to each member. The mother had criticised Jane for not helping at home. Jane may not have been aware of what was expected of her. It was decided to explore this avenue.

> *Psychologist*: As I see it, you don't seem to be giving Jane a chance to help.
>
> *Mother*: I don't know – what help . . . What could she do, would she do?
>
> *Psychologist*: Ask her.
>
> *Mother*: I don't know what to ask.
>
> *Psychologist*: I'll ask her for you. Jane, I want to talk to you. Your mother is going through a bad time at the moment, as I think you know. As I understand it, she's saying that you don't really understand what she's going through and don't want to help out at home.
>
> *Jane*: I don't understand.
>
> *Psychologist*: Well, she *says* that you don't want to help her.
>
> *Mother*: Yes, when I tell you to help clean up the mess and maybe help wash the dishes or something. Not just you, the rest of them too. But you're the oldest and you could get Sally to help, too. I get home, the music's blaring, you and your friends are having a good time and the house is a mess. How do you think I feel when I come in to that going on and I'm already upset? You're the eldest, you're 17, you should get the other children to clear their mess up and if they don't . . .
>
> *Psychologist*: Hold on a moment, give her a chance to answer.
>
> *Jane*: What do you want me to say?
>
> *Psychologist*: Well, your mother says that she wants some help with the house. She wants you to get Sally to help. Do you want to do these things?
>
> *Jane*: Yeah, but they never listen. If they're not going to listen then I'm just not going to bother.
>
> *Psychologist*: Who doesn't listen?
>
> *Jane*: Well, they listen some of the time but not usually.
>
> *Psychologist*: So, you would like to help clean up and get the others to help?
>
> *Jane*: Yeah. I mean, sometimes I've been in the house on my own and just got on with it. Then when Mum comes home she just goes up to her room and shuts the door. But sometimes they make me so mad I just don't want anything to do with them. They don't listen, you know.

Psychologist: Who doesn't listen to you?

Jane: None of these three, none of them listens.

Psychologist: OK. Your mother mentioned Sally a few moments ago. Doesn't she listen to you?

Jane: I don't know, I don't know why she doesn't listen to me.

Psychologist: Why don't you find out? Ask her.

Jane: Sally, why don't you listen to me? (Turns to psychologist.) See. I just can't ask her any questions.

Psychologist: Now it's my turn not to understand. Why can't you ask your younger sister why it is that she doesn't listen to you?

Jane: It's just strange, that's all. I've never done anything like that.

Psychologist: Fine, but you are her older sister and your mother has put you in charge. Your mother has asked you to help clean the house and told you to get Sally to help.

Jane: I do tell her, but she just tells me to go and boil my head.

Psychologist: Ask her now. Your mother has said that you can ask her. Ask her why she doesn't listen to you.

Jane: Why don't you listen to me when I ask you to help clear up?

Sally: 'Cause you're always shouting at me.

Psychologist: Go on, talk to her about it.

Jane: How do I always shout at you, Sally?

Sally: Because, before Mummy gets home, you keep saying to clean up the house and you keep making me wash the dishes for you.

Jane: Wait. I keep making you wash the dishes or I ask you to wash the dishes?

Sally: You tell me to wash the dishes. (Jane is exasperated and ready to stop talking.)

Psychologist: Go on.

Jane: That's all.

Psychologist: You haven't worked anything out with her. You have a problem, now sort it out with her. Talk to her about it.

Jane: But I don't know what to ask. I mean, I've just asked her why she doesn't listen and she says that I shout at her. Well, I don't think I shout at her. I just say, 'Sally, go and do whatever it is,' and she says 'Don't you tell me what to do. Mummy isn't here, you know.'

Psychologist: Well, get her to reply to what you've just said.

Jane: Why when I tell you to do something do you always say, 'Don't tell me what to do, Mummy isn't watching,' and then when she gets home you tell her I said something else?

Discussion

The psychologist proceeded to encourage Jane to talk about her frustration in her attempts to communicate with her sister Sally. She tried

to help the mother become aware of her daughter's difficulties in dealing with Sally and the rest of the children. The mother felt burdened
by the fact that she could not count on Jane, who in turn could not
count on Sally. Jane did not know how to request help, in the same
way that her mother had the same difficulty asking her for help. How
do you think Jane could remedy the situation?

Tennant (1993) says that the importance of the family system has been de-empha-
sised by community psychiatric nurses in planning and delivering mental health services,
but that there are exceptions to the rule. This is a long exercise, but in this instance, actually performing and acting out the roles gives a better insight into the dynamics of family
interaction than setting out a theoretical discourse. By representing the series of events
in this way, one can get an idea of treating the family as a whole and not just a set of
individuals. You may like to construct your own scenario based on the principles and
issues outlined.

Summary

Here a number of concepts relating to the nature of social influence were introduced.
I have explored the nature of groups – why people tend to form groups and how those
groups influence the behaviour of the individual. Some factors which influence conformity to social norms have been discussed. They included cohesiveness, size, gender and
having an ally. Other concepts are social facilitation and social loafing. Studies on social
facilitation have shown that group presence is less likely to have a positive effect on the
performance of complex tasks than on the performance of simple tasks. Social loafing is
a concept used to describe the behaviour of those individuals within a group who make
the least effort necessary to maintain their membership of the group.

An example has been given of a method of observing group dynamics in the process
of decision making. The studies from which this example has been drawn explained the
tendency to greater polarisation in group decision making in terms of diffusion of
responsibility for more extreme decisions. A range of techniques have been suggested as
ways in which nurses might reduce bias in group decision making.

Towards the end of the chapter I have focused on the family as an example of one
specific type of group. The family is described as a system of social relationships, with
each family member influencing the others in either positive or negative ways. Different
patterns of parenting have been related to a range of behavioural responses in children,
and a cultural perspective has been brought to bear on family life and parenting behaviour. Lastly the chapter gives a detailed example of family therapy which attempts to
show how maladaptive family communication systems might be restructured.

? Questions for further consideration

1 Do individuals or groups make the riskier decisions?
2 What factors influence conformity in a group?
3 Discuss the processes involved in social facilitation.
4 Are there different styles of parenting?
5 In what ways can a knowledge of group dynamics be applied to case conferences?

References

Anderson, K. E., Lytton, H. and Romney, D. (1986). Mothers' interactions with normal and conduct-disordered boys: who affects whom? *Developmental Psychology, 22,* 604–609.

Argyle, M. (1988). *Bodily Communication.* 2nd edn. London: Methuen.

Asch, S. E. (1951). Effects of group pressure upon the modification and distortion of judgement. In Guetzkow, H. (ed.) *Groups, Leadership, and Men.* Pittsburgh PA: Carnegie.

Bales, R. F. (1958). Task roles and social roles in problem-solving groups. In Maccoby, E. E., Newcomb, M. and Hartley, E. L. (eds) *Readings in Social Psychology.* 3rd edn. New York: Holt Rinehart and Winston.

Baron, R. A. (1986). Self-presentation in job interviews: when there can be 'too much of a good thing'. *Journal of Applied Social Psychology, 16,* 16–28.

Baumrind, D. (1977). Socialisation Determinants of Personal Agency. Unpublished paper presented at the biennial meeting of the Society for Research in Child Development, New Orleans.

Belsky, J. (1981). Early human experience: a family perspective. *Developmental Psychology, 17,* 3–23.

Belsky, J. (2006). *Transition to Parenthood.* New York: Delacourt.

Belsky, J. and Isabella, R. A. (1985). Marital and parent–child relationships in family of origin and marital change following the birth of a baby: a retrospective analysis. *Child Development, 56,* 342–349.

Crandall, C. S. (1988). Social contagion of binge eating. *Journal of Personality and Social Psychology, 55,* 588–598.

Crockenberg, S. (1987). Predictors and correlates of anger toward punitive control of toddlers by adolescent mothers. *Child Development, 58,* 964–975.

Crutchfield, R. A. (1955). Conformity and character. *American Psychologist, 10,* 191–198.

Dalgas-Pelish, P. L. (1993). The impact of the first child on marital happiness. *Journal of Advanced Nursing, 18,* 437–441.

Davis, J. H., Stasson, M., Ono, K. and Zimmerman, S. (1988). Effects of straw polls on group decision-making: sequential voting pattern, timing, and local majorities. *Journal of Personality and Social Psychology, 55,* 918–926.

Duck, S. (1992). *Human Relationships.* 2nd edn. London: Sage.

Dunn, J. and Kendrick, C. (1982). *Siblings: Love, envy, and understanding.* Cambridge MA: Harvard University Press.

Eagly, A. H. and Carli, L. (1981). Sex of researchers and sex-typed communications as determinants of sex differences in influence-ability: a meta-analysis of social influence studies. *Psychological Bulletin, 90,* 1–20.

Glen, S. and Corland, (1993). The family. In Hinchliff, S. M., Norman, S. E. and Schober, J. E. (eds) *Nursing Practice and Health Care.* 2nd edn. London: Edward Arnold.

Goldberg, W. A. and Easterbrooks, M. A. (1984). Role of marital quality in toddler development. *Developmental Psychology, 20,* 504–514.

Goldenberg, I. and Goldenberg, H. (1980). *Family Therapy: An overview.* Monterey CA: Brooks Cole.

Harkins, S. (1987). Social loafing and social facilitation. *Journal of Experimental Social Psychology, 23,* 1–18.

Holmes, C. A. (1992). The drama of nursing. *Journal of Advanced Nursing, 17,* 941–950.

Janis, I. L. (1982). *Groupthink: Psychological studies of policy decisions and fiascos.* 2nd edn. Boston MA: Houghton Mifflin.

Knox, R. E. and Stafford, R. K. (1976). Group causation at the racetrack. *Journal of Experimental Social Psychology, 12,* 317–324.

Lamb, M. E. (1981). *The Role of the Father in Child Development.* New York: Wiley.

Loasa, I. M. (1981). Maternal behavior: sociocultural diversity in modes of family interaction. In Henderson, R. W. (ed.) *Parent–Child Interaction: Theory, research, and prospects.* London: Academic Press.

McCauley, C. (1989). The nature of social influence in groupthink: compliance and internalization. *Journal of Personality and Social Psychology, 57,* 250–260.

Miller, B. C. and Sollie, D. C. (1986). Normal stresses during the transition to parenthood. In Moos, R. H. (ed.) *Coping with Life Crises.* New York: Plenum.

Morris, W. N., Miller, R. S. and Spangenberg, R. (1977). The effects of dissenter position and task difficulty on conformity and response to conflict. *Journal of Personality, 45,* 251–266.

Moscovici, S. and Zavalloni, M. (1969). The group as a polarizer of attitudes. *Journal of Personality and Social Psychology, 12,* 125–135.

Niven, N. (1994). *Health Psychology* 2nd edition. Edinburgh: Churchill Livingstone.

Niven, N. (2000). *Health Psychology: An introduction for health care professionals.* 3rd edn. Edinburgh: Churchill Livingstone.

Norman-Jackson, J. (1982). Family interactions, language development, and primary reading achievement of Black children in families of low income. *Child Development, 53,* 349–358.

Ogbu, J. U. (1981). Origins of human competence: a cultural-ethological perspective. *Child Development, 52,* 413–429.

Paulus, P. B. (ed.) (1989). *Psychology of Group Influence.* 2nd edn. Hillsdale NJ: Erlbaum.

Pederson, F., Anderson, B. and Cain, R. (1977). An Approach to Understanding Linkages between Parent–Infant and Spouse Relationships. Unpublished paper presented at the biennial meeting of the Society for Research in Child Development, New Orleans.

Robbins, S. P. (1989). *Organizational Behavior: Concepts, controversies, and applications.* 4th edn. Englewood Cliffs NJ: Prentice Hall.

Sanna, L. J. and Shotland, R. L. (1990). Valence of anticipated evaluation and social facilitation. *Journal of Experimental Social Psychology, 26,* 82–92.

Stasser, G., Kerr, N. L. and Davis, J. H. (1989). Influence processes and consensus models in decision making groups. In Paulus, P. B. (ed.) *Psychology of Group Influence.* 2nd edn. Hillsdale NJ: Erlbaum.

Steiner, I. D. (1976). Task-performing groups. In Thibaut, J. W., Spence, J. T. and Cardon, R. C. (eds). *Contemporary Topics in Social Psychology.* Morristown NJ: General Learning Press.

Stewart, R. B. and Marvin, R. S. (1984). Sibling relations: the role of conceptual perspective-taking in the ontogeny of sibling caregiving. *Child Development, 55,* 1322–1332.

Stoner, J. A. F. (1961). A comparison of individual and group decisions involving risk. In Brown, R. (ed.) *Social Psychology.* New York: Free Press.

Tanford, S. and Penrod, S. (1984). Social influence model: a formal integration of research on majority and minority influence processes. *Psychological Bulletin, 95,* 189–225.

Tennant, D. (1993). The place of the family in mental health nursing: past, present and future. *Journal of Advanced Nursing, 18,* 752–758.

Weisner, T. S. and Gallimore, R. (1977). My brother's keeper: child and sibling caretaking. *Current Anthropology, 18,* 169–190.

Zajonc, R. B. (1965). Social facilitation. *Science, 149,* 269–274.

Zajonc, R. B., Heingartner, A. and Herman, E. M. (1969). Social enhancement and impairment of performance in the cockroach. *Journal of Personality and Social Psychology, 13,* 83–92.

Further reading

Duck, Steve (1998). *Human Relationships.* London: Sage. Duck is concerned with presenting social psychology in a context that is relevant to the reader as opposed to a more formal academic structure. I think he succeeds because he maintains academic rigour whilst discussing issues in a very readable fashion. In this sense the book is similar to Baron and Byrne, but I think he goes outside standard social psychological structures.

Le Guin, Ursula K (2002) *The Birthday of the World.* London: Gollancz. In a series of stories Le Guin examines the possibilities of relationships and in doing so gives us insight into our own.

Miell, Dorothy and Dallos, Rudi (1996) *Social Interaction and Personal Relationships.* London: Sage. Rudi Dallos has been working in the field of family therapy and personal relationships for many years now and here, alongside Dorothy Miell, he presents six interesting chapters on different aspects of relationships.

4

Child Health Development

> ## A practice conundrum
>
> 'To parent a disadvantaged child successfully you need to understand child development, children as people and your own reactions to problems.' This observation is made by Raymet and Neil, whose 17-year-old son Samuel was born blind. Raymet and her husband aren't bitter but they do observe that they would have benefited from a lot more guidance on what lay ahead in those early days when, as a young baby, Samuel's diagnosis was made. As Neil reflects, 'It wasn't just about growing up using other senses that you needed to know about, we needed to know about how we could help Sam become a person in his own right.' Over a number of years Sam had a series of contacts with health care professionals. At first these were associated with attempts to improve his sight. Later the contacts were with nurses who specialised in challenging child behaviour. Sam had become periodically aggressive and at other times dismissive of his personal worth.
>
> Before proceeding with this chapter prepare a three-column table using the following headings:
>
> - Problems (those affecting Sam and his parents).
> - Origins (where or how might the problems arise).
> - Practice implications.
>
> Use Chapter 4 to help you fill in the first two of your columns, identifying how Sam's situation contrasts with the norm of sighted child development. Discuss what such problems might mean for practice by reviewing this case study with your colleagues.

In the previous chapters it has been assumed that the patients in our investigations have been adults; however, much of nursing is concerned with the care of children. The question arises as to whether there are differences in children's health behaviour according to age. Studies of human development have found many changes in behaviour throughout the life span, and these can be divided into two categories:

- *Quantitative changes* (differences in amount). Children may not know how you catch a cold because they have never been told about colds.
- *Qualitative changes* (differences in essence/nature). Children find it impossible to understand about catching a cold no matter how hard you try to explain.

This chapter investigates both quantitative and qualitative changes in child development and examines some of the important issues facing nurses when caring for children. One of the main factors that helps children understand the world around them is the development of a framework. If children have a basic plan or pattern of events, not only can they slot present information into the scheme, but they can go on to investigate variations on basic themes. The purpose of this chapter is the same: to provide a basic framework for the nurse to understand child development and then investigate further.

The neonate

Many people believe that babies are born into the world with no ability to understand what is happening around them. This supposition is not new and was in fact proposed by John Locke, a British empiricist philosopher, in the seventeenth century. He saw the neonate's mind as a blank slate ready to receive information from the outside world, but with no preset ability to comprehend it. Research over the last thirty years has indicated that Locke was wrong. Infants are born with a number of abilities or acuities that enable them to make a limited but nevertheless functional sense of their environment.

Sensory acuities

Vision

- *Visual acuity*. This refers to how well the neonate can see. At birth the visual acuity of the newborn is thirty times worse than that of an adult (Bremner and Slater, 2003). Adult acuity is about 20/20 or 6/6, depending on the system used, whereas the acuity of the neonate is about 20/150. This means that a newborn infant can see an object at 20 ft (6 m) as well as an adult can see the object at 150 ft (45 m).
- *Focusing*. The neonate has difficulty focusing properly. The ciliary muscles are unable to operate and manipulate the lens correctly at this stage, so the infant has an optimum focal point of about 8–10 m (200–250 mm). Any object presented to the infant outside this range will appear blurred. Thus toys placed too far away from the baby will not stimulate the child as much as those placed about nine inches away.
- *Physiology*. The eye of the neonate is about half the size of an adult's eye but is anatomically complete. It is slightly 'squashed' in appearance because some parts of the eye mature at a faster rate than others. The optic tract that transmits messages from the eye to the brain is partially myelinated, indicating that information is

getting to the brain but not as quickly or as efficiently as it will do when a full myelin sheath has been formed (Kessen *et al.,* 1970).

Thus the infant's visual system is active from birth. There are operational difficulties, as mentioned, but the baby is equipped to engage in the active exploration of his or her environment.

Haith (1980), using research from a number of studies, has tried to look at the world through the eyes of the neonate and has described a typical pattern of visual search.

- If I'm awake and alert, and the light is not too bright, open eyes.
- If I'm in darkness, maintain a controlled, detailed search.
- If there is light but no form to the figure, search for the edges.
- If an edge is found, terminate the broad scan and stay in the vicinity of the edge.

Some researchers have argued over the precise make-up of these 'rules', but they do indicate the active nature of the neonate's visual system. Bremner and Slater (2003) summarise the research in this area by saying:

Nevertheless, there is general agreement that the newborn is biologically prepared to explore the environment and is able to actively seek out and to attend to some forms of stimulation in preference to others.

Implications

There are two main implications from the research:

- Babies need appropriate levels of stimulation.
- It may be useful to parents if the nurse explains to them how a baby sees the world.

As Slater points out, infants tend to prefer some forms of perceptual stimulation to others. Fantz (1961) showed babies a series of pictures and measured the amount of time they spent looking at each one. He found that the babies spent much more time looking at patterned pictures than they did looking at plain ones and nearly twice as much time looking at a picture of a mother's face. The preference for pattern can be explained by the fact that the black-and-white contrast contained in the patterns stimulates more cells in the retina and is thus more 'exciting'. The preference for a mother's face is not so easily explained. Some researchers have suggested that the neonate is programmed to respond to a face pattern (Dannemiller and Stephens, 1988) while others have suggested that, in the absence of experience of faces, neonates do not show a preference for the face pattern (Small, 1990). Bremner and Slater (2003) provide a tentative solution to the controversy by suggesting that immediately after birth black-and-white contrast 'will easily swamp any specific response to facedness'. However, the human face does seem to have special significance for babies from birth onward.

Colour vision also forms part of the infant's early visual environment. Aslin (1987) found that whilst very young infants could see red, green and yellow, blue was not part of their visual repertoire until they were four months old.

Hearing

The ear, like the eye, is fairly well developed at birth. Keith (1975) found that the middle ear is free from mucus a few hours after birth and therefore able to operate, but there are certain limitations to the neonate's perception of pitch. Babies respond more to high-pitched sounds in the region of 4000 Hz (the highest note on a piano is about 4,180 Hz), and many adults speak to babies in a high-pitched voice because babies are more responsive to sounds at the top end of the spectrum.

Eimas (1985) found that newborns could distinguish between the sounds 'pa' and 'ba', but probably the most startling findings in relation to audition come from studies by Anthony De Casper and his colleagues. De Casper and Spence (1986) asked twelve pregnant women to read a passage from a children's story, *The Cat and the Rat,* to their unborn babies twice a day for the last six weeks of their pregnancies. A few days after birth the neonates were played tape recordings of two stories, the one they had heard *in utero* and a new story. The researchers found that the babies were able to modify their sucking rate whilst listening to the *Cat and the Rat* story but not to the new one, suggesting that:

- the babies could discriminate between the two stories;
- the babies could hear in the womb;
- the babies could learn and memorise before birth.

Smell

The ability of newborn children to discriminate between smells is quite weak at birth, but after a few weeks they can tell the difference between their mother's and a stranger's odour. Macfarlane (1977) presented ten-day-old babies with pads which had been placed inside their own mother's bra and pads which had been placed inside that of a stranger. He found that the babies turned significantly more often to their own mother's pad. Interestingly, Cernoch and Porter (1985) found that this discriminatory skill was only true of breast-fed babies; bottle-fed babies showed no evidence of recognition. However, bottle-fed babies can tell the difference between the odours of lactating and non-lactating females (Makin and Porter, 1989), but, maybe owing to lack of contact, are not able to differentiate subtle differences between mothers' smells.

Taste

Neonates can tell the difference between water and sugar solutions, even discriminating between sucrose and glucose (Engen *et al.,* 1974). Evidence exists of an innate ability to distinguish between certain flavours. Ganchrow *et al.* (1983) placed flavoured water in the mouths of babies who had never been fed before. The facial responses of the babies to the different tastes were observed and recorded on video machines. The sweet water produced a relaxed expression; the sour liquid was met with pursed lips; and the bitter solution produced an arched mouth with the sides turned down and an expression of disgust. The researchers concluded that the different expressions in reaction to the water solution indicated that the neonates could taste the difference.

Touch

The fact that neonates can experience touch is evidenced by reflexive responses. Placing a finger in the palm of a baby's hand will elicit the *grasp reflex* and stroking the cheek will cause the baby to turn in the direction of the touch (the *rooting reflex*). Many of the reflexes described may have their origins in species survival; the clinging and grasping may have been important in times of danger. The majority of reflexes disappear after a few months when the brain starts to exert more cortical control (Kalat, 1981).

Intersensory co-ordination

A number of studies have found that neonates have a better integrated intersensory system than older children. Bower (1989) showed that blind babies could 'see with their ears,' and young children were much better than older children at this task. Using ultrasonic devices, waves are bounced off objects and picked up by a device which transfers them to the baby's ear, so that pitch indicates object distance, loudness the size of the object, clarity the texture of the object and right/left the location of the object.

Bower found that infants between the ages of five and sixteen months were able to reach accurately for objects using this apparatus and the younger ones adapted much quicker than the older ones. Bower suggests that the babies do not treat the information they receive as sound but are in fact seeing with their ears, that is, responding to sound in much the same way as sighted infants do to light. It seems that the sensory world of the neonate is much less differentiated than that of older infants or adults.

There does not seem to be much doubt that the neonate comes into the world with sensory acuities which are operational. Whilst the efficiency of the sensory system is still limited, babies can make a certain sense of their environment. A knowledge of what babies can and can't do will enable nurses and parents to provide an appropriate level of stimulation and an awareness of the importance of the environment.

Parent–child interaction

During the course of infancy an emotional bond develops between children and parents. Bowlby (1951) went so far as to suggest that the lack of opportunity for the development of such a bond could result in 'affectionless psychopathy' – the inability to have deep feelings for another person. Many have taken issue with Bowlby over these statements (see Rutter, 1981) since his findings were based on studies that possessed a number of methodological flaws (Pinneau, 1955). However, the feeling still remains among many people that disruption of the parent–child relationship can lead to problem behaviour later on in the child's development. In order to examine the accuracy of such feelings it is necessary to investigate the processes involved in parent–child interaction.

Early influences

Some factors that have been put forward as potential hazards to successful parent–child interaction include: infant temperament; pre-term birth; postnatal depression.

Infant temperament

One obstacle to the development of an appropriate relationship between parents and their babies might be the temperament of the baby. Thomas *et al.* (1970) conducted a large-scale study into the nature of infant temperament. They wanted to find out if infants had different temperaments and whether these temperamental qualities remained stable throughout childhood.

Thomas and his colleagues interviewed 141 parents about the behaviour of their babies from the age of two months to 10 years old. They found nine temperamental characteristics to be consistent throughout this period of time (see Table 4.1). Patterns of interrelationship between the characteristics were also found, so that an active baby was often rated as less cuddly and more irritable and restless than a placid baby. Three basic clusters of traits were identified:

- *Easy babies* (40 per cent of sample)
  Regular in natural functions.
  Positive approach to new objects and events.
  Mild in intensity or reaction.
  Adjusted easily to change.
- *Difficult babies* (10 per cent of sample)
  Irregular sleeping/eating patterns.
  Difficulty negotiating new events.
  Intense reactions.
  'Fussy' mood.
- *'Slow to warm up' babies* (15 per cent of sample)
  Low activity level.
  Passive resistance to new objects and people.
  Low threshold of responsiveness.
  Once new situations adapted to – positive response.

Table 4.1 *Consistent temperament characteristics*

Activity level. Ranging from very fidgety and active to relatively still and passive

Quality of mood. Can range from predominantly positive, happy, and contented to mainly negative, fretful and miserable

Approach versus withdrawal tendencies. The child, when exposed to new features of the environment, reacts either positively or negatively to particular types of stimulation or sensory stimulation, such as taste or touch, or to new people

Rhythmicity. Habits of, for example, eating, sleeping, bowel movements, relatively predictable rather than erratic or unpredictable

Adaptability. Child settles down relatively easily rather than resisting change when exposed to new routines or situations.

Threshold of responsiveness. Child is hypersensitive to sounds, touch, versus relatively insensitive

Intensity of reaction. Some babies may cry loudly and intensely, while others react more moderately to stimuli

Distractability. Some children attend to things for considerable periods of time, while others flit from one thing to another

Persistence. Some babies are very 'singleminded' and stick to 'goals' with great persistence

Thomas and his colleagues said that these clusters might prove useful in counselling new parents about the nature of their babies' temperamental qualities; knowing that some babies are born with a 'difficult' temperament could perhaps reduce feelings of inadequacy in parents. Further, Gennaro *et al.* (1992) investigated three studies of pre-term, low-birth-weight infants and found that they were significantly more difficult than comparison groups of full-term infants.

However, there are a number of problems with Thomas's research: a large proportion of the sample (35 per cent) did not seem to fall into any of the clusters, and the study did not consider the effects of the parents' temperament on the behaviour of the children. Rutter (1978) found that infants' temperamental qualities affect the way adults respond to them, so that difficult babies may be punished more frequently, leading to frustration in the children, which in turn makes them even more difficult. Sameroff (1991) sums up the transactional nature of parent–child interaction by saying:

> The mother's anxiety during the first months of the child's life may have caused her to be uncertain and inappropriate in her interactions with the child. In response to such inconsistency the infant may have developed some irregularities in feeding and sleeping patterns that give the appearance of a difficult temperament. This difficult

temperament decreases the pleasure that the mother obtains from the child and so she spends less time with the child.

There is little doubt that babies possess different temperamental qualities; whether these are due to genetic factors, or are the result of the child's response to the parent, they *can* be changed. The 'difficult' child does not have to remain so. Nurses should stress to parents that they have a significant role to play in their child's development. Rather than labelling the child 'difficult', nurses should be a good role model and indicate to parents how to interact appropriately with their children. As such, an analysis of parent–child interaction is of more use than a categorisation of temperament.

Prematurity

Generally, premature infants can be categorised into two groups:

- *Small-for-their-date babies.* Infants born below the weight expected for their gestational age. Some are born at their normal term; others earlier.
- *Pre-term infants.* Birth weights are appropriate for gestational age but they are born early.

Both groups of infants produce problems for parent–child interaction since the babies spend long periods of time in isolation from their parents. Brazelton *et al.* (1987) have suggested that premature babies are less responsive and more irritable then full-term infants. These characteristics, and the accompanying isolation, disrupt the normal parent–child interaction sequences.

One answer to the problem has been to provide the infants with extra stimulation whilst they are in hospital (Oehler, 1993). An early study by Solkoff *et al.* (1969) found that premature babies given extra tactile stimulation in the hospital by nurses experienced increased weight gains as compared to a similar group of babies who did not receive stimulation. In addition to extra handling, Korner (1987) found that extra stimulation in the form of objects to look at and music to listen to leads to improvements in many areas of development. Other forms of stimulation apart from touching are extremely important for very small babies (those weighing less than 1,500 g), as their skin is very sensitive.

However, extra stimulation in the hospital is not the only answer to the problem. Parents need to be given information about the amount and quality of stimulation that their babies will need once they return home. Not only can too much stimulation be as bad as too little, but parents also have problems with the quality of interaction with premature infants. Crnic *et al.* (1983) found that mothers and their babies have difficulty maintaining eye contact with one another. The mothers also had difficulty in finding the correct level of stimulation, resulting in the babies becoming either over-excited or bored.

Slater (1991) has suggested that extreme care should be taken in providing correct levels of stimulation for premature babies. For instance, in many neonatal units there are high levels of lighting which may cause harm to the babies' visual system, since the pupillary reflex can be inoperative at this stage. Slater recommends that if high levels of lighting are needed, then infants should have their eyes protected by lubricated goggles in order to guard against any possible damage to vision.

The Brazelton scale

One method of teaching parents how to interact with their babies is to have them watch or take part as the Brazelton Neonatal Assessment Scale (NBAs) (see Table 4.2) is administered to their child (Myers, 1982). This scale is particularly good for teaching parents, as it is designed to elicit from the child pleasing characteristics such as smiling, cooing and gazing. As the test proceeds, parents see how their child can respond positively to other people, and they will learn how to elicit these behaviours themselves. Hopefully the success of these exchanges between parents and child will promote greater understanding and lead to feelings of increased competence. Widmayer and Field (1980) found that Brazelton training for the premature babies of teenage mothers led to increased responsiveness in comparison with a control group who did not receive the training. Parents who had received the training were more knowledgeable about infant behaviour, more confident in their caretaking abilities, and more satisfied with their infants than the control parents were.

Parents do have fears and worries about interacting with their premature infants, and the role of the nurse must be to allow parents to come to terms with these feelings in such a manner that they do not feel failures.

Postnatal depression

Difficulties in establishing desirable parent–child interaction patterns may be due to unresponsive parents. Williams and Carmichael (1985) looked at a sample of Australian women who had just had their first baby. Those mothers who were depressed reported significantly more problems than the non-depressed mothers. The types of disturbances identified were:

- Failure to establish a relationship with the infant on the postnatal ward.
- Difficulty in developing a routine pattern of management of the baby.
- At home the infant was said to cry a lot, feed poorly, sleep irregularly and was difficult to soothe.
- The behaviour of the infant caused the mother to become frustrated and angry.
- Some mothers experienced depression weeks after delivery, with similar interaction problems.

These were the mothers' perceptions, and may have been distorted by their depressive state. However, further evidence of disrupted parent–child interaction caused by

Table 4.2 *The twenty-six categories on the Brazelton Neonatal Behavioral Assessment Scale*

1 Response decrement to repeated visual stimuli.
2 Response decrement to rattle.
3 Response decrement to bell.
4 Response decrement to pinprick.
5 Orienting response to inanimate visual stimuli.
6 Orienting response to inanimate auditory stimuli.
7 Orienting response to animate visual stimuli – examiner's face.
8 Orienting response to animate auditory stimuli – examiner's voice.
9 Orienting responses to animate visual and auditory stimuli.
10 Quality and duration of alert periods.
11 General muscle tone – in resting and in response to being handled, passive and active.
12 Motor activity.
13 Traction responses as he or she is pulled to sit.
14 Cuddliness – responses to being cuddled by examiner.
15 Defensive movements – reactions to a cloth over his or her face.
16 Consolability with intervention by examiner.
17 Peak of excitement and capacity to control self.
18 Rapidity of build-up to crying state.
19 Irritability during the examination.
20 General assessment of kind and degree of activity.
21 Tremulousness.
22 Amount of startling.
23 Lability of skin colour – measuring autonomic lability.
24 Lability of states during entire examination.
25 Self-quieting activity – attempts to console self and control state.
26 Hand-to-mouth activity.

postnatal depression comes from Murray and Trevarthen (1985). They found that 'unnatural disruptions' produced distressed patterns of infant response. When maternal behaviour was interrupted quite naturally by, for example, a conversation with someone else, the baby responded with no distress. If, however, an unnatural disruption was arranged by the mother, such as adopting a blank face, or mistiming interaction sequences, the baby very quickly appeared disturbed. Investigations of the behaviour of 'depressed' mothers have indicated that unnatural disruptions can cause significant distress in young infants, leading to subsequent behavioural problems.

Guidelines for detecting postnatal depression

Murray and Stein (1991) have suggested some guidelines for the detection of postnatal depression:

> It may be possible to identify those mothers at risk of postnatal depression antenatally. Nurses should pay attention to such factors as: social and economic stress, lack of close relationships, and a previous psychiatric history. All these factors have been associated with postnatal depression.
>
> Predictions based on antenatal risk will never be entirely accurate, so attention has to be directed towards behaviour on the postnatal ward:
>
> (i) strong adverse maternal reactions to the infant after delivery may affect the mother's future relationship with the baby.
> (ii) feeding difficulties are frequently experienced by those who become depressed;
> (iii) severe feelings of low mood ('four-day-blues') have been associated with a full depressive episode postpartum;
> (iv) absence of social support may be another risk factor. Lack of visitors on the postnatal ward or difficult relationships with those who do visit may indicate imminent problems.
>
> It should be stressed that none of these factors on its own need indicate any concern, but taken together they may indicate a risk of postnatal depression.

Since the majority of marital and personal stress often occurs weeks or months after the birth of the child (Miller and Sollie, 1986), attention has to be paid to the identification of postnatal depression in the community. Cox *et al.* (1987) developed a self-report questionnaire to detect postnatal depression which can be administered to mothers at a six-week postnatal check. There is evidence that it works and also seems to be acceptable to mothers (Murray and Stein, 1991).

The nurse also has a significant role to play in the management of postnatal depression. Holden *et al.* (1989) trained health visitors to give non-directive counselling to depressed mothers. This approach emphasised viewing the situation through the eyes of the mother. A supportive, counselling approach alongside practical advice can reduce maternal depressive symptoms and may also be perfectly appropriate for parents who are not depressed but are experiencing problems at home.

Attachment behaviour

During the course of the first year after birth the infant develops a relationship with his or her parents. Through the process of parent–child interaction, a bond develops between the child and parents. This is called the *attachment bond*. The main interactive processes contributing to the development of this bond are the *social signalling processes,* two of the most important being crying and smiling.

Crying

The main psychological function of crying is to bring someone, usually the caregiver, into close proximity with the child so that interaction can take place. Wolff (1969) identified three different types of cry:

● The *basic/hungry cry* follows the rhythmical pattern of cry, silence, breath in, silence, cry.
● The *mad/angry cry* follows the same pattern but the length of the elements differs. (The mad/angry cry was labelled as the 'fussy cry' by Fuller (1991) and found to be less tense than the hungry or pain-induced cry.)
● The *pain cry* – a loud, long cry, a long silence, followed by a series of short, sharp inhalations.

Both parents and non-parents are able to distinguish between these cries (Gustafson and Harris, 1991) although they tend to react differently. After a few months the infant learns that pleasant consequences often accompany crying behaviour and the 'attention please' cry develops. The question of whether continually responding to a baby's crying rewards the behaviour, thus producing more was examined by Ainsworth and her colleagues (Ainsworth *et al.,* 1991). She found that mothers who were quick to respond to their babies' cries had infants who cried very little. Why should this occur? Sensitive caregivers who respond to an infant's cries are usually also responsive to other social signals such as the smiling and babbling that infants are likely to emit when they calm down. Gradually alternative modes of attention seeking are reinforced to replace crying.

Sometimes babies cry for no readily identifiable cause. If they have just been fed and still cry mothers often assume it is because their nappy is wet or that they are cold. Wolff (1969) had nurses change the nappies of crying babies just after they had been fed, when a wet nappy was more than likely. Half the babies actually had their nappy changed, while the other half did not – the nurses went through all the motions but put the wet nappy back on. Most of the babies in both groups stopped crying. This suggests that it was the handling and stimulation the babies received rather than the change of nappy that made the difference.

Many studies have investigated how to sooth fussy crying in babies. These include:

● picking them up and holding them to the shoulder or breast in an embrace (Korner and Thoman, 1972);
● rocking, patting, cuddling and swaddling (Campos *et al.,* 1989);

- sucking on a pacifier (dummy) (Field and Goldson, 1984);
- listening to tapes of low-pitched rhythms like heartbeats (Brackbill, 1975);
- rhythmic (up and down) movement of three inches, sixty per minute (Ambrose, 1969).

In general it seems that fussy behaviour in babies may be reduced through a combination of touch and rhythmic stimulation.

Smiling

If the purpose of crying is to bring the adult into contact with the infant, then the function of smiling is to maintain that contact. Initially, young infants will smile indiscriminately at things they see and hear, and will even smile in their sleep (Emde and Robinson, 1979). However, after a few months social smiling develops, and the infant will initiate a sequence of interaction with the parent by using the *greeting response* (Bell, 1974). The greeting response is characterised by the child seeing the parent and responding by opening his or her eyes and mouth in a distinctive shape, making a sort of cooing sound and smiling. The parent typically reacts by smiling, touching and talking to the child. The infant finds this behaviour rewarding and responds by smiling even more, and so on. A mutual reward system has been created whereby the parent is rewarded by the infant's smiling response and is thus encouraged to engage in more touching, cuddling and talking, which in turn the baby finds rewarding. It is this type of interaction process that leads to the development of an attachment between child and parents.

The attachment bond

The process of mutual conditioning and interaction results in the development of a bond between the child and his or her parents. To determine the nature of this bond it is necessary to look at situations where the child is separated from his or her parents. Schaffer and Callender (1959) investigated separation responses by studying the effects of short-term hospitalisation on infants aged between one month and one year old. Separation upset was measured by the amount of crying, responsiveness to the mother during her visits, and attitude towards nurses. The researchers found the behaviour of the children changed when they reached the age of about seven months. Those infants above seven months reacted to the separation with protest, a negative attitude towards the nurses, by becoming withdrawn, and, on returning home, a period of insecurity with the mother. Infants under seven months of age showed no protest and the nurses were accepted as mother substitutes. A brief upset was observed when the infants returned home but this was put down to a change in environment rather than to the mother's renewed presence. Schaffer and Callender suggested that a bond had developed between the children and their mothers at about the age of seven months old and the intensity of this bond remained consistent until the end of the child's first year.

Many hospitals provide rooming-in facilities for parents so that they can be with their children during hospitalisation. Alexander *et al.* (1988) have commented not only on the positive effects of rooming-in for the hospitalised child, but also on the positive effects for the parents. However, attention should be directed at non-rooming-in fathers who may be left with children to look after at home, in addition to experiencing high stress levels engendered by separation from the hospitalised child.

A study investigating the development of the attachment bond in home environments was conducted by Schaffer and Emerson (1964). They asked mothers to observe their infants' separation responses in a variety of everyday separations such as the child being left alone in a room or left with a stranger. There were sixty infants in the study and they were examined from birth every month for a year and then again at the age of eighteen months. Again, the experimenters found age differences in separation responses above and below about seven months. They also found that babies above seven months were upset by strangers approaching them, whereas the younger children had no such apprehension. These and previous findings led Schaffer and his colleagues to conclude the following points about the attachment bond:

- The average age for its development in a child is at about seven months.
- It is characterised by separation anxiety and fear of strangers.
- The child can develop a bond with more than one person.

Most of the children initially formed an attachment to one person, but after eighteen months most had developed other bonds with fathers, grandparents, aunts, siblings and other caregivers. Furthermore, one-fifth of the infants had formed strong attachments to people such as the fathers who did not take part in feeding the child and were absent for the majority of the day. In these cases the fathers were noted to engage in intensive, stimulating interaction with the child on returning home, indicating that the quality of interaction is more important than feeding the child or spending long periods of time with him or her. Indeed, Jones and Thomas (1989) found that fathers appeared to be highly sensitive to the stimuli involved in interacting with their children.

Mary Ainsworth made extensive studies of children and their mothers, and then, together with her colleagues, developed a method of studying attachments called 'the strange situation'. This consists of a sequence of eight episodes, each lasting three minutes, in which the mother/father and a stranger enter and leave the room. Trained observers record the child's behaviour during these episodes, and on the basis of this, the children are categorised into three groups: Securely Attached; Insecurely Attached–Avoidant; and Insecurely Attached–Ambivalent (Ainsworth *et al.* 1978).

Maternal deprivation

> Separation *per se,* whether it lasts a month, a year, or is permanent, has not been found to have any direct long-term effects on development.
>
> Tizard (1991)

Many people have taken exception to Bowlby's theory of the 'affectionless psychopath' (see p. 106–7). His views were based on his psychoanalytic background and evidence from some studies of poorly run children's institutions in the 1940s. Not surprisingly, the concept of maternal deprivation has, according to Rutter (1981), outlived its usefulness; there is no indication of whether maternal deprivation refers to no mother or to lack of her presence at certain times. And what about separation from the father? A more useful exercise is to examine Tizard's statement and look at the effects of short-term and long-term separation on the development of children.

Short-term separation: hospitalisation and 'working mothers'

One of the main studies investigating the long-term effects of hospitalisation was carried out by Douglas (1975). He carried out a national survey of children born in 1946, noting the number and length of stays in hospital they had. When the children reached adolescence, he found significant correlations between number and length of hospital admissions and troublesomeness, poor reading, delinquency and unstable job history. From this he concluded that there was a direct link between hospital admission in the pre-school years and later behavioural problems.

Quinton and Rutter (1976) questioned some of the methodology used in the Douglas study, and in attempting to replicate it found no long-term psychological consequences following single hospital admissions of less than a week. They did, however, find that multiple or recurrent admissions were linked with later disorders.

Problems of data interpretation

It might seem, on the basis of the research presented, that frequent separations due to hospitalisation can cause problems in later life. Not so. One must beware of every study where the terms 'relationship' or 'correlation' are used. For instance, it might conceivably be true that there is a significant correlation between drowning and ice cream consumption, since both tend to occur at the seaside. But to say that eating ice cream causes drowning would be erroneous.

Let us re-examine the separation data. There is a link between multiple and recurrent admissions to hospital and psychological problems later on in a child's development, but what caused these multiple admissions? Could it be the case that the factors responsible for the child being admitted to hospital were the same ones that caused the child to have psychological problems in adolescence? Could conditions in hospital, such as the quality of nursing care, be a factor? The answer is 'maybe'; we really cannot tell but we should always refrain from making causal inferences from correlational studies.

'Working mothers'

Of course all mothers work, but here the term refers to those women who work away from the home as well as in it. When Bowlby's report was published in 1951, many seized upon the implications of his findings for the employment of women. A World Health Organisation report in the same year stated that mothers who went out to work and placed their young children in day nurseries would cause 'permanent damage to an entire generation'. With the advent of child care books in the 1950s and 1960s, such as Dr Spock's, it became 'common knowledge' that it was essential for children to be reared by a loving mother at home. Even among nurses the accepted wisdom was that women who had children under 3 and who went out to work put the children at serious risk. Tizard (1991) states:

> Few people now realise that British nursery schools until the 1950s took children from the age of two, and that full-day school was seen as important to allow for the valuable social experiences of communal meals, rest and a balanced day.

During the last four decades there has been a wealth of research indicating that short-term separations *per se* have no adverse psycho-logical consequences. A number of the primary attachment figures in the Schaffer and Emerson (1964) study were, in fact, fathers who went out to work and saw their children only when they returned home. Children may form attachments to caregivers, but they normally show an overwhelming preference for their parents. There is some evidence that children from 'unstimulating' environments can actually benefit from attendance at day nurseries (Andrews *et al.*, 1982). A review of this topic by Clarke-Stewart (1991) concluded that the issue of the psychological consequences of short-term separation is complicated by extraneous variables such as the quality of parental care. However, quality of care outside the home can make a crucial difference to the child's development. It seems that it is the quality of care at home and in the nursery which is important for the child's emotional and intellectual development, not the fact that the mother goes out to work.

Long-term separations: divorce and death

Both divorce and death involve a similar element of separation. Thus, according to Bowlby's hypothesis, there should be no differences in the psychological consequences, as both involve disruption of affectional bonds. Rutter (2002) summarised the research and concluded that there is no correlation between the death of a parent and deviant behaviour. There was a correlation between divorce and personality problems, but only if the divorce was accompanied by marital discord. In his studies of delinquency and deviance he found that marital discord or disharmony was the main factor involved in the development of 'problem children', rather than parent–child separation. Divorces which occurred under more amicable circumstances were found to prove less harmful than those relationships that remained intact and unhappy. There was an association between separation from parents and antisocial behaviour in boys, but this occurred only in those homes where the marital relationship was difficult and strained. Hetherington (1989) conducted a long-term study of the effects of divorce on children's behaviour in the United States and found ho simple pattern. Whether children of divorced parents develop psychological problems depends on their personal characteristics, events following the breakdown of the relationship, and the child's ability to turn to other social relationships.

The child's life is inevitably disrupted by divorce and death, economic problems, the emotional state of the parent and long illnesses which can precede death. All these can produce difficulties for the children, leaving Rutter (1976) to conclude that 'The present findings suggest that separation as such is of negligible importance in the causation of delinquency.'

Institutionalisation

Long-term separation due to institutionalisation has been investigated by Barbara Tizard and her colleagues (Tizard, 1977; Hodges and Tizard, 1989). Again, the main problems are related to the nature of care rather than to the degree of separation from the parent. Whilst the twenty-five institutions studied provided good physical care for the children, their psychological provision appeared deficient. Close relationships in all the nurseries were discouraged, so the children were unable to form attachments. This resulted in attention-seeking behaviour which seemed to persist even for those children who were subsequently adopted.

> The nurseries thus provided an environment for the children which was very different from that found in any private family. While considerable attention was given to the children's health and education, their care passed through the hands of rather young girls, who attempted to remain emotionally detached from them.

The absence of stable close relationships results in an inability to consummate attachment behaviour, which is represented by attention seeking in later development.

Implications

Many parents are worried if they have to be away from their children for even short periods of time. Often it is assumed that the separation will result in some form of psychological deficit. Nurses should be able to identify the real causes of children's difficulties and act accordingly. This highlights the importance of nurses having a knowledge of children's development and underlines the need for greater continuity in the management of child care. It is also appropriate to dispel some of the myths that surround the quality of care provided by the 'working mother'.

Children's understanding of health and illness

Bibace and Walsh (1979) in their study of children's conceptions of illness asked 4 and 5-year-olds about the purpose of the stethoscope. Among the children's responses were that it was to discover 'if I have a heart', which 'is what makes me live'. Niven (2000) asked a similar question of 5-year-old children and their response was that the stethoscope was for listening to your heart to see if it had stopped. Then, on enquiring as to whether this was important, he obtained the reply 'Uh-huh, very important to your whole body . . . Don't you know about this?'

Clearly, children can have different ideas from adults about health and illness, but we need to know the extent to which these differences are due to a lack of knowledge or to inability to understand health concepts. If nurses are to communicate effectively with children they need to be able to phrase their words at a level which is meaningful to the child. Therefore, it may be useful at this point to:

- examine the differences between adult and children's concepts of health and illness;
- determine whether any differences are due to inability to understand;
- investigate ways in which nurses might use research findings to facilitate communication and health promotion.

Differences between children's and adults' perceptions of illness

In the context of pain, Eland (1985) says that adults are able to realise that the pain associated with an injection is only transitory and will result in practical benefits. She says that children do not make a similar association and may sincerely believe the injection to be unnecessary.

> If a nurse's response to an adult's admission of pain were striking the patient with a baseball bat, the patient would deny all pain from that moment. To a young child, the shot [injection] is the baseball bat.

Children have more difficulties than adults with ambiguous words. 'Sick' can mean feeling ill or it can mean vomiting. A colleague related a conversation with his 4-year-old son which started with his son asking him one morning whether God used their bathroom often. This question took him quite by surprise, until, after some thought, he realised why his son had asked such a question. The day before he had shouted upstairs to the occupier, 'Oh God, when are you going to come out of that bathroom?' His son had taken the request literally.

Table 4.3 *Cognitions of illness (from Bibace and Walsh, 1979)*

1 What does it mean to be healthy?
2 Do you remember anyone who was sick? What was wrong? How did he or she get sick? How did he or she get better?
3 Were you ever sick? Why did you get sick? How did you get sick? How did you get better?
6 What is a cold? How do people get colds? Where do colds come from? What makes colds go away?
8 What is a heart attack? Why do people get heart attacks?
9 What is cancer? How do people get cancer?
11 Have you ever had pain? Where? What is pain? Why does it come? Where does it come from?
12 What are germs? What do they look like? Can you draw germs? Where do they come from?

In Bibace and Walsh's study of age differences in the conceptions of illness they asked children aged between 3 and 13 years old twelve questions on health and illness (see Table 4.3). The children's answers were analysed and allocated to categories according to the sophistication of their response.

Stage 1 Children aged approximately under 7 years

- *Incomprehension.* The child gives irrelevant answers or evades the question.

    'What is a heart attack?'
    'A heart attack is on vacation.'
    'Why?'
    'Can I have a pencil?'

- *Phenomenism.* Illness is usually a sight or sound that the child has, at some time, associated with the illness.

    'What is a heart attack?'
    'A heart attack is falling on your back.'
    'Why do people get heart attacks?'
    'A heart attack is from the sun.'

- *Contagion.* Illness is usually a person or an object that is close to, but not necessarily touching, the ill person. It can also be an activity that occurs before the illness.

    'Where does a cold come from?'
    'From other people.'
    'How do you get a cold from other people?'
    'You're just playing with them.'

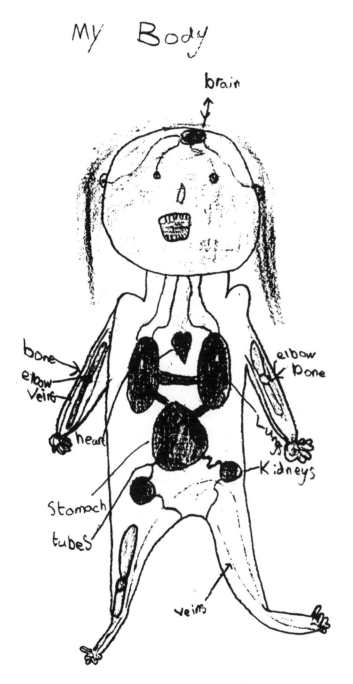

Figure 4.1 A 7-year-old child's perception of her body

Stage 2 Children aged approximately 7 to 11 years old

- *Contamination* – the child cannot distinguish between mind and body, thus bad or immoral behaviour can cause illness as well as contact with germs.

  > 'What is cancer?'
  > 'Cancer is when you are very sick and you have to go to hospital and you throw up a lot, and stuff.'
  > 'How do people get cancer?'
  > 'From smoking without their mother's permission. You shouldn't do it, it's bad.'

- *Internalisation.* Illness is within the body and the cause comes from outside.

  > 'How do people get colds?'
  > 'From germs in the air, you breathe them in.'
  > 'How does this give you a cold?'
  > 'The germs, they get in your blood.'

Stage 3 Children aged approximately 11+

- *Physiological.* The child can now describe the functioning of internal organs, and illness is often perceived as some malfunctioning part of the body.

  > 'What is a heart attack?'
  > 'A heart attack is when the heart stops pumping blood to the rest of the body. A person faints, stops breathing, and collapses.'

- *Psychophysiological.* An additional cause of illness is perceived, namely a psychological cause. Feelings can now affect the functioning of the body.

  > 'What is a heart attack?'
  > 'It's when your heart stops or doesn't work right.'
  > 'How do people get heart attacks?'
  > 'A heart attack is being all nerve-racked and weary.'

There is support for classifying conceptions of illness in this way from the studies of Perrin and Gerrity (1981) and also Fielding (1985), but there are advantages and disadvantages to such an approach.

- *Advantages.* This approach gives an indication of the sort of mistakes children make about health and illness. Furthermore, the stages give information about the ages at which children can understand specific concepts.
- *Disadvantages.* This approach gives little indication of why children think in this way. It implies that children in one stage will not be able to understand concepts in another. The relevance and meaningfulness of the questions given to the children must be challenged.

Understanding

Donaldson (1978) has shown that children can understand concepts above their stage if they are phrased in a way that is meaningful. According to her research, it would be wrong for nurses to assume that because the child was a specific age he or she would be unable to comprehend certain concepts of health and illness.

An alternative way of representing the development of children's understanding of health and illness is provided by the work of Katherine Nelson (1986). She suggests that as a result of participation in routine day-to-day events, children construct a kind of plan. This plan she calls a *script*, and this specifies the people involved, the roles they play, the objects used, and the sequence of actions that make up the event. Children grow up inside other people's scripts and thus experience an environment that has been prepared by their parents and culture. Nelson proposes that scripts have three functions:

- They are guides to action that tell children what is likely to happen next in familiar circumstances. If they lack scripted knowledge, close attention has to be paid to detail. This mental effort can lead to mistakes.
- They allow people within a given group to co-ordinate and communicate more effectively.
- They provide a framework within which abstract concepts can be acquired.

Maniulenko (1975) asked a group of Russian 4-year-olds to stand still with their hands by their sides for as long as they could. They understood what was required of them but found it virtually impossible to stand still for more than a few seconds. Maniulenko then asked the children to pretend they were part of the guard of honour at the entrance to the tomb of Lenin. Every Soviet child knew how still those soldiers stood. When this request was part of a pretend game, the children's ability to stand still increased dramatically. Here the utilisation of a common script through play enabled children to put into practice a relatively abstract concept.

Children's concepts of health and illness will thus be determined by the scripts they have experienced and constructed during their everyday lives. The nature of these scripts will be influenced by parents and by the child's culture. Although some scripts from different cultures may have the same label, they may have different contexts, and therefore care should be taken in generalising across cultures.

Nursing interventions: socio-dramatic play

Whilst children between the ages of 4 and 10 years will experience an average of four to six illnesses a year (Parmalee, 1986), one does not have to wait for actual events to happen before giving children an idea of their contents. Socio-dramatic play has an extremely important role to play in the acquisition of new scripts, as the use of play can significantly influence children's concepts about health, illness and hospital (Gillis, 1989).

Goodman and Adams (1989) say that the more healthy children understand about hospital the less anxiety they will have on future contact. Even so, they propose that there is little research on how the children themselves feel about hospital. Accordingly they asked about 100 children to list the first ten words which came to mind when the word 'hospital' was mentioned. The result was an overwhelmingly negative response. (The words they produced are the ones used in Exercise 4.1 and the frequencies are given at the end of the chapter.) If parents, teachers and nurses do not give similar responses, then obviously the children's common hospital scripts are different from adults'. It is therefore important to try to look at hospital through the child's eyes. In this particular study, the common script was produced by the children's actual contact with hospital, as only three children had had no contact at all.

Exercise 4.1 *Children's responses to hospital*

About 100 children aged between 11 and 12 from two Newcastle schools were asked to write down up to ten words describing a hospital. Only three of the children had had no contact with a hospital. The most frequently occurring words chosen were

Pain	Smell
Anxiety	Food
Needles	Operations
Boredom	Loneliness
Fear	Noise
Blood	Bedclothes
Sad	

Try to put yourself in their shoes and rate the words according to how you think the children responded. If you think that the word 'Operations' was the most commonly given rate it first and so on. One word was nearly twice as important as the others – can you guess which it was? The answers are given at the end of this chapter.

Some care should be taken in interpreting the results, as although anxiety and fear are treated separately, when put together they represent the most frequent comment (see answers at the end of this chapter). Also, the word most frequently mentioned is not necessarily the one the children 'hate the most', it is merely the one that is mentioned more often.

One way of reducing children's anxiety about illness and hospital is to develop 'health scripts' through play. Eiser and Hanson (1989) conducted a school-based intervention preparing children for hospital. The children came from a rural primary school and had little or no experience of hospital. There were forty-two children aged 5 and twenty-four children aged 8. The children played in groups of three with a 'play hospital' comprising a reception area, ward, x-ray room, and surgery. The play sessions were facilitated by a school nurse and teacher. The children were filmed at the start of the experiment and then again one month later. During the sessions a wide range of 'hospital equipment' was used and there were visits to a hospital and from hospital staff.

Eiser and Hanson observed differences in the children's play behaviour in the second filming session. The children seemed to have empathy with the patient's role and were careful to warn patients of impending pain. They were also more aware of the equipment and techniques used in hospital. Interestingly, and perhaps unfortunately, the authors report that during the first play session the 'nurses' cared for patients, whereas by the time of the second session the 'nurses' were involved much more in administrative tasks.

The study was not able to investigate whether these play sessions subsequently helped children who were admitted to hospital, but it does suggest that a greater knowledge of hospitals would reduce anxiety.

The children in this type of play session, whether it takes place in school or in hospital, develop a sequence of hospital scripts. They are able to develop a framework which accommodates the scenarios presented to them in hospital. Understanding what is going on around them produces less anxiety; there might be fear, but not fear of the unknown.

Play can be used for many other purposes in the hospital as well as in the school. It can be used just as successfully for health education, using different scripts. Nurses should try to enter the world of the child and construct scenarios that will provide a basic framework for the child to go out and develop a better understanding of his or her health environment.

Summary

The focus of this chapter has been on children and the nursing implications of both the qualitative and the quantitative changes associated with child development. Neonatal development has been described in terms of the range of basic sensory abilities which enable the infant to explore and gradually make sense of the environment. Attachment and bonding have been explored in terms of early parent–child interaction, as well as the effects of parental separation on the process of bonding and mental health in adult life. In particular, this chapter has examined the arguments which currently exist in relation to the effects of maternal deprivation and the conditions under which such deprivation can be detrimental to the child. Studies exploring the effects of institutionalisation on children suggest that problems for the child are more likely to arise as a result of the nature of the care given, rather than as a direct effect of separation from the parents.

I have explored the child's understanding of health and illness in relation to both the amount of knowledge the child acquires at different developmental stages and the ability of the child to understand concepts relating to health and illness. It is important to see the world from the child's perspective, and to understand the mistakes they may make, if effective communication about health and illness is to occur. The use of familiar scripts to help children understand abstract concepts will develop the range of scripts available to the child and influence the child's concepts of health and illness. Effective communication has been found to reduce the child's anxiety about illness and hospitalisation.

Conundrum revisited

Sam's situation impresses upon us just how profoundly a sensory difficulty impacts upon psychological development and well-being. Moreover, it highlights the challenges facing parents who try to create a supportive environment within which the child can develop. Parents protect their child from what Raymet called 'the insults, hurts and idiocies of the world'. In so doing they may unwittingly contribute to the developmental problems faced by the child, for instance by insulating the child from opportunities to learn through experience.

Babies and very young children are highly dependent upon sight for the gathering of information about the world, establishing a bond with their parents, the development of a secure psychological environment and, from that, a sense of self worth. Chapter 1 highlights the importance of self-esteem and motivation. Sam suffered from sensory deprivation that influenced his ability not only to learn (for instance by reading and interpreting pictures), but also to form a satisfying relationship with his parents. In the absence of sight, other means of communication had to be substituted (touch and sound) and as early as possible. As Raymet put it, 'I wanted to stimulate Sam as much as possible, but only in ways that he could recognize as loving. I knew he didn't know how to understand some of that because he couldn't see me smile.'

Significantly, in the earliest stages the problem of distress lies with the parents. Deprived of a reference norm (how things should seem when you are born) Sam was unaware of what it meant not to be sighted. The challenge was to parent Sam in ways that maximized his opportunity to develop (by using music, familiar sounds and then words combined with cuddles) whilst minimizing the risk that Sam was learning to despise his situation. Sam (like other children) had his own unique temperament, something which Raymet and Neil found hard to interpret. It was difficult for Sam to read subtle situations as visual information often supplements that learned through other senses. Sam learned to focus upon hearing and touch comparatively quickly, but understandably he was much more dependent upon familiar approaches and signals. His tolerance of new situations was very limited and learning opportunities were consequently diminished.

At the time when Sam was born family support was less developed and there was little appreciation of the emotional effort involved in responding to a child who had to develop using fewer senses. Neil recalls, 'We were told to listen to Sam, to sense what he was feeling, and we got better at that. But no one told us how draining the effort would be. At times I am sure that we were both depressed as a result.' Raymet stayed at home and developed a close relationship with her son, but the bond with Neil deteriorated. Later, Sam concluded that his father was uninterested in him.

By the time Sam was 10 Raymet had accompanied him several times to hospital and both parents had resigned themselves to fulfilling different needs for their son. Neil would work longer hours to supplement the family income and leave child care to his wife. Sam exhibited anxieties regarding the possible separation from his mother should she spend more than a short time away from him. The psychologist asked Sam, 'What does it mean, not to be able to see?' He replied, 'My mum sees. She tells me what is there.' Persisting, the psychologist replied, 'Yes, I understand. But how do you feel about using your ears instead of your eyes?' Sam retorted angrily, 'Dad said I'm always earwigging. He says I listen in too much.'

In this conundrum the challenge is to work with what is known about the development of child senses, the importance of parental bonding and the need to establish a supportive environment within which a child may become incrementally more independent. Periods of time spent in hospital, the normal stressors that can affect families and human relations need to be anticipated as tests that can affect the child's sense of security. It then becomes important to elect what sorts of stimulation and support might effectively help a child develop self-esteem and the belief that he or she can solve problems. Just who provides the support may be equally important if the child is to learn to become adaptable in future.

? Questions for further consideration

1 'The infant is born into a world of buzzing, blooming confusion' (William James). Discuss.
2 To what extent can a knowledge of infant sensory acuities be helpful to parents?
3 In what ways can a nurse influence the psychological development of a premature baby?
4 Describe the processes involved in parent–child interaction.

5 Mothers who go out to work cannot care for their children as well as mothers who stay at home. Discuss.

6 To what extent does delinquency have its roots in lack of mothering?

7 A 6-year-old child cannot understand concepts of health and illness. Discuss.

8 How can a nurse facilitate young children's understanding of hospital?

Answers to Exercise 4.1

Word	No. of times word used by children
Pain	19
Anxiety	29
Needles	19
Boredom	15
Fear	36
Blood	15
Smell	67
Food	15
Operations	22
Loneliness	13
Noise	11
Bedclothes	7
Sad	20

References

Ainsworth, M. D. S., Bell, S. M. and Stayton, D. J. (1991). Infant–mother attachment and social development: 'socialisation' as a product of reciprocal responsiveness to signals. In Woodhead, M., Carr, R. and Light, P. (eds) *Becoming a Person.* London: Routledge and Open University.

Ainsworth, M. D. S., Blehar, M. C., Walters, E., and Wall, S. (1978). *Patterns of Attachment: a psychological study of the strange situation.* Hillsdale NJ: Erlbaum.

Alexander, D., Powell, G. M., Williams, P., White, M. and Conlon, M. (1988). Anxiety levels of rooming-in and non-rooming-in parents of young hospitalized children. *Maternal–Child Nursing Journal, 17,* 79–99.

Ambrose, J. A. (1969). Discussion contribution. In Ambrose, J. A. (ed.) *Stimulation in Early Infancy.* London: Academic Press.

Andrews, S. R., Blumenthal, J. B., Johnson, D. L., Kahn, A. J., Ferguson, C. J., Lasater, T. M., Malone, P. E. and Wallace, D. B. (1982). The skills of mothering: a study of parent child-development centers. *Monographs for the Society for Research in Child Development, 47,* 1–83.

Aslin, R. N. (1987). Anatomical constraints on oculomotor development: implications for infant perception. In Yonas, A. (ed.) *Twentieth Minnesota Symposium on Child Psychology.* Hillsdale NJ: Erlbaum.

Bell, R. Q. (1974). Contributions of human infants to caregiving and social interaction. In Lewis, M. and Rosenblum, L. A. (eds) *The Effect of the Infant on its Caregiver.* London: Wiley.

Bibace, R. and Walsh, M. E. (1979). Developmental stages in children's conceptions of illness. In Sone, G. C., Cohen, F. and Adler, N. (eds) *Health Psychology.* New York: Jossey Bass.

Bower, T. G. R. (1989). The perceptual world of the new-born child. In Slater, A. and Bremner, G. (eds) *Infant Development.* Hove: Erlbaum.

Bowlby, J. (1951). *Maternal Care and Mental Health.* Geneva: World Health Organisation.

Brackbill, Y. (1975). Continuous stimulation and arousal level in infancy: effects of stimulus intensity and stress. *Child Development, 46,* 364–369.

Brazelton, T. B., Nugent, K. J. and Lester, B. M. (1987). Neonatal behavioral assessment scale. In Osofsky, J. D. (ed.) *Handbook of Infant Development.* 2nd edn. New York: Wiley.

Bremner, G. and Slater, A. (eds) (2003). *An Introduction to Developmental Psychology.* Oxford: Blackwell.

Campos, J. J., Campos, R. G. and Barret, K. C. (1989). Emergent themes in the study of emotional development and emotion regulation. *Developmental Psychology, 25,* 394–402.

Cernoch, J. M. and Porter, R. H. (1985). Recognition of maternal axillary odors by infants. *Child Development, 56,* 1593–1598.

Clarke-Stewart, K. A. (1991). Infant day care: maligned or malignant? In Woodhead, M., Light, P. and Carr, R. (eds) *Growing up in a Changing Society.* London: Routledge and Open University.

Cox, J. L., Holden, J. M. and Sagovsky, R. (1987). Detection of postnatal depression: development of the ten-item Edinburgh Postnatal Depression Scale. *British Journal of Psychiatry, 150,* 782–786.

Crnic, K. A., Rogozin, A. S., Greenberg, M. T., Robinson, N. M. and Basham, R. B. (1983). Social-interaction and developmental competence of preterm and full-term infants during the first year of life. *Child Development, 54,* 1199–1210.

Dannemiller, J. L. and Stephens, B. R. (1988). A critical test of infant preference models. *Child Development, 59,* 210–216.

De Casper, A. J. and Spence, M. J. (1986). Prenatal maternal speech influences newborn's perception of speech sounds. *Infant Behaviour and Development, 9,* 133–150.

Donaldson, M. (1978). *Children's Minds.* London: Fontana.

Douglas, J. (1993). *Psychology and Nursing Children.* Leicester: BPS Books (The British Psychological Society) and Macmillan.

Douglas, J. W. B. (1975). Early hospital admissions and later disturbances of behaviour and learning. *Developmental Medicine and Child Neurology, 17,* 456–480.

Eimas, P. D. (1985). The perception of speech in early infancy. *Scientific American, 204,* 66–72.

Eiser, C. and Hanson, L. (1989). Preparing children for hospital: a school-based intervention. *The Professional Nurse,* March, 297–300.

Eland, J. M. (1985). The role of the nurse in children's pain. In Copp, L. A. (ed.) *Perspectives on Pain.* Edinburgh: Churchill Livingstone.

Emde, R. N. and Robinson, J. (1979). The first two months: recent research in development psychobiology. In Noshpitz, J. and Call, J. (eds) *Basic Handbook of Child Psychiatry.* New York: Basic Books.

Engen, T., Lipsitt, L. P. and Peck, M. B. (1974). Ability of newborn infants to discriminate sapid substances. *Developmental Psychology, 10,* 741–746.

Fantz, R. L. (1961). The origin of form perception. *Scientific American, 204,* 66–72.

Field, T. and Goldson, E. (1984). Pacifying effects of non-nutritive sucking on term and preterm neonates during heelstick procedures. *Pediatrics, 74,* 1012–1015.

Fielding, D. (1985). Chronic illness in children. In Watts, F. (ed.) *New Directions in Clinical Psychology.* Chichester: Wiley and BPS Books (The British Psychological Society).

Fuller, B. F. (1991). Acoustic discrimination of three types of infant cries. *Nursing Research, 40,* 156–160.

Ganchrow, J. R., Steiner, J. E. and Daher, M. (1983). Neonatal facial expression in response to different qualities of intensities of gustatory stimuli. *Infant Behaviour and Development, 6,* 189–200.

Gennaro, S., Medoff-Cooper, B. and Lotas, M. (1992). Perinatal factors and infant temperament: a collaborative approach. *Nursing Research, 41,* 375–377.

Goodman, S. and Adams, D. (1989). Uncumphortable. *Nursing Times, 85,* 28–31.

Gustafson, G. E. and Harris, K. L. (1991). Women's responses to young infants' cries. *Developmental Psychology, 26,* 144–152.

Haith, M. M. (1980). *Rules that Babies Look By.* Hillsdale NJ: Erlbaum.

Hetherington, E. M. (1989). Coping with family transitions: winners, losers and survivors. *Child Development, 60,* 1–14.

Hodges, J. and Tizard, B. (1989). Social and family relationships of ex-institutional adolescents. *Journal of Child Psychology and Psychiatry, 30,* 77–97.

Holden, J. M., Sagovsky, R. and Cox, J. L. (1989). Counselling in a general practice setting: controlled study of health visitor intervention in treatment of postnatal depression. *British Medical Journal, 298,* 223–226.

Jones, L. C. and Thomas, S. A. (1989). New father's blood pressure and heart rate: relationships to interaction with their newborn infants. *Nursing Research, 38,* 237–241.

Kalat, J. W. (1981). *Biological Psychology.* Belmont CA: Wadsworth.

Keith, R. W. (1975). Middle ear function in neonates. *Archives of Otolaryngology, 101,* 375–379.

Kessen, W., Haith, M. M. and Salapatek, P. (1970). Human infancy: a bibliography and guide. In Mussen, P. H. (ed.) *Carmichael's Manual of Child Psychology.* 3rd edn. London: Wiley.

Korner, A. F. (1987). Preventive intervention with high-risk newborns: theoretical, conceptual, and methodological perspectives. In Osofsky, J. (ed.) *Handbook of Infant Development.* New York: Wiley.

Korner, A. F. and Thoman, E. (1972). The relative efficacy of contact and vestibular proprioceptive stimuli in soothing neonates. *Child Development, 43,* 443–454.

Macfarlane, A. (1977). *The Psychology of Childbirth.* London: Open Books.

Makin, J. W. and Porter, R. H. (1989). Attractiveness of lactating females' breast odors to neonates. *Child Development, 60,* 803–810.

Maniulenko, V. V. (1975). The development voluntary behaviour in preschool-age children. *Soviet Psychology, 13,* 65–116.

Miller, B. C. and Sollie, D. C. (1986). Normal stresses during the transition to parenthood. In Moos, R. H. (ed.) *Coping with Life Crises.* New York: Plenum.

Murray, L. and Stein, A. (1991). The effects of postnatal depression on mother–infant relations and infant development. In Woodhead, M., Carr, R. and Light, P. (eds) *Becoming a Person.* London: Routledge and Open University.

Murray, L. and Trevarthen, C. B. (1985). Emotional regulation of interaction between two-month-olds and their mothers. In Field, T. M. and Fox, N. A. (eds) *Social Perception in Infants.* Norwood NJ: Ablex.

Myers, B. J. (1982). Early intervention using Brazelton training with middleclass mothers and fathers of newborns. *Child Development, 53,* 462–471.

Nelson, K. (1986). *Event Knowledge: Structure and function in development.* Hillsdale NJ.: Erlbaum.

Niven, N. (2000). *Health Psychology: An introduction for health care professionals.* 3rd edn. Edinburgh: Churchill Livingstone.

Oehler, J. M. (1993). Developmental care of low birth weight infants. *Nursing Clinics of North America, 28,* 289–301.

Parmalee, A. H. (1986). Children's illnesses: their beneficial effects on behavioural development. *Child Development, 57,* 1–10.

Perrin, E. C. and Gerrity, P. S. (1981). There's a demon in your belly: children's understanding of illness. *Pediatrics, 67,* 841–849.

Pinneau, S. (1955). The infantile disorder of hospitalism and anaclitic depression. *Psychological Bulletin, 52,* 429–452.

Quinton, D. and Rutter, M. (1976). Early hospital admissions and later disturbances of behaviour. In Clarke, A. M. and Clarke, A. D. B. (eds) *Early Experience.* London: Open Books.

Rutter, M. (1976). Parent–child separation: psychological effects on children. In Clarke, A. M. and Clarke, A. D. B. (eds) *Early Experience.* London: Open Books.

Rutter, M. (1978). Early sources of security and competence. In Bruner, J. S. and Garten, A. (eds) *Human Growth and Development.* Oxford: Oxford University Press.

Rutter, M. (1981). *Maternal Deprivation Reassessed.* Harmondsworth: Penguin.

Rutter, M. (2002). Nature, nurture and development: from evangelism through science toward policy and practice. *Child Development, 73,* 1–21.

Sameroff, A. J. (1991). The social context of development. In Woodhead, M., Carr, R. and Light, P. (eds) *Becoming a Person.* London: Routledge and Open University.

Schaffer, H. R. and Callender, W. M. (1959). Psychological effects of hospitalisation in infancy. *Pediatrics, 24,* 528–539.

Schaffer, H. R. and Emerson, P. E. (1964). The development of social attachments in infancy. *Monographs of the Society for Research in Child Development, 29*(3) (whole No. 94).

Slater, A. (1991). Unpublished personal communication.

Slater, A. and Bremner, G. (eds). (1989). *Infant Development.* Hove: Erlbaum.

Small, M. (1990). *Cognitive Development.* San Diego CA: Harcourt Brace Jovanovich.

Solkoff, N., Jaffe, S., Weintraub, D. and Blase, B. (1969). Effects of handling on the subsequent development of premature babies. *Developmental Psychology, 1,* 765–768.

Thomas, A., Chess, S. and Birch, H. G. (1970). The origin of personality. *Scientific American, 223,* 102–109.

Tizard, B. (1977). *Adoption: A second chance.* London: Open Books.

Tizard, B. (1991). Working mothers and the care of young children. In Woodhead, M., Light, P. and Carr, R. (eds) *Growing up in a Changing Society.* London: Routledge and Open University.

Widmayer, S. and Field, T. (1980). Effects of Brazelton demonstrations on early inter- actions of preterm infants and their teenage mothers. *Infant Behaviour and Development, 3,* 79–89.

Williams, H. and Carmichael, A. (1985). Depression in mothers in a multi-ethnic urban industrial municipality in Melbourne: aetiological factors and effects on infants and pre-school children. *Journal of Child Psychology and Psychiatry, 26,* 277–288.

Wolff, P. H. (1969). The natural history of crying and other vocalisations in early infancy. In Foss, B. M. (ed.) *Determinants of Infant Behaviour* IV. London: Methuen.

Further reading

Bee, Helen and Boyd, Denise (2003) *The Developing Child.* Boston MA: Allyn and Bacon. A comprehensive and well written text on child development that has stood the test of time.

Douglas, J. (1993). *Psychology and Nursing Children.* Leicester: BPS books (The British Psychological Society) and Macmillan. This book has three sections: care of chil- dren in the community, caring for sick children and caring for the carers. It inves- tigates the particular health requirements of children in hospital and in the community, using a psychological framework.

Slater, Alan and Lewis, Michael (2002) *Introduction to Infant Development.* Oxford: Oxford University Press. In contrast to Bee and Boyd this is a British text with up- to-date research presented in an easily comprehensible style.

Adolescence, Adulthood and Ageing

A practice conundrum

In Chapter 9 we discuss the conundrum of how best to prompt people to give up cigarette smoking. This conundrum though poses a deeper question about psychological well-being and how this can be assured as people progress through the different stages of their lives. If cigarette smoking is considered a physical health risk what are the psychological health risks as we grow and age? What might nurses do to back up their claim that they deliver holistic health care, supporting psychological as well as physical well-being?

One way to conceive of this issue is to think of a triangle of risks, demands and expectations at three stages of life (adolescence, adulthood and old age). At the centre of the triangle is the individual who tries to manage each of these in order to sustain a psychological equilibrium. For this conundrum take three A3 sheets of paper and reproduce the above triangle on each of them. One of these should be labelled adolescence, one adult life and the third old age. Now annotate each triangle with the risks, demands and expectations that might tax psychological well-being. With colleagues add in (using a different coloured pen) the nursing interventions that assist people to sustain psychological well-being. Chapter 9 details a wide range of psychological changes associated with ageing. How many of these did you recognise and use in your mapping exercise?

- *Barbara*: aged 16, looks anorexic, seems to get on well with her parents, has no boyfriend but two reasonably close friends, exams imminent, took a bottle of paracetamol plus half a bottle of vodka, found by her mother in a pool of vomit.
- *James*: aged 44, works too hard, has problems with his teenage son, knows he should do something about the pains in his chest (will see someone next week); his wife's father is intolerable at weekends, which is causing problems with his wife, thinks 'Must walk the dog more often.'

● *Edith*: aged 72, used to be very good at her job, and good at crosswords too, but her memory has been getting very bad; thinks that she has become a real nuisance to everyone because of it; also gets disoriented and will not keep still, is in hospital for a back operation.

If you took away the ages of the people described above you would still be able to make a reasonable guess as to how old they were. This is because there are certain stages in our lives at which some things are more likely to happen than others. The 'world' of the adolescent is different from that of his or her father or mother, and older people do face different problems to those of their children. The purpose of this chapter is to highlight the differences in behaviour that occur at particular stages in the life span.

Adolescence

This stage in human development is often associated with storm and stress, although some adolescents experience relatively few and minor difficulties (Rutter, 1976). Nonetheless, it is a time of potential 'crisis', and having a sense of the sorts of difficulties facing people at this time will facilitate nursing care.

Adolescence is made up of a series of sub-stages: early, middle, and late. The problems facing the 12-year-old are not necessarily the same as those facing the 15-year-old, and therefore the term 'adolescence' must be used in a broad context, covering a range of years from 11 to 18. Some problems may be described as physical (for example, those connected with puberty), some as psychological (identity crises) and some as social (such as those associated with changing or leaving school). Table 5.1 gives some examples of these problems.

Table 5.1 *Physical, psychological and social factors that can influence both males and females at different stages of adolescent development*

| | | Adolescence | |
Factors	Early	Middle	Late
Physical	Puberty	Body image	Body image
Psychological	Sexuality	Identity: parental problems	Identity: career/ beliefs
Social	Peer problems	Becoming an adult?	Leaving home

Puberty and body image

The term 'puberty' comes from the Latin *pubertas,* meaning 'age of manhood' or, literally, 'to grow hairy'. It may be defined as the point at which a person reaches sexual maturity. Accompanying puberty is the *adolescent growth spurt,* which is a rapid increase in physical growth, and the *menarche,* the first occurrence of menstruation. For most girls, puberty begins at about 11 years old and the average female reaches the menarche within six months of her thirteenth birthday. For boys, sexual maturation begins at about 11–11½ years old, and the penis is fully developed at about 14½–15 years of age. At this time girls may spend a great deal of time worrying about how other people will respond to them (Greif and Ulman, 1982). They are concerned with their height and weight, the condition of their hair, the size of their ears, breasts, noses and hips, but tend to be ambivalent about their first menstruation.

Boys also have worries about their bodies, even if some of them would have us believe differently. Flaming and Morse (1991) interviewed twenty-two boys who were at least 15 years old about their experience of pubertal changes. They found that a basic social psychological process for minimising embarrassment emerged. The process was comprised of four stages:

- *Waiting for the change.* Boys developed expectations by listening to others.
- *Noticing the change.* The boys looked at older males and imagined what the changes might be like.
- *Dealing with the change.* They compared their physical changes with others and their own expectations.
- *Feeling comfortable with the change.* If the boys felt they were different, they worried about the difference.

Puberty can occur over a wide range of time, and the rate of maturation has been found to influence behaviour. Jones and Bayley (1950) followed the development of thirty-two male late and early developers over a six-year period. The late maturers were rated as less masculine and less physically attractive than the early maturers. Jones (1965) followed up the previous study and found the sixteen late maturers, now in their early 30s, to still be less sociable, less confident, less responsible and less popular with their peers. However, the late maturers were found to be less rigid and more innovative in problem-solving. For late and early maturing females, the situation is more complex, as there is evidence that early maturing females have more problems than late maturing females. Early maturing females tend to be less confident, outgoing and popular than late maturers (Aro and Taipale, 1987). However, Faust (1960) found these disadvantages to be short-lived, and early maturers were very popular in late adolescence.

Exercise 5.1 *Rates of maturity*

Try to account for the following findings.

1 Why should male early maturers have such positive characteristics as opposed to male late maturers?
2 Why should the opposite be the case with females?
3 Why should early maturing females become popular in late adolescence?

Possible answers

1 People may react positively to the adultlike appearance of the early maturing male, giving him privileges and responsibilities normally reserved for older males. Parents have higher educational and achievement aspirations for their early maturing sons, and this positive, even harmonious, atmosphere may promote self-confidence. Conversely, if parents, teachers and other adolescents treat late maturers as unsophisticated and naive, they may well become unsure of themselves and feel rejected.
2 Early maturing females may get teased a lot by their female classmates and by immature boys. Parents report more conflicts with early maturing females, and thus a brusque, defiant attitude may develop which can affect relations with other females.
3 Faust (1960) suggests that as females in late adolescence develop a strong interest in relationships with males, they discover that early maturing females are very popular with boys and thus the early maturing female's popularity is boosted with her peers, although jealousy can also occur.

Body image continues to be of great concern throughout adolescence. Females are generally more sensitive to body image in themselves and in others too. Even minor accidents producing small changes in physical appearance can result in high levels of stress for adolescents (Newell, 1991).

Perceptions of body image

Price (1990, 1999) has produced a model designed to assist nurses to plan and deliver body image care that is based on five central concepts.

● *Body reality.* This is the body as it really exists. It is the body not as we would like to see it, but as it exists or may be described in a physical examination. Threats to the body image include such events as malignant change, degenerative conditions, infection, inflammation or poisoning.

- *Body ideal.* This is the picture in one's head of how the body should look, and is influenced by societal and cultural norms through advertising and changing attitudes to fitness and health. It is threatened by conditions such as anorexia nervosa, bulimia nervosa, pregnancy, obesity, incontinence, pain, attachment to ventilators, and intravenous infusions.
- *Body presentation.* The reality of our bodies rarely meets our ideal, resulting in an attempt to make the two converge by presenting our bodies in a particular way. Dress, grooming, walking and the use of aids such as walking sticks or hearing aids affect the way the body is presented. Threats to our body presentation include alopecia, abnormal gait, body odour, and attachments such as a stoma bag.
- *Coping strategies.* Direct coping requires the patient to view the body image threat in a similar way to onlookers. Indirect coping occurs when the body presentation is adjusted to support body reality, as in the case of the patient with burns accepting analgesia in order to undergo wound toilet. Palliative coping (that which gives relief but does not cure) often relieves immediate stress but does not affect long term recovery. As the formation of a new body image may take months, the coping strategies adopted by the patient are very important.
- *Social support network.* Family and friends can provide an environment conducive to the integration of the patient's new body image into society. Thus patients with an active social support network are liable to make better progress. Support can be expressed in different ways including practical aid, sympathetic listening, boosting self-esteem and acceptance into society.

Price says that through the steps of the nursing process – assessment, diagnosis, care planning, intervention and evaluation – the nurse is able to use the model 'to specify care needs more accurately and to own the means to effect improvement in body image'.

Eating disorders

Anorexia nervosa

This is an eating disorder characterised by insistence on abnormally low body weight and fear of becoming fat. As a result, individuals experience an altered body image and amenorrhoea (absence of menstruation) often occurs in women.

The disorder is most common in adolescent women from middle-income families. Although the term means 'nervous loss of appetite', anorexics rarely lose their appetite and can literally starve themselves to become thin (Palmer, 1988). The main problem of adolescent anorexics is their denial of the existence and severity of their condition. The causes of anorexia nervosa are complex. A theory proposed by Bruch (1974) is linked with one of the effects of starvation. This leads to the switching off of the part of the system involving the reproductive organs, resulting in a pituitary response similar to that of pre-puberty. Thus the anorexic can be seen as simply starving herself to deny womanhood, and using the results to delay maturation. It is arguable, however, whether adolescent girls are aware that their periods will stop when they practise self-starvation.

Another factor associated with the development of the disorder is parental control. Anorexia is most prevalent in middle-income families, and the fathers and mothers of anorexics are usually in professional or managerial occupations. There may be conflict between the parents' goals for their offspring and the needs and wishes of the children. Bruch tells the story of the young Spaniard who preferred to sit and starve rather than do any work. When asked why he did not get up and find himself some work, he replied, 'In hunger, I am king.'

Whilst dieting itself is not a cause of anorexia, it can act as a trigger. Losing a few pounds can develop into a mania for thinness, especially when set in the context of society's emphasis on the ideal body shape as being slim.

In a study of 715 adolescent girls Steiger *et al.* (1992) found that mood and eating symptoms were related to an abnormal psychological profile; there were concerns about body shape and family relationships indicating that more than one factor was involved in their condition.

The treatment for anorexia is concerned with the restoration and maintenance of a normal healthy weight, and hospitalisation is usually required in order to gradually increase the calorific intake. At this stage skilled nursing care is needed to provide emotional support and also to help implement behavioural therapy which is often used at this stage in the treatment programme. The weight maintenance phase frequently involves a cognitive-behavioural approach which concentrates on the links between the patient's feelings, behaviours and thoughts (see Chapter 10).

Bulimia nervosa

This is a related eating disorder marked by recurrent episodes of binge eating followed by self-induced vomiting or the use of laxatives and diuretics. Sometimes fasting or vigorous exercise is used to counter the binge eating but these techniques are not so popular, as they take time to take effect (Palmer, 1988). Bulimics share the anorexics' concern with weight and body shape but are not necessarily underweight. Some also tend to experience bouts of depression. Bingeing and purging can result in a sore throat, kidney damage, menstrual problems, hair loss, erosion of tooth enamel and loss of sex drive (Szmukler, 1989). Fairburn and Beglin (1990), reviewing the studies of the epidemiology of bulimia, found that approximately 1 per cent of adolescent women suffer from the disorder but also point out that the figure may be higher, since bulimics are known to be unco-operative with these types of survey.

There are several treatments for bulimia nervosa, including individual cognitive-behaviour therapy to help the patient understand the causes of bingeing and how to control such episodes; family therapy in which members of the family learn how to provide support which can lessen the chances of the patient using food counterproductively; and group therapy to utilise group dynamics in the restoration and maintenance of normal eating behaviour. Meades (1993) suggests that community psychiatric nurses are well placed to observe and supervise people with eating disorders who are potentially vulnerable to relapse following discharge from hospital (see Milne, 1993).

Social and cultural factors

In the United Kingdom a 16-year-old is allowed to make one of the most responsible decisions of life – to get married and have a family. Yet this same person is not allowed to vote, drive a car or view a film rated '18' at the cinema. It is no wonder adolescents feel some confusion if society is so ambiguous about their adult status.

Although the concept of adolescence can be found in ancient civilisations, it was only during the nineteenth century that it became seen as a distinct phase of human development. When formal schooling was introduced on a mass basis it led to a long delay in young people becoming economically self-sufficient or being given responsibilities. However, this lack of prescribed adult behaviour is not apparent in all cultures. Condon (1987) notes that among the Inuit Eskimos the young women were considered to be adult at menarche ,when they were likely to be married and ready to start bringing up children of their own. The boys achieved adult status somewhat later when they were able to build a snowhouse and fend for themselves.

Sexual behaviour

Many of the problems of adolescence revolve around lack of knowledge about what is the right thing to do in new circumstances. This can be seen in the area of sexual relations, where questions like 'How far should I go?' and 'Can I ask him to wear a condom?' are common. Seifert and Hoffnung (1991) state that the greatest increase in cases of gonorrhoea is among adolescents aged between 10 and 14 years, and one in five adolescents will contract either syphilis or gonorrhoea. Although the reported cases of AIDS in adolescents aged between 13 and 21 years old was only 1 per cent of all reported cases in 1987, the percentage is doubling each year (Brooks-Gunn *et al.,* 1988). Further evidence of adolescents' lack of knowledge about AIDS comes from Bozzi (1988), who found that in sexually active adolescents aged between 14 and 19 only 2 per cent of girls and 8 per cent of boys reported using condoms during intercourse, even though they believed that using condoms was effective in reducing the risks of catching sexually transmitted diseases.

A good example of how culture can determine what is right and wrong in adolescent sexual relations is given by Worthman and Whiting (1987). The Kikuyu people of Kenya have strict rules for the sexual behaviour of males and females before marriage. Girls may visit boys at a special hut used as a meeting place for the young men. If there are more boys than girls, the girls select a partner. Intimate friends are not usually selected, as that is considered selfish. The boy ushers the girl to a bed and undresses. The girl takes her top off, but retains her soft leather apron which she passes between her legs and ties to her waist, providing an effective barrier. The two lie together with their legs entwined to restrict movement of the hips. They then fondle each other and engage in 'love-making conversation' until they finally fall asleep. The girls and boys do not engage in sexual intercourse because they are taught that if their genitals touch they will become polluted and will be ostracised by their peers.

Kikuyu society has clear rules about how adolescents should behave. Contrast this with adolescents in our society who are not provided with such guidelines.

Self-identity

Erikson (1968) characterised the main problem of adolescence as the need to achieve a secure sense of identity. Each individual's ability to form a sense of their own identity depends on the following judgements.

- What you think about other people.
- What others think of you.
- Your rating of the way others judge you.
- The ability to evaluate others as members of social groups. The following example looks at identity formation.

Example:

> Julie was really stupid to get caught with a bottle of vodka in her bedroom by her parents.

A statement such as this would be an example of the first judgement – what you think about other people. But according to Erikson, this is not enough. In order to develop a true sense of identity the other three categories need to be considered. Thus further statements might include: 'Wait a minute, I've had the odd illicit drink. Does that make me stupid too?' 'What does Julie think about the way I always come home late? Maybe she thinks that's worse' or 'Maybe parents think coming home late is worse than drinking vodka.'

The process of identity formation is difficult and *can* put strains on the adolescent's friends and family, but the idea of a generation gap between parents and adolescents seems to have been overemphasised. Coleman (1980) said that there are disagreements between parents and their children, but that they do tend to agree on what the important issues are, such as planning for the future, developing a good reputation, and so on.

Csikszentmihalyi and Larson (1984) asked adolescents to carry a 'beeper' with them from when they got up in the morning to when they went to sleep at night. The adolescents were beeped randomly and asked to fill in a form about what they were doing and feeling at the time. The experimenters found that conflicts between parents and adolescents seemed mainly to be about matters of taste. Parents on the whole thought these to be trivial, whereas adolescents found them very important.

Extending Erikson's theme of identity conflict, Marcia (1966) distinguished four patterns of coping used by adolescents to deal with the task of identity formation.

- *Identity achievers.* These individuals have gone through a period of decision making about their lives and have decided on a particular course of action: 'I have thought through the advantages and disadvantages, and I definitely want to be a nurse.' These adolescents then actively pursue their preference of occupation, politics and religion.
- *Foreclosers.* These adolescents are similar in that they too actively pursue goals. The difference between foreclosers and identity achievers is that foreclosers did not go through the decision-making stage: 'I'm a farmer because my Dad's a farmer,' 'I vote Conservative because my family always have.'
- *Moratoriums.* This category refers to adolescents who are deciding on issues and have not made up their minds: 'I'm not sure whether it is right or wrong to live together before marriage.'
- *Identity diffusions.* These adolescents have often tried a number of different 'identities' and rejected them all. This can result in a cynical attitude to the issues that have been considered and discarded: 'Politicians and political parties are all the same. I stopped thinking about them ages ago.'

As adolescents grow older there is a shift from *identity diffusion* to *identity achievement* although the level of identity achievement differs for the issue in question; for instance choice in politics has a lower identity achievement level than vocational choice.

Health

Although studies suggest an overall decrease in adolescents' use of most drugs (Johnston *et al.,* 1988), high rates of experimentation are still common among the adolescent population. The type of drug used tends to vary with the age of the adolescent. Johnston and colleagues noted that among young adolescents (those under 15) smoking (45 per cent) and drinking (56 per cent) were the most common form of drug use, with 30 per cent admitting to having used at least one illicit drug. In older adolescents (those over 15) the figures were: drinking (92 per cent), marijuana (50 per cent), with 57 per cent having used an illicit drug.

Apart from the physiological and psychological harm caused by drug abuse, drugs can also produce behaviour and altered states of consciousness responsible for many accidents. In males below the age group of 10–14 years old, deaths per 100,000 due to accidents were about twenty, and deaths due to suicide about two. From 10–14 years old onwards the rates soar. At the age of twenty, deaths per 100,000 due to accidents were eighty-five, and due to suicide twenty-seven. Females also show an increase in deaths by accident and suicide at the age of 20, but the curve is not so severe. Females seem to attempt suicide more than males but are less likely to succeed (Holden, 1986).

Suicide

Gibbs (1990) said that nurses may experience a number of potential difficulties in communicating with those who are being assessed following an unsuccessful suicide attempt. The potential difficulties may be due to different attitudes towards suicide being held by patient and carer.

Exercise 5.2 *Attitudes to suicide*

Which of the following is true?

1 People who talk about suicide don't tend to kill themselves.
2 Only certain types of people commit suicide.
3 Suicide among young people is decreasing.
4 When a person talks about suicide, you should change the subject to get his or her mind off it.
5 Most people who kill themselves really want to die.

(For the answers, see the end of the chapter.)

Nursing adolescents

Adams (1983) says that there are a number of problems facing those nurses who come into contact with adolescent patients. The main problems are:

- *Communication difficulties.* Communication may be made difficult by the patient's lack of mature social skills, concern about being ill and the stress of hospitalisation. An affinity needs to be developed between the nurse and the adolescent, based on an understanding of the young person's condition.

- *Over-identification.* Adams argues that empathy with the adolescent should not be achieved at the expense of over-identification, as the nurse's experiences may be out-of-date and thus irrelevant. Further, care should be taken to avoid lapsing into a 'parental role', as advice from a person only a few years older can seem patronising. The nurse should appear a concerned, mature professional person.
- *Confidentiality and privacy.* If assurances about the confidential nature of the information given by the adolescent are not forthcoming, important details may be missed. Therefore the nurse should give due care to planning the setting of any interview.

Coleman (1980) sums up the adolescent stage of development by saying:

> Adolescence is not an either/or phenomenon, but, as the evidence shows, is a period in the life cycle which contains difficulties and where stress is experienced, though of a minor rather than a major nature. There is conflict with parents, over mundane domestic issues, rather than fundamental values. Many young people experience feelings of unhappiness but on the whole these go unnoticed by parents and teachers. Adolescents do worry over their future identity as they become older but these worries rarely cause an identity crisis.

Adulthood

Whilst it is difficult to put ages to stages of development, in order to make a 'working distinction' early adulthood may be defined as 18 to 40 years of age and mid-adulthood as 40 to 65 years of age. Of course many people who are in their early 40s may consider themselves to be young adults, and a number of 'thirty-somethings' may act a lot older than their physical age, but in general terms age markers act as a working guide to distinguish between the two main adult stages of development.

Early adulthood

Early adulthood is a period during which physical characteristics reach their peak. Males and females reach their maximum height by 20 and 18 years respectively, and young adults are in their prime as far as speed and strength are concerned. Muscle structure and internal organs achieve their maximum physical potential between the ages of 18 and 25, but after that period the body begins to slow down. The discs of the spine settle and thus there is a slight decrease in height. The body's fatty tissue increases, with a consequent increase in weight. Muscle strength declines and reaction times level off.

As with physical functioning, mental activity reaches its prime during this stage. Some researchers have suggested that young adults go through stages of intellectual and ethical development (Perry, 1981), while others have been unable to discern any clear-cut progression of stages (Belenky *et al.*, 1986). Perry (1981), in a study based on males aged between 17 and 22, proposed that intellectual and ethical development progress through nine stages divided into three categories.

- *Dualism*
  1 Essentially, the world is made up of things which are either right or wrong. Right answers are obtained by going to the appropriate person or authority for advice.
  2 Some uncertainty exists owing to the fallibility of some authorities.
  3 Sometimes authorities may not know the answer yet, but have the ability to find it out.
- *Relativism*
  4 Anyone can have an opinion and it is possible to disagree on certain issues.
  5 Simple right and wrong explanations are relatively rare. Knowledge and values exist in different contexts.
  6 It is necessary to make some commitment to an idea or a concept.
- *Commitment*
  7 Starts to choose commitments to specific areas such as choosing to become a nurse, or joining a group such as Greenpeace.
  8 Experiences the implications of commitments and explores issues involved.
  9 Identity is confirmed through commitments made.

The process through these stages can be smooth or delayed, depending on the specific circumstances encountered by young adults. The advantage of this approach is that it provides a commonsense account of the types of issues and solutions facing young adults during the years 17–22. However, it should be stressed that the theory was based on a study of males only, and thus is unrepresentative of all young adults. However, it did lead to a series of studies on female young adult development.

Belenky *et al.* (1986) set out to determine whether females went through different stages of intellectual and ethical development from males. The experimenters interviewed 135 women from a wide range of socio-economic backgrounds and found five ways in which these young women represented their environment.

- *Silence.* These women feel passive and dependent. They describe themselves as 'deaf and dumb'. The thinking is similar to Perry's first stage of development; however, the women state that they don't even know the rules about what constitutes right and wrong. They had often experienced lives of abuse, chaos and violence.
- *Received knowledge.* These women report that they learn by listening and quietly accept as truth all that they are told by figures of authority. Again the women in this group seem similar to the men in Perry's first stage, but with one main difference – whilst the men felt a strong association with their authority, the women felt a sense of awe.

- *Subjective knowledge.* These women adopt the notion of multiple truths and base their selection on their 'gut' reactions. First-hand experiences are seen to be the important determinants of truth. Sometimes a crisis of male authority has produced a marked distrust of objective sources of knowledge.
- *Procedural knowledge.* These women distrust both subjective and objective knowledge. There is an interest in form rather than content, and how something is said is seen as more important than what is said. A feature of this category is a heightened sense of control and an analytical approach to truth.
- *Constructed knowledge.* This is an integration of subjective and procedural ways of knowing. Women in this stage examine and test ways of constructing knowledge. There is a high tolerance of ambiguity and internal contradictions in other people's arguments.

The work of Belenky and her associates, alongside others such as Kohlberg (1981) and Gilligan (1982), represents an attempt to structure the ethical/intellectual development of women into distinct stages. It should not be assumed, however, that all women will fall neatly into each specific category, and as Belenky *et al.* (1986) point out, there is no evidence of clear-cut progression from one stage to another. Nevertheless, it does provide a useful description of different types of women's thought during young adulthood.

Sexuality and love

Adult sexuality has been investigated in a number of different ways. Some researchers have concentrated on the development of 'sexual scripts' (Gagnon and Simon, 1987); others have looked at the motivations that underlie sexual behaviour (Mitchell, 1972); and yet others have viewed sexuality from a sociobiological perspective (Wilson, 1978).

Sexual scripts

Just as in Chapter 3 where children were seen to use scripted behaviour in their development, so adults use sexual scripts in their social interaction. In Gagnon and Simon's (1950) view, culture and society play a crucial role in determining how sexuality should be portrayed. Specific sexual scripts are learned in adolescence from parents, the media and, probably most commonly, older adolescents. During development, these scripts are gradually refined until they represent a culturally defined characterisation of sexuality. Thus the manifestation of sexuality through sexual behaviour will vary from culture to culture accordingly and is represented by the presence of specific sexual scripts.

Motivation for sexuality

Mitchell (1972) put forward six motivations for human sexuality expressed in the form of needs, desires and curiosity.

- *Needs.* There are two main needs, intimacy and belonging, and Mitchell regards these as two of the most basic motives for human sexuality. Sometimes these needs may conflict with other needs, such as independence, but if intimacy and belonging are absent from relationships, depression and loneliness can often occur.
- *Desires.* Power, submission and passion constitute the basic desires of sexual motives. In a maladaptive form, power manifests itself as domination and manipulation; in a constructive context, power may be viewed as control over the course of the relationship. Submission is a complementary need to power and relates to a need to feel cared for and looked after by someone. Finally, passion and ecstasy (from the Greek *ekstasis,* 'to be outside of oneself') suggest the need to experience emotional euphoria with other people.
- *Curiosity.* Just as there is a need to know more about life in general, there is also a specific curiosity about sex. Many adults are curious about their own sexuality and whether the sexual feelings of others are similar to their own.

Love

Although often conceived of as one emotion, love may in fact be many. Maslow (1970) thought that there was 'being love', which was positive and implied a certain degree of independence, and 'dependency love' which, as the name implies, involves dependence and need. Another distinction, provided by Berscheid and Walster (1974), is between 'passionate love' and 'companionate love'. Passionate love is the sort that took place between Romeo and Juliet, and is characterised by passion and desire; companionate love is the sort that exists between parents and their children or sometimes between people who have been together for a long time. This love is based on commitment rather than intense physiological arousal.

Lee (1973) suggests that there are six types of love which can be combined to produce complex interactions.

- *Eros or romantic love.* People who score highly on Eros are attracted to partners on the basis of physical characteristics. They are sensitive to physical blemishes and often believe in love at first sight. Love for these individuals is almost totally sensuous.
- *Ludus or game-playing love.* Ludus people like to flirt. They tend to keep their partners guessing about their degree of commitment to the relationship. They often enjoy teasing their lovers and get over affairs quickly, especially when they cease to be fun.
- *Storge or friendship love.* This type of love is based on caring rather than passion. It grows over a period of time and is related to the development of respect and consideration for the other person. Friendship love is typically resistant to long separations and based on mutual interests.
- *Pragma or logical love.* People in this category believe that love has to work. They are concerned whether they themselves or their partner will make good parents and are

willing to work at their relationship. Pragmatism and realism are central to this type of love.

- *Mania or possessive love.* This is an anxious, uncertain type of love, where lovers often get very jealous and do stupid things if they feel the relationship is in jeopardy. Illness is sometimes used to gain attention if their partner ignores them or takes them for granted.
- *Agape or selfless love.* This type of love deals with compassion and seeks to love everybody without qualification. Agapic lovers would claim to maintain their love despite their partner's numerous transgressions.

Perhaps not surprisingly, there is a degree of controversy as to whether these six types of love form distinct styles (Davis and Latty-Mann, 1987) or at best represent a potential to express love in a particular way. Duck (1992) provides a useful summary of love's typologies by saying:

> I suspect that researchers of love ought to look less at the presumed single-minded and enduring aspect of the person who feels love (as psychologists tend to do when they explore love attitudes or love styles). Instead they should pay more attention to the circumstances and rhetorical/social/interpersonal contexts or situations where love is communicated in everyday life.

A somewhat different view of love is that it is based either on principles of reinforcement or on misattribution. Kenrick and Cialdini (1977) propose that we come to love someone because they do things to us that we like and we do things to them that they like. In other words, love stems from a schedule of mutual reinforcement. Another view is that whenever we feel aroused we seek to attach a label to our feelings. When we look down from a twelve-storey building we label the emotion 'anxiety'; when we get food spilled over us at a restaurant we label the emotion 'anger/frustration', and so when we are in the presence of an attractive person we label the emotion 'love'. Whilst neither view represents a comprehensive explanation of love, there is evidence that both misattribution and reinforcement do play a role in the perception of love (Walster and Walster, 1978).

Finally, can love be measured? Zubin (1970) said that it could and to illustrate his point constructed the Love Scale (see Table 5.2). This is a series of nine statements concerning the person towards whom you (or someone else) feel love. Participants are required to indicate on a scale from 1 to 9 whether they agree or disagree with the statement. One is equivalent to 'disagree strongly', and 9 to 'agree strongly', with 5 implying ambivalence. Obviously, the nearer your score is to 81, the person in question is probably very important to you; if your score is closer towards 9, the person is probably of little relevance to you.

Rubin (1970) would not suggest that his scale is a perfect measure of love; however,

Table 5.2 *The Love Scale (adapted from Zubin, 1970)*

1 I feel that I can confide in X about virtually everything.
2 I would do almost anything for X.
3 If I could never be with X, I would feel miserable.
4 If I were lonely, my first thought would be to seek X out.
5 One of my primary concerns is X's welfare.
6 I would forgive X for practically everything.
7 I feel responsible for X's well-being.
8 I would greatly enjoy being confided in by X.
9 It would be hard for me to get along without X.

there is some evidence that couples who scored high on this scale spent more time gazing into each other's eyes than couples who scored low on the scale!

Parenthood

Helen Deutsch, a leading psychoanalyst in the 1930s and 1940s, viewed having a baby thus:

> Pregnancy is the fulfilment of a woman's deepest yearnings: . . . it is a calm, partly dream-like period during which women can give up all other demands and pressures and devote themselves to the forthcoming child.
>
> (Deutsch, 1947)

These views of Deutsch may seem misplaced in the context of present-day attitudes to pregnancy, yet they were not seen as anything strange at the time. Indeed, it is true to say that the views are an accurate reflection of the society in which she lived and its attitudes to women. Pregnancy and motherhood were seen as positive events in a woman's life. Unfortunately this 'idealisation' of motherhood denied women the right to express doubts and negative feelings about the event. If they did exhibit conflicting emotions, it was often assumed that they were not going to become 'good' mothers. A number of studies began to appear illustrating the period of pregnancy as a time of mixed feelings and doubts.

Bibring (1959) was so surprised at the amount of psychiatric problems experienced by women during pregnancy that she turned to Erikson's theory of normative developmental life crises. She suggested that pregnancy, childbirth and parenthood were times of 'normative crisis', where women could be expected to experience emotional disturbance and feelings of rejection. This view gave recognition to the difficulties that women experience during this period but implicit in Erikson's theory of normative life crises is the need to go through the crisis and resolve it in order to move on to the next stage.

Thus women who do not experience emotional difficulties are 'abnormal' because they are either denying or repressing the underlying emotional trauma. They have to 'come clean' about their emotions in order to resolve the crisis and establish a stable female identity. So the question arises: do women experience emotional difficulties during this period of their lives?

Studies in the 1960s produced equivocal findings. Caplan (1960) found that 85 per cent of a sample of women having a baby for the first time (primiparous) admitted feelings of marked disappointment and anxiety when they found out that they were pregnant. Cobliner (1965) found that 47 per cent of a sample of women in New York openly stated at the beginning of the pregnancy that they did not want the child. However, Cartwright (1976) conducted a survey of primiparous women in Britain and found that 67 per cent were pleased that they became pregnant when they did. These different findings can be explained first by reference to the time during the pregnancy when interview was conducted. Attitudes to the birth may change during the course of the pregnancy, particularly when the mother, and father, are able to feel the presence of the baby in the womb (quickening). Second, pregnancies that were planned may have different psychological correlates from those that were unplanned.

Wolkind and Zajicek (1981) conducted a longitudinal study of ninety-six primiparous women from the East End of London. They investigated attitudes to the pregnancy, emotional and physical health and self-concept development.

Attitudes to pregnancy

Women were asked about their feelings about the pregnancy: 68 per cent had planned to become pregnant and 32 per cent had not. Feelings that were felt at the beginning of the pregnancy were compared with feelings felt after seven months.

The results indicate that only a small percentage of women who planned their pregnancies had changed their attitudes after seven months, whereas a larger percentage of women who had not planned their pregnancies at first changed their attitudes at seven months, largely in the positive direction. The authors suggest that these findings support the work of Caplan (1960) and Cobliner (1965), who found that negative reactions at the beginning of pregnancy are often transformed owing to quickening. Wolkind and Zajicek (1981) summarise their findings on women's attitudes to their pregnancy as follows:

> Data described thus far gives us a picture of a group of married women, most of whom welcomed pregnancy and felt positive about it, who seemed to cope with the reality and the prospect of fairly major life changes in a calm, rational way, and who were preparing themselves, as far as possible, for the experiences to come.

In order to get a better idea of whether pregnancy is associated with any form of crisis, it is necessary to look at emotional reactions and physical symptoms expressed by this sample of women.

Emotional and physical health

Women were given an extensive psychiatric examination after seven months of their pregnancy. It was found that 75 per cent showed no disturbance all, 11 per cent had only mild emotional difficulties and 14 per cent were diagnosed as having disorders that would definitely handicap them in some way.

Sorts of problems mentioned were tearfulness, anxiety and depression, but the authors note that there was no evidence of the 'full-blown psychotic disorder' described by Bibring (1959). Physically the women seemed to be in good health. After seven months of pregnancy, 68 per cent had no physical problems, 11 per cent reported minor difficulties and 20 per cent had complaints that required medical treatment. The most common physical problem at seven months into the pregnancy was pre-eclampsia, which is a hypertensive disorder in pregnant primiparous women.

In order to gain some information regarding the sorts of physical discomfort pregnant women experience during their pregnancy, twenty-one common symptoms of pregnancy (described in an obstetrics textbook) were presented to the women and they were asked whether they suffered from them. The symptoms were also presented to a sample of non-pregnant women with children and a sample of student nurses. The most common symptoms were indigestion (43 per cent), lack of energy (68 per cent), breathlessness (46 per cent), cramp (68 per cent), backache (48 per cent), tired legs (55 per cent) and the need to go to the toilet quickly (66 per cent). Many of the other 'symptoms' did not seem to bother the pregnant women. Also, whilst 68 per cent of the pregnant women complained of lack of energy, 59 per cent of the non-pregnant women complained of the same thing. Other similar experiences were backache and tired legs. The nurses scored lower on just about all the measures (lack of energy 1 per cent) except on items 5 (poor appetite) and 17 (itching in the private parts).

To get some idea of pregnancy as a crisis period it was decided to compare those women who had at first wanted to become pregnant (planned pregnancy + positive feelings first) with those who did not want to become pregnant (unplanned and not initially positive). At seven months into the pregnancy there were significant differences between the two groups. Those who had not wanted to become pregnant had not begun to make preparations, had not read any books, felt that their lives would not be positive and expected to have more financial problems. There were no differences between the groups regarding such things as physical problems, psychiatric problems and disrupted family background.

Since quickening has been found to be an influential factor in changing attitudes to pregnancy, it was decided to investigate those women who did not react positively to their pregnancy even after quickening had occurred. The authors found that women who were negative at seven months were significantly more likely to have had psychiatric problems during the pregnancy and period problems in the past. They were also more likely to resent the restrictions imposed by pregnancy. Wolkind and Zajicek (1981) summarise their findings with respect to crisis as follows:

The conflict about being pregnant which occurs at the beginning of pregnancy results in lack of preparation for the birth and feelings that having the child will cause problems. However, many such women seem to resolve their conflicts by seven months of pregnancy and tend to react positively at that time. Conflicts about being pregnant which occur later during pregnancy are not related to whether or not pregnancy was planned and whether the women originally felt pleased to be pregnant. They are conflicts which seem to arise directly from the psychophysical experiences of pregnancy which are perhaps linked to more general reactions to womanhood.

Is interesting to note that 61 per cent of a sample of primiparous women questioned by the authors felt that they had been changed in some way by the pregnancy. This suggests that the process of pregnancy, childbirth and parenthood is a developmental stage marking a transition from adulthood to parenthood. However, only 8 per cent of women felt that the pregnancy was a significant milestone in their lives. This latter finding lends credence to the suggestion that pregnancy is not necessarily a period of crisis, but a transitional period involving some degree of upheaval and change.

Fathers

Although Wolkind and Zajicek (1981) examined the effects of pregnancy and childbirth on fathers, unfortunately they did not actually speak to the fathers themselves, but assessed the wives' perceptions of their spouses' attitudes. In the same year, May (1981) published research targeting fathers themselves. Twenty first-time expectant fathers were interviewed about their involvement in their wives' pregnancy and their attitudes to it. May identified three phases of 'father involvement': the announcement phase, the moratorium and the focusing phase.

- *Announcement phase.* This is the period when the pregnancy is first suspected. The length of the phase varies according to individual circumstances; sometimes it is a few hours, some-times a few creeks. It seems that men are not oblivious to the early signs of pregnancy and typically report the time where the diagnosis of pregnancy is in doubt as stressful and uncomfortable, regardless of whether the pregnancy was wanted or not. After the pregnancy has been confirmed and starts to have a noticeable impact on the woman, the fathers in the sample reported they seemed to be lagging behind their wives in experiencing the pregnancy.
- *The moratorium phase.* This phase usually occurs between the twelfth and twenty-fifth weeks of the pregnancy and is characterised by the expectant fathers becoming emotionally distant from the pregnancy. This period can be a quite stressful experience, since the man does not experience the physical changes of the woman and thus has a different perspective on the event. The emotional distance allows the man to 'work through' his feelings about the pregnancy and the changes in lifestyle that are likely to occur as a result. The man's ambivalence towards the

pregnancy can result in problems between the expectant couple. The woman may feel that her partner does not care in the same way she does about the new baby and the man may not give adequate support to the woman because he does not see that it is necessary.

● *Focusing phase.* This ends the moratorium. One man described his realisation: 'It is like measles, you get exposed, but it takes a while before you catch on that you have got it.' The phase begins around the twenty-fifth to thirtieth weeks, although it may begin sooner if the man is particularly prepared for the pregnancy. The man focuses on his own experience of the pregnancy, redefines his role *vis-à-vis* his future status and becomes much more sensitive to his wife's needs. Men report that they feel fatherly and start to have mental images of themselves with the prospective child. May (1981) concludes that preparation during the focusing phase may relate to 'constructive' parenting after the birth of the child.

Parents

Finally, Miller and Sollie (1986) looked at the experiences of both parents during their transition to parenthood. The study consisted of 120 couples that were required to complete and return questionnaires when the wife was in mid-pregnancy, when the baby was about six weeks old and when the baby was between six and eight months old. The questionnaire was concerned with measures of personal well-being, personal stress and marital stress. New parents reported higher personal stress scores after they had become parents than during the pregnancy period. Wives' personal stress scores were lower than their husband's during the pregnancy, but considerably higher afterwards. Personal well-being scores declined steadily throughout the three time periods, indicating that the time when the baby was one month old was harder than the pregnancy and eight months postpartum was more difficult than one month postpartum. Marital stress increased. steadily from pregnancy to eight months postpartum for the mothers, but there was no change in the fathers' marital stress scores with time.

Miller and Sollie (1986) suggest that becoming a parent for the first time involves a slight decline in personal well-being and some increase in personal stress over the first year of parenting. Mothers feel these changes more acutely than fathers, and wives are more likely than their husbands to view the marriage as changing in a negative way. Coping with the stress of a baby puts a certain amount of strain on the parents' relationship. Adaptation to stress involves two major kinds of family resources. The first is internal, the second is external (community and social support). Levitt *et al.* (1986) highlighted the importance of the husband in providing emotional support. They interviewed mothers of thirteen-month-old infants about the degree of emotional support they received from family and friends. Mothers reported an average thirteen persons in their social networks, but support was provided primarily by the husband. It seemed to be the case that the mothers turned to friends for support only if the relationship with their husband was strained.

Much of the research indicates that becoming a parent is stressful and that the greatest stress occurs after the baby has been born. Many parenthood classes are childbirth preparation classes that fall short in helping prospective parents after the child is born. Whilst there are postnatal support groups, there is no tuition along the lines of the prenatal classes with husbands present. There are practical problems in bringing new parents together, but it would seem that post-parenthood classes, with both parents present, could provide support after the birth of a first child.

Middle adulthood

Mention the term 'middle age' and people will probably immediately think of the mid-life crisis. Such was the popularisation of this feature of middle adulthood during the 1970s that it has come to represent the main concern of people in this age bracket. But what age bracket? Some people place middle adulthood firmly between the ages of 40 and 60. However, a few people may act as if they are well into their middle adulthood by the time they are 35, and some 65-year-olds may act and behave as if they were twenty years younger. Therefore, to provide an age framework for middle adulthood it is advisable to say that it begins between the ages of 35 and 40, and ends between the ages of 60 and 65.

Part of the difficulty in defining middle adulthood stems from the fact that it is a relatively new phenomenon. Until the end of the nineteenth century people were expected to die in what we now call middle age and the average life expectancy was 50. Nowadays people can expect to live a good twenty years longer. Further, the mid-life crisis is but one of the issues that have developed from research on middle age. Havighurst (1972) proposed that there were seven specific developmental 'tasks' faced by middle-aged people in our culture (see Table 5.3). As research into middle age has concentrated on many of Havighurst's developmental tasks, it is appropriate to use them as a framework for examining the main issues of middle adulthood.

Table 5.3 *Havighurst's developmental tasks*

1 Accepting and adjusting to the physiological changes of middle age.
2 Reaching and maintaining satisfactory performance in one's occupation.
3 Adjusting to ageing parents.
4 Assisting teenage children to become responsible and happy adults.
5 Relating to one's partner as a person.
6 Assuming social and specific responsibility.
7 Developing leisure time activities.

Physiological changes and health

Middle adulthood is a time when the body experiences a number of changes and it is also a time when certain diseases begin to develop. Two areas of physiological change that have received a great deal of attention are the *decline in sensory acuities* and the *menopause*.

Sensory acuities

- *Vision.* The most significant changes in the visual system occur after the age of 50. The lens of the eye becomes increasingly dense and develops a yellowish tinge, making the shades of blue and green in the eye difficult to discern. The ciliary muscles, responsible for manipulating the lens correctly, lose their efficiency and decrease in size. There is also a decrease in pupil size and the retina becomes less sensitive (Schulz and Ewen, 1988). These changes result in an overall loss of visual acuity or ability such that the closest point at which the eye can see an object without blurring gets further and further away. When this point becomes further than the arms can stretch to hold a book or read a newspaper, it is often realized that glasses are needed. Increasing age also brings with it a greater susceptibility to eye diseases such as glaucoma, which is progressively more common after the age of 40. Finally, cataracts (cloudy formations on the lens of the eye) start to become a problem about the age of 60, but are more prevalent in older people of 70 and 80.

- *Audition.* After the age of 40 the ability to hear sounds starts to decrease. In the inner ear there is a degeneration of sensory receptor cells, loss of auditory nerve cells and a decrease of flexibility in the cochlear partition, which is responsible for the transmission of vibrations from one chamber to the other. The result of these changes is a progressive decline in the ability to hear high-frequency tones. This is known as *presbyacusis*. To get an idea of what it might be like to suffer from presbyacusis, on a hi-fi system turn the treble right down and the bass right up, and note that the muffled sound is not improved by turning up the volume. Speaking loudly to patients experiencing this type of hearing dysfunction does not improve their hearing ability, and merely causes frustration.

- *Smell.* Whilst Stevens and Cain (1987) suggest that the sense of smell declines slowly around the age of 50 and decreases rapidly after age 70, Engen (1977) and Rovee *et al.* (1975) reported no such changes. A possible resolution of these different findings may come from the contribution of factors such as disease and smoking to the sense of smell. Many of the studies reviewed did not take into consideration the extent to which the participants had contracted mild forms of disease which may affect the sense of smell. Nevertheless, whether due to age, disease, smoking or other factors, becoming less sensitive to certain odours can have embarrassing social consequences.

- *Taste.* Unfortunately the sense of taste has received little attention in the research literature. Schiffman (1977) noted that the sense of taste begins to decline around the age of 50. However, Spence (1989) found that there is a decline in the ability to detect weak tastes but a retention of the ability to discriminate between familiar medium-strength tastes. Much more research needs to be done in this area, especially a consideration of cultural differences with respect to both taste discrimination and preference.

The menopause

In most women, the menopause occurs between the ages of 41 and 59 years, with wide individual differences in onset and cessation. The ending of the monthly menstrual period is part of a longer process known as the *climacteric* where women make the transition from the reproductive to the non-reproductive stage of life. In addition to menstruation becoming increasingly irregular in timing and the amount of blood flow, other physical symptoms include hot flushes and dryness of the vagina. However, McElmurry and Huddleston (1987) say that textbook descriptions of the severity of symptoms experienced during the menopause can be highly exaggerated. In fact some women experience no symptoms at all, apart from cessation of the menses. In one study (Goodman, 1982), the symptoms reported by menopausal women were barely more numerous than those reported by women of a similar age who were still menstruating. Some of the symptoms attributed to the menopause may in fact be part of a much wider psychological adjustment to becoming middle-aged.

There is no physical equivalent of the female menopause for males.

Heart disease and Type A behaviour

Another common problem of mid-adulthood is coronary heart disease (CHD). Coronary heart disease occurs when the coronary arteries narrow to such an extent that not enough blood can get through to supply the muscles of the heart with sufficient oxygen and nourishment. Factors known to affect the incidence of CHD include a high-cholesterol diet; smoking; obesity; high blood pressure; physical inactivity and family history. Although these factors are major determinants of heart disease, they are totally absent in nearly 50 per cent of all new cases (Sheridan and Radmacher, 1992). These research findings have shifted attention to an examination of psychological risk factors. Two cardiologists, Friedman and Rosenman (1959), found an increased prevalence of CHD in men who exhibited what they termed a 'coronary-prone behaviour pattern'. This consisted of extreme competitiveness; a high need to achieve; aggression; impatience and time-hurry behaviour; restlessness; hyperalertness; a feeling of being constantly under pressure and a need to be in control of events. They labelled this behaviour pattern Type A.

In a study of 3,454 men aged between 39 and 59 years, Friedman and Rosenman found evidence of a relationship between Type A behaviour and CHD. The Type A men had six and a half times the incidence of coronary heart disease as men who did not show Type A behaviour patterns. Some later studies failed to find any connection between

Type A behaviour and CHD (Shekelle *et al.,* 1985), but this may have been due to sampling errors and measurement problems. Certainly, Chesney *et al.* (1988) have obtained evidence that hostility, competitiveness and time urgency are strong predictors of coronary heart disease.

The modification of Type A behaviour can be very difficult. Behaviour patterns that have been built up over many years are not easy to change. Indeed, many people in mid-adulthood do not see any reason to change their habits, especially if they believe that their Type A lifestyle has helped them reach high levels of attainment. Prevention programmes need to emphasise the possibility of maintaining current levels of work whilst reducing the physical and psychological cost. Roskies (1988) has developed a multimodal programme based on modifying physiological, behavioural and cognitive responses to stressful situations. Over a fourteen-week training programme, she claims to have significantly reduced the incidence of Type A behaviour in 'at risk' individuals. Chapter 8 will examine this and other stress management programmes in more detail.

The mid-life crisis

The term 'mid-life crisis' was popularised in an article by Elliot Jaques (1965) on the careers of artists. In almost every case he studied, he found a dramatic change occurred in the artist's life at about 35. Some artists started to work at this time (Gauguin), while others gave up and some died. Since that time Levinson (1978), Sheehy (1976) and Gould (1978) have all proposed crises occurring in mid-life. Levinson (1986) suggests that there are three tasks associated with this period.

● a reappraisal and review of achievements since young adulthood;
● a move towards accepting middle age;
● dealing with sources of conflict.

Levinson (1978) says:

> For the great majority of men this period evokes tumultuous struggles within the self and with the external world. It must involve emotional turmoil, despair, the sense of not knowing where to turn or of being stagnant and unable to move at all.

There are several shortcomings to these studies of mid-life crises. First, the samples are taken largely from small numbers of white, middle-income men. Second, they use the same cohort. Therefore generalising to other generations, women and people from different social and cultural backgrounds is limited. Further, McCrae and Costa (1984) point out that mid-life crisis research is totally based on interview data, with little attempt at statistical analysis.

An alternative view was taken by Neugarten (1968). She proposed that mid-adulthood is a time of transition where men and women may well look back at what they have achieved during their lives. If the children have left home it may be a time to reassess one's purpose in life. However, these events are not necessarily traumatic nor need they involve a crisis. Many women are in fact pleased when the children leave home, as it gives them the opportunity to do things that were previously impractical. However, there may be genuine anxieties about returning to work or taking on new roles. Gottfredson (1977) found that over 80 per cent of workers aged between 41 and 55 remained in the same job category over a five-year period. Of those who did change jobs, 60 per cent changed to a job within the same occupational category. Julian *et al.* (1992) examined the correlates of psychological well-being for seventy-five middle-aged men. They found that the best predictors of men's well-being at mid-life were perceived closeness to children, perceived closeness to spouse, adjustment to the husband role and the number of close friends.

In summary, mid-adulthood often offers the opportunity for reflection and change; how this is managed will determine the degree of psychological conflict.

The 'sandwiched people'

It was Davis (1981) who said that middle-aged adults were 'sandwiched' between adolescent children and ageing parents. Care of ageing parents has only recently become widespread, mainly owing to significant increases in life expectancy, but the idea that the adult children of ageing parents can hardly wait to pack them off to a home is misplaced. Brody (1990) points out that for every disabled person in a nursing home there are two or more equally disabled elderly people living with their families. Thus caring for aged parents has become a normative part of mid-adulthood. In the absence of a spouse, the most likely people to care for the elderly are adult daughters, and since many middle-aged women go out to work, caring for aged parents as well as their own families can prove a substantial strain.

Horowitz (1985) isolated a number of types of support that adult children can provide their parents with:

- When a parent is worried or feeling low, their children can provide emotional support by cheering them up.
- Children can provide direct support by doing the shopping, running errands, taking care of the bills and, for the less mobile, bathing them and cooking for them.
- They often act as a 'buffer' between the support services and the elderly person. They can fill in forms, arrange meals on wheels or negotiate for home helps.
- Children can, and sometimes do, provide financial support.
- Children may have their elderly parents to live with them.

Not surprisingly, support of the elderly may bring with it strains and stresses, the most common being emotional concern about their health and safety. There are also restrictions on leisure time and almost inevitably family conflicts arise. Whilst there are also benefits, such as increased feelings of self-satisfaction and respect, care of the elderly can take its emotional toll. Therefore it is important that nurses consider support for the carers as well as for the elderly patient.

Late adulthood

With the advances that have been made in the treatment and prevention of diseases, the life expectancy of both males and females has increased dramatically over the last fifty years. In Britain, over 14 per cent of the population is aged 65 and above; in the United States the figures are nearly as high, with about 11 per cent aged above 65. (This compares with only 4 per cent of the total US population aged 65 and above in the 1930s.) Not always has an increase in life expectancy led to better quality of life. It can be argued that, as a society, we have paid scant regard to the needs of our elderly population, and too many have spent their last years poor, dependent and ill. Therefore it is important to determine the nature of the ageing process and, perhaps more important to investigate ways of increasing the quality of life for people in their late adulthood.

Theories of ageing

Bacteria are able to continue living indefinitely as long as they have a sufficient supply of food and space but most animals have a life span limited to their reproductive ability. Although the human life span extends way beyond the end of reproductive ability, it is still limited to an average of 69 years for males and 75 years for females. Why is it that we cannot live for ever?

Heredity

One theory of human ageing states that the life span of any species is set by genetic or hereditary characteristics which have evolved over thousands of years. As females are likely to live for at least twenty-five years after going through the menopause, it is not clear what evolutionary function is served during this period of time. There may, however, be a social function. The anthropologist Margaret Mead (1970) suggested that in some tribal societies old people were extremely important for the survival of the group, since it was they who could remember where food and water had been found during a drought that had occurred many years before.

External factors

Obviously accidents curtail the life span regardless of genetic factors. But other factors known to affect longevity include marriage, rural living, being overweight, smoking and disease (Jones, 1956). Based on the work of Jones (1956) and Schulz (1978) it is possible to estimate prospective life spans (see Table 5.4).

Table 5.4 *Prospective life spans (based on the work of Jones and Schulz)*

If you are male start with a score of 69 years. If you are a female start with a score of 75 years. Add or subtract years according to the following 'external' factors.

1 Subtract one year for every 10 lb you are overweight.
2 Add three years if you engage in regular exercise two or three times a week.
   Subtract three years if your job involves a lot of sitting down.
   Add three years if you have an active job.
   If you sleep more than nine hours per day, subtract five years.
3 If you are married add four years.
   If you are over 25 and not married, subtract one year for every unwedded decade.
4 Subtract three years if you think you have been poor for most of your life.
5 If you smoke over forty cigarettes a day, subtract eight years.
   If you smoke twenty to forty cigarettes a day, subtract four years.
   If you smoke less than twenty cigarettes, a pipe or cigars, subtract two years.
6 If you have regular medical and dental check-ups, add three years. If you are often ill, subtract two years.
7 If you have lived most of your life in a rural environment, add four years.
   If you have lived most of your life in an urban environment, subtract two years.
   If your house is hardly ever warmer than 20°C, add two years.
8 If you are Type B (relaxed and easy-going), add two years.
   If you are Type A, subtract two years.
   Add between one to five years according to how content and happy you are with life.
   Subtract one to five years according to how often you feel unhappy, worried or guilty.
9 Add five years if two or more of your grandparents lived to the age of 80 or more.
   Subtract four years if any grandparent, parent, brother or sister died of a heart attack or stroke before 50.
   Subtract two years if anyone died of these diseases before 60.
   Subtract three years for each case of diabetes, thyroid disorders, breast cancer, cancer of the digestive system, asthma or chronic bronchitis among parents or grandparents.
10 Add two years if you are a light drinker (one to three units per day). Subtract five to ten years if you are a heavy drinker. Subtract one year if you are a teetotaller.

Please note that the figure you end up with is only a very rough estimate. Many things can happen between now and old age that will probably have a great influence on the number of years you will live. The exercise gives a reasonable indication of how your present life style is contributing to longevity, but should by no means be taken as an absolute indication of your life span.

Wear and tear theory

This view of ageing sees the body rather like a machine. Over a period of time the organs of the body gradually wear out, just like the parts of an old engine. However, there is no conclusive evidence that hard work alone is responsible for reducing the life span (Curtis, 1966). It seems that 'spare part' surgery will not prove to be the answer to the ageing process, as it is the interrelation of the various systems of the body that is involved in the ageing process rather than the failure of any particular organ.

Homeostatic imbalance

Homeostatic mechanisms are responsible for the maintenance of physiological balance in the body, controlling such things as the pH and sugar levels in the blood. Shock (1977) has suggested that the ability of the homeostatic mechanisms to maintain equilibrium decreases with age, and thus it is more difficult for old people to maintain body temperature during exposure to heat and cold than it is for their younger counterparts. Strains on the homeostatic mechanisms are easier to tolerate when young, and homeostatic inefficiency can result in a risk of death for older people. However, rather than being an explanation of ageing, homeostatic imbalance is probably better viewed as a contributing factor to the ageing process, and as we shall see, other factors are also involved.

Accumulation of metabolic waste

As organisms age, the functioning of their cells is affected by the accumulation of waste products of metabolism. Collagen, a fibrous protein linked with the wrinkling of the skin and the slowness of wound healing, builds up with age and is eliminated only very slowly if at all. Another group of substances, the lipofuscins, also builds up with ageing and leads to pigmentation. However, Curtis (1966) believes that the accumulation of metabolic waste is more a symptom of ageing than a cause.

Autoimmunity

Animals reject their own tissues when autoimmune antibodies are produced. The frequency of this occurrence increases with age and has been associated with diseases such as rheumatoid arthritis. Further, Makinodan (1977) has noted that the thymus gland tends to degenerate with age. As this gland is responsible for normal immune processes, there may be a decline in certain immune responses with age. Whilst some leading causes of death have been linked with autoimmune reactions, autoimmunity is still more of a symptom than a cause of ageing.

Cellular ageing

Some of the cells in the body rarely, or never, reproduce (for example, brain cells, muscles). Most cells reproduce themselves, however, and theoretically there is no reason to suppose why this process should not go on for ever. One of the reasons put forward to account for the inability of cells to reproduce indefinitely is the presence of 'chemical noise' within the cell. Faulty transcription of information from DNA (deoxyribonucleic acid) leads to errors which hamper or deflect cell function and division. Chemical noise may also be created by a gradual build-up of random replication errors (Medvedev, 1964). At the moment it is not clear whether the errors of replication are genetically programmed or are random events that accumulate with age; nevertheless, this theory seems to provide one of the best explanations so far of the physiological process of ageing.

Intellectual and psychological functioning

As the age structure of society shifts upwards, there has been increasing concern about the changes in intellectual functioning which occur with age. In some occupations it is believed that one's intellectual contribution declines after the age of 60, whilst High Court judges are deemed to be intellectually able well into their 70s. One of the factors that has confused the issue regarding the nature of intellectual functioning in late adulthood is the presence of disease. It is important to distinguish between those changes in ability that result from disease and those that result from ageing.

Birren *et al.* (1963) examined a sample of forty-seven men aged between 65 and 91 who were classed as healthy. They were given a battery of medical, physiological and psychological tests, and two groups emerged. One group of men (group A) was found to have optimal health. Another group (group B), whilst having no clinical disease, was found to have mild diseases. When measures of the cerebral blood flow of the group A men were compared with those of a sample of 21-year-old men, there were no significant differences. However, when measures of the cerebral blood flow of the group B men were compared with the same sample of young men, significant differences were found. Thus even a mild, or subclinical, degree of disease may affect the efficiency of brain functioning in late adulthood.

Electroencephalograph (EEG) readings of both groups were taken and both groups were found to have a slower frequency spectrum than normal. This would indicate that there is a slowing down of electrical activity in the brain with age, and this may be one reason why some old people need longer to perform certain tasks.

Both groups of men were given twenty-three tests of intellectual performance and group B gave poorer results on twenty-one out of twenty-three tests. Group B were particularly bad at retrieving stored information. Both groups took longer than average to complete the tests, and thus we can see that a genuine feature of the ageing process is a slowing down of performance.

Several 'personality' tests were administered to both groups of participants. Subclinical disease was found to affect such things as the ability to terminate social interaction appropriately and showing ordered sequences of thought. A significant finding was the effects of loss of performance on both intelligence and personality measures. If a person had just lost someone close, the ability to think and interact with others was seriously affected.

Birren summarised their findings, reporting that mild disease plays a greater role in performance deficits than ageing; there is a slowing down of reaction time with age; social loss significantly affects psychosocial and cognitive abilities.

Eleven years later, a follow-up study was carried out on the same participants by Granick and Patterson (1971). Not surprisingly, half the men had died. Most (70 per cent) of group B had died, whereas most (63 per cent) of group A had survived. Some of the factors that were related to survival were higher intelligence, faster reaction time and lower social loss. Two items were found to predict 80 per cent of the survivors and non-survivors. These were:

- not smoking;
- the organisation and planning of daily events.

Not smoking may be an obvious factor related to longevity, but why should organisation and planning be important?

Toffler (1970) proposed that a major problem for the elderly was that they were now living in a society which was totally different from the one in which they grew up. Changes have taken place so fast that the elderly person has not had a chance to 'catch up'.

> This means, generally speaking, that the child reaching teenage in any of these societies is literally surrounded by twice as much of everything newly man-made as his parents were at the time he was an infant. It means that by the time today's teenager reaches age thirty, perhaps earlier, a second doubling will have occurred. Within a seventy-year lifetime, perhaps five such doublings will have taken place – meaning, since the increases are compounded, that by the time the individual reaches old age the society around him will be producing thirty-two times as much as when he was born.
>
> (Toffler, 1970)

Under these circumstances it is clear that a degree of organisational and planning ability is necessary to cope with the increased number of 'things to do' in everyday life. In one of the few longitudinal studies in this area, Willis *et al.* (1992) investigated everyday task competence in the elderly. They examined 102 white community-dwelling older adults (sixteen males, eighty-six females) whose average age when the study started was 76.9 years. Everyday task competence was assessed in 1979 and again in 1986. The results indicated a significant mean level decline in competence over this period. However, wide individual differences were apparent, as 62 per cent of the sample remained stable or improved in competence over the seven-year period. Those who declined in ability had particular difficulty with everyday problems which required 'new' solutions; these were particularly troublesome for the elderly if they attempted to apply routinised or stereo-typical responses. It seems that, for a certain proportion of elderly people, cognitive set (see Chapter 7) is a problem. Some old people attempt to apply plans and strategies that have worked in the past without thinking about whether they are applicable to present circumstances.

Where there is cognitive decline, it is not necessarily irreversible. Schaie and Willis (1986) found that simple training programmes could reverse cognitive decline in a substantial number of adults. They conclude that:

> For at least a substantial proportion of the community dwelling elderly, observed cognitive decline is not irreversible, is likely to be attributable to disuse, and can be subjected to environmental manipulations involving relatively simple and inexpensive training programmes.

The ageing 'executive brain'

The term 'executive brain' comes from Goldberg (2002) and refers to a particular part of the brain – the frontal lobes. He says that 'The frontal lobes perform the most advanced and complex functions in all the brain, the so-called executive function. They are linked to intentionality, purposefulness and complex decision making.' He likens the relationship between the frontal lobes and the brain to that of a conductor with an orchestra. They co-ordinate neural structures and are a critical feature of organisation and planning ability. They are also particularly affected by the dementias.

Consider again the work of Toffler (1970) and what he actually said thirty-five years ago on what he termed 'future shock'.

> In France in the twenty years between 1910 and the outbreak of the second world war, industrial production rose only 5 percent. Yet between 1948 and 1965, in only seventeen years, it increased by roughly 220 percent. Today growth rates of from 5 to 10 percent per year are not uncommon among the most industrialised nations. There are ups and downs of course but the direction of change has been unmistakable. Thus for the twenty-one countries belonging to the Organization for Economic Cooperation and Development the average annual rate of increase in gross national product in the years 1960–1968 ran between 4.5 and 5 percent. The United States grew at a rate of 4.5 percent and Japan led the rest with annual increases averaging 9.8 percent. What such numbers imply is nothing less revolutionary than a doubling of the total output of goods and services in the advanced societies about every fifteen years – and the doubling times are shrinking. This means, generally speaking, that the child reaching teenage in any of these societies is literally surrounded by twice as

much of everything newly manmade as his parents were at the time he was an infant. It means that by the time today's teenager reaches thirty, perhaps earlier, a second doubling will have occurred. Within a seventy- year lifetime, perhaps five such doublings will take place – meaning, since the increases are compounded, that by the time the individual reaches old age the society around him will be producing thirty-two times as much as when he was born.

Essentially, these two pieces of information are saying that as we grow older we are faced with more and more 'things' in our lives and more and more decisions and choices to make. This is compounded by governments whose main aim is to provide even more choice. At the same time the parts of our brains responsible for being able to deal with all this are becoming susceptible to disease. For Toffler, older people are living in a different society, hence not culture shock but future shock, and for Goldberg we are placing more importance on the successful functioning of our frontal lobes than ever before. Goldberg (2002) provides a solution in what he terms cognitive exercise. He suggests that exercising the brain in particular ways can prevent cognitive decline and reduce the affects of disease. However he is particularly 'cagey' about the nature of this cognitive exercise other than as he uses it in his clinical programmes.

In studies I conducted many years ago (Niven, 1977) I found that there were particular types of executive planning abilities that were related to other types of cognitive functioning such as psychological differentiation. One of these abilities I called Critical Path Planning ability. It refers to the ability to order events into a system whereby a sequence of events can take place simultaneously. This is done by looking at each event, selecting the one that will take the longest (the critical path) and sequencing each event to correspond to the time limit of the critical path. A simple example would be making a cup of tea. What do you do if you are a critical path planner?

- Select the longest event – the critical path – which would be boiling the kettle.
- Work out the timing of all the other events (getting the cups, milk, warming the pot, etc.).
- Start with the longest and then the next and the next to construct a flow diagram.

This is a very simple example of what can be a very complex process but it illustrates perhaps how particular kinds of thinking can help with organising and dealing with a whole range of events. Thus as we are faced with more and more to do, these sorts of planning skills can help manage the load. There are individual differences in such ability and it can be easily measured using the eggtimer test (Niven, 1977). However, the importance is in the training rather than the assessment.

These research findings have a number of implications for nurses who have frequent contact with elderly people:

- Intellectual competence does not necessarily decline with age and there is every chance that if people have been intellectually active during early adulthood they will continue to be so in late adulthood.
- A general feature of the ageing process is the need to take more time to perform tasks. Therefore, elderly patients should not be hurried into making decisions, but should be given adequate time to make up their minds.
- Where there is some deterioration in cognitive functioning, it may be necessary to provide simple training sessions in such things as planning and organising everyday events.

Overall, it is important to make the elderly feel competent to cope with the stresses and strains of everyday life, by reinforcement, training and understanding.

Senile dementia

Dementia is a term used to describe various different brain disorders that have in common loss of brain function which is usually progressive and and eventually severe. There are over 100 different types of dementia. The most common are Alzheimer's disease, vascular dementia and Lewy body dementia. People with dementia have particular problems with their short-term memory. They consistently forget things that they have just said or done, even though they can often recall clearly events that happened many years ago. Their sense of time and place is typically lost. They may develop problems with finding words and it becomes increasingly difficult for them to learn new information and to do new things. As time goes on, people with dementia need help to perform even the most basic tasks of everyday living, including washing, dressing and eating. Eventually, people with dementia may become uncommunicative and incontinent. Sometimes there are severe behavioural problems. Most people with dementia eventually require twenty-four-hour care.

Alzheimer's disease is the commonest type of dementia, accounting on its own for about half of all cases. There are, however, quite a number other types of dementia. Among these other types of dementia, all but vascular dementia, which is the second commonest type of dementia, are rare.

Types of dementia other than Alzheimer's disease include:

- vascular dementia, which results from brain damage due to tiny strokes;
- Lewy body dementia, which some people regard as a variant of Alzheimer's disease or Parkinson's disease;
- fronto-temporal dementia, for example Pick's disease, in which there are striking changes in behaviour before the memory problems appear;
- Huntington's disease, also called Huntington's chorea, which is characterised by jerky movements in addition to dementia;
- AIDS-related dementia;

- dementia that sometimes occurs together with Parkinson's disease;
- Creutzfeld Jakob disease, or CJD;
- dementia due to a brain tumour;
- normal pressure hydrocephalus, due to a build-up of fluid in the brain;
- dementia due to an excessive intake of alcohol over an extended period of time;
- dementias due to various treatable causes, including vitamin deficiency, hormone deficiency and syphilis.

Dementia refers to an overall decline in intellectual functioning associated with pathological changes in the brain. If a patient is younger than 65 the term 'pre-senile dementia' is used. Holden and Woods (1982) estimated that there were 700,000 sufferers of senile dementia in the United Kingdom, with most of them (75 per cent) living in the community. Senile dementia is characterised by a wide range of symptoms, including the following:

- *Difficulty in remembering* information and the layout of the environment. Thus people with dementia find new environments such as the hospital ward particularly confusing and are apt to wander around, unsure of their bearings. Further, forgetting what they intended to do can lead to aimless meandering because the real purpose has been forgotten.
- The *disorientation* that can result from loss of memory produces feelings of helplessness and uselessness. The disruption in behaviour that occurs with dementia often leads to a reduction in self-esteem and in feelings of social worth. These beliefs and emotions are particularly prevalent in people who are mildly affected by the condition, since they are able to understand the full implications of their situation.
- The *behaviours that generally accompany senile dementia* are restlessness and a need for activity. Some of the uneasiness results from memory problems; however, in some cases there is a genuine desire to be active. Incontinence can result from a urinary tract infection, or it may be due to inability to remember where the toilet is. Aggression and hostility may occur, often due to exasperation at declining competence or sometimes simply to cover up mistakes.

Not all dementia sufferers will show all these symptoms; indeed, there are large individual differences in the nature and degree of impairment. However, there are some important guidelines to consider when nursing patients with senile dementia.

Guidelines to consider in the nursing of patients with dementia

Self-care

A dilemma facing the nurse is how much help to give senile dementia patients. Doing everything for them ensures success, but reinforces feelings of inadequacy; allowing them to care for themselves may result in failure and consequent feelings of incompetence. Orem (1985) suggests that the role of the nurse should be to compensate for any lack of self-care ability. This may be achieved by identifying a patient's specific strengths and weaknesses and then supplementing appropriate maladaptive behaviours whilst reinforcing adaptive ones. Hence a patient who has difficulty washing may find it difficult to start but once having begun is able to finish without further help. In this instance the role of the nurse would be to help direct the hands at the beginning of the washing sequence and then leave the patient to finish the process.

Reality orientation

Communication is essential for keeping one's 'feet on the floor'; it enables us to maintain contact with external reality. Unfortunately, dementia can interfere with a person's ability to maintain social relations and hinder communication. It is therefore extremely important for nurses to communicate effectively with patients suffering from dementia, utilising all the techniques discussed in the first chapter. Armstrong-Esther and Browne (1986) found that nurses tended to communicate less with confused than with coherent patients, and thus every effort should be made to increase the opportunities to communicate with patients burdened by dementia.

Holden and Woods (1982) suggest three ways to improve communication by discouraging rambling talk.

- If the patient is blatantly incorrect in what he or she says, it is appropriate to gently disagree and put him or her right. For example, 'I understand that you'd like me to fetch your wife/husband but I'm afraid she/he isn't upstairs. You're in hospital because you've not been well and she/he is at home. She'll/he'll be coming to see you this evening after tea, though.'
- Distraction is often useful. To break rambling talk you could change the topic of conversation or point out something that is happening close by. For example, 'They're just about to start dishing up your lunch. Shall we go and see what there is to eat?'.
- Disregard what is being said and concentrate on any feelings that are expressed. For example, 'You must really miss your wife/ husband while you're in hospital.'

A second feature of reality orientation is the provision of a structured environment. The use of easily seen clocks and calendars helps confused people keep track of time. Colour-coding rooms and doors, using large signs and noticeboards can help to aid memory for everyday tasks. But most important is training the person to be able to take full advantage of the structured environment. Merely placing a person in a 'tailored habitat' and hoping that they will get on with it is not good enough; they need to be taught how to benefit from the environmental cues (Begert and Jacobsson, 1976). Not surprisingly, even people with mild dementia have difficulty in orientation when moved from their familiar home environment to new surroundings such as a hospital ward. Thus reality orientation provides the nurse with a useful combination of techniques that can be tailored to fit the needs of individual patients.

Isolation and belonging

Old people may become separated from family and friends for a number of reasons. Sometimes isolation may be due to sons and daughters moving away from the area where the elderly person lives, but there is also a tendency for old people to leave their families and friends to enjoy their retirement in 'a little cottage in the country' or 'a little bungalow by the sea'. Unfortunately, if new friendships are not developed, elderly people may experience loneliness and as a consequence their self-esteem may be reduced. Kahana (1982) said that the availability of intimate contacts was positively related to psychological well-being. Thus, if elderly people do decide to move from their 'home environment', it is important to have structures for local integration should they choose to make use of them. Lowenthal and Haven (1968) interviewed 280 elderly people aged over 60 years and found that life crises such as a bereavement were a lot easier to deal with if there was someone close in whom to confide.

Disengagement or activity

Cumming and Henry (1961) proposed that, rather than wanting to maintain close relationships, elderly people seek to disengage themselves from social contacts (disengagement theory). Based on a study of a small number of elderly residents in Kansas, the researchers found that their participants tended to gradually decrease their social contacts and slowly fade out of the social scene. They suggested that old people are happiest when allowed to disengage themselves from society and that this process is inevitable and universal. On the other hand, *activity theory* (Havighurst *et al.*, 1968) states that the elderly have the same need of social interaction in old age as they had in earlier life. Circumstances may have transpired to isolate the elderly from social interaction, but this is not of their choosing and they would prefer to retain their active lifestyle.

Clearly, there is a dilemma posed by these two perspectives. Should nurses encourage the elderly to detach themselves from social interaction or should they actively encourage it? Neugarten (1980) reviewed the evidence for the two theories and found that social participation did tend to decline with age and that there were losses of occupational roles. Further, some individuals withdrew voluntarily from participation in social interaction. However, some of those individuals who appeared to be disengaged in later life were found to have been disengaged in earlier life as well, and had been relatively uninvolved in social interaction throughout their lives. Also, it was found that those with a relatively low level of social activity and involvement did not necessarily enjoy themselves any less than other people of similar ages. Carstensen (1987) provides a useful assessment of disengagement by saying that if people are forced to withdraw from social interaction by ill health, bereavement or relocation, they will not be likely to appreciate disengagement. But if people chose to withdraw to concentrate on a few aspects of life such as their closest friends or their favourite activities, then disengagement can become the optimal pattern of ageing.

The social network approach

Disengagement theory and activity theory describe some patterns of ageing but a successful analysis of the ageing process needs to take account of the variability of personality and situational factors. One of the problems associated with the study of interpersonal relations in elderly people is the scarcity of objective measures of social interaction and isolation. It may be the case that an apparently disengaged person is in fact quite socially active. A technique that has been developed to measure the exact nature of the relationships between elderly people, their family and acquaintances is called *social network analysis*. A social network refers to the group of people with whom one is likely to have contact over a specified period of time. Network analysis was originally used by social anthropologists to aid them in their investigations of community familial and social relations. A network is similar to a communication diagram and indicates the nature of the associations between people. Lopata (1975) states:

> An individual's social network can be seen as a support system involving the giving and receiving of objects, services, social and emotional supports defined by the receiver and the giver as necessary or at least helpful in maintaining a style of life.

There are two sets of criteria which are used to define social networks.

- *Interactional criteria.* These refer to the frequency of interaction, duration of interaction, direction of flow of conversation, content of interaction and uniplex or multiplex relations. A uniplex relationship involves a link with only one content, such as interacting with the postman who delivers your mail. However, if a postman were to deliver mail, provide emotional support, help with the groceries and give advice about health care then the relationship would be multiplex, involving more than one content.
- *Morphological criteria.* These are the size, density and clustering of a network. Density refers to the ratio of actual to potential links; clustering refers to areas of high density.

The advantage of constructing social networks for a population of elderly people has been demonstrated by Cohen and Sokolovsky (1979) in a community context, and by Powers (1992) in an institutional context. Cohen and Sokolovsky used network analysis to investigate a sample of elderly residents who lived in a series of mid-Manhattan 'single-room-occupancy hotels'. These hotels, or hostels, house large numbers of people with a wide range of psychological and physical problems. In one neighbourhood, 31 per cent had a history of chronic alcoholism or mental illness, 15 per cent were homebound and 50 per cent were estimated to need substantial help from social and health services. Whilst the majority of the residents were in need of some form of care, the majority were reluctant to have any contact with the community services. Social network analysis can prove a useful descriptive tool in this context for the following reasons.

- It introduces community nurses to the idea that their patients are not always socially isolated, but often have intact, functioning support networks. Ninety-six per cent of the hotel residents had average contacts of 7.5, with more than half of them multiplex.
- It enables nurses to view behaviour as the interaction of an individual with their environment. The tendency to interpret behaviour as a product of the individual was examined in Chapter 2 in the context of the fundamental attribution error. Network analysis helps focus attention on the environmental context.
- It identifies what resources are needed; when and where. In the mid-Manhattan project, males had much larger social networks *outside* the hotels, whereas females had larger networks *inside* the hotels. Further, elderly males who became ill tended to have fewer family links than healthy males. Therefore, as part of the project, it was decided for males to concentrate on facilitating family links and for females to work on links inside rather than outside the hotels.
- In many cases where old people form themselves into groups a 'leader' emerges. These leaders often take responsibility for providing the group members with such things as food, support and places to meet. Considerable influence can be exerted over the group by these individuals and they are usually receptive to carers. In cases where the elderly refuse to have anything to do with nurses, leaders can be a useful source of access. Providing the leaders with information and resources is one way of helping to ensure adequate provision for the other members of the group.
- Degree of physical illness should not necessarily be equated with ability or inability to live in a non-institutionalised environment.

  Mr L had a number of problems, including emphysema and heart disease, and could only walk a few yards. However, he regularly met a group of other men for drinks and to play cards. Mr A acted as a leader to Mr L and to another man, Mr D, who was the same age as Mr L but had better health. Mr A would get both men groceries and help them with such things as filling in forms. Then Mr A left. Mr L still had a fully functioning support network who were able to take on responsibility for his needs; Mr D did not. Thus, even though the health of Mr L was worse than the health of Mr D, he had an intact support group and was able to stay in a non-institutionalised environment.
- Disruption of a social network may occur if a well intentioned intervention by a nurse results in a shift of care. Offering to give an individual help can result in that

person being ostracised by the other members of the support network. Offering one form of help may also lead to the extinction of other forms of help. For example, handing out money may result in the discontinuance of ties with people who not only lend money but provide important emotional support as well. Inadvertent intervention may interfere with a functioning network and result in dependence on the nurse.

Steinbach (1992) examined the effects of social networks on institutionalisation and mortality among 5,151 non-institutionalised people aged 70+. Social networks decreased the likelihood of institutionalised mortality. Also, elderly people who participated in some form of social activity were less likely to become institutionalised.

Formal, or informal, analysis of social networks is useful in a wide variety of contexts, as it can establish the true nature of interpersonal relationships. Rather than concentrating on disengagement theory or activity theory, a more fruitful approach is to focus on the establishment and maintenance of functioning support networks for the elderly (see also Chapter 11).

Baltes (1991) has said that we should be moving towards a psychological culture of old age. He puts forward a model of good psychological ageing which focuses on the dynamic interplay between three processes: *selection, optimisation* and *compensation.* He illustrates the three processes by relating a television interview with the famous 80-year-old pianist Artur Rubenstein. When asked how he succeeded in continuing to be a successful concert pianist Rubenstein mentioned three factors:

- He noted that he maintained his ability and coped with ageing by reducing the scope of his repertoire and playing fewer pieces. (An example of selection.)
- He spent more time at practice than earlier in his life. (An example of optimisation.)
- He used special tricks such as slowing down his playing before fast segments to give the appearance of playing faster. (An example of compensation.)

The combination of these factors with a society that reflects the many faces of ageing leads to a psychological culture of old age. Baltes says:

Providing resources for a positive culture of old age requires a society that extends its values beyond economic criteria and is willing to allocate to old age more resources than is justified by old people's past productivity or strategies of investment in the future.

In concluding his paper he quotes the Chinese proverb 'Don't be afraid of walking more slowly. Be afraid only of coming to a halt.'

Summary

Differences in behaviour occur at particular stages in the life span, extending beyond infancy and childhood. This chapter has described some factors associated with adolescence, adulthood and old age in the light of psychological studies and the nursing implications which can be drawn from them.

Particular attention has been paid to body image, eating disorders, identity formation and suicide in relation to adolescence. Adulthood has been considered in terms of continuing cognitive development, physiological characteristics, sexuality and love as it relates to the early years, and the developmental tasks associated with middle adulthood. Finally, this chapter has explored theories of ageing and the psychological problems most commonly associated with old age.

Conundrum revisited

Reading Chapter 9 is likely to have prompted you to think about quite a wide range of psychological well-being issues at each of the three stages of life under discussion. What is challenging, though, is to decide how to translate a concept into a professional practice context (for instance, as a need) and then to identify a nursing response. The issue of different kinds of love, for example, is broadly informative but requires a little imagination to convert into a 'so what?' practice implication. Consider, though, how the quest for different forms of love and expression of love in different ways may shape human relations and the perceived level of self-fulfilment or happiness of individuals. Divorce, isolation, depression and even aggression may be bound up with 'love' when people seek it in various ways and expect different things of human relationships.

Now compare your triangles with the summary information that we have included in Table 5.5. Our information is illustrative rather than comprehensive, but we wonder whether you are now surprised just how widely nurses are engaged in psychological health care!

? Questions for further consideration

1 To what extent is adolescence a time of crisis?
2 Is there such a thing as a generation gap?
3 What are the main problems associated with nursing adolescents?
4 Can young adulthood be said to be relatively free from stress and anxiety?
5 Is there intellectual decline in old age?
6 Is it true that as we get old we want to 'disengage' ourselves from other members of society?

Table 5.5 *Risks, demands and expectations*

Risks (R)/Needs (N) and Expectations (E) Nurse contributions

Adolescence

Achieving a satisfactory body image (cathexis) (N)	Most nursing contributions are tertiary, we work with patients who suffer from an altered body image, for instance patients coping with anorexia or bulimia nervosa, with those that feel stigmatised owing to physical disfigurement. There is, though, scope for nurses to contribute health promotion teaching on the development of a satisfying body image associated within public and social education curricula within schools. This may relate to avoiding or managing obesity, promoting self-esteem or the understanding of sexuality
Discovering a personal identity (N) (E) (feeling loved/respected and worthwhile)	Nurses work with youth groups, families and individuals to develop adolescents' self- esteem in the face of adversity, for instance associated with poor housing. This work is especially important in a society where the expectations of adolescents and the expectations imposed upon adolescents by others are so prominent and in some instances unrealistic
Becoming a sexual being/managing sexual health risks (N) (R)	The risks of sexually transmitted diseases and the confusions and anxieties of developing a sexual identity are both problematic. Nurses work in clinics, with schools and youth groups and as individual counsellors or community mental health nurses to deal with identified difficulties
Avoiding the risks of drug abuse (including alcohol) (R)	Nurses work as health educators and counsellors, helping adolescents to avoid or manage the difficulties associated with drugs

Table 5.5 *(continued)*

Being individual and a part of the group (E)	Adolescents may struggle to understand, form or sustain satisfactory human relationships. Nurses for instance work with adolescents who have attention deficit problems or autism and assist them to understand the needs of others and their own behaviour in order to enable patients to engage in social interaction
Adulthood Feeling and being responsible, making healthy decisions (R) (N) (E) (e.g. regarding work and relationships or parenting)	The choices that adults face day to day may seem far removed from the work of nurses, until we recall that decisions often have psychological consequences (e.g. regret/guilt/depression/anxiety). Whilst they would be ill advised to act as prescriptive 'lifestyle gurus' they are experienced in understanding the consequences of decisions and the problems that can arise. Sometimes the two most telling questions that the nurse might pose are 'Do you need to make the decision immediately?' and 'What compels you to see this as something requiring a decision?'
Sustaining satisfying/meaningful sexual relationships (N)	Some nurses are formally employed in association with sexual health practices but many more provide support and guidance in association with childbirth, surgery, general practice and well woman clinics. No one has told patients that they cannot talk about intimate matters to someone they trust in places beyond the right 'clinic'
Completing developmental tasks (feeling adequate) (R) (E) (middle adulthood)	Mid-life crisis is a familiar and variously described social phenomenon. Nurses usually encounter it in work associated with the consequences, in the Accident and Emergency department, associated with alcohol abuse management or

mental health more generally. Nurses have the potential though to work more proactively and to question the criteria of human adequacy or dignity developed within societies, the factors that may lead to damaged self-esteem and confusion

Dealing with physiological changes (e.g. the menopause or deteriorating sexual prowess) (R) (N)

Did you identify how nurses work in community practice, through health promotion or well woman and well man clinics to assist adults dealing with the discomfort or anxiety of changing physical function or ability?

Managing the work/personal life balance (R)

Problems associated with this psychological challenge cost health services millions of pounds annually. Depression, anxiety, alcohol and other drug abuse, heart disease and hypertension, mental and physical exhaustion are all part of the complex issue. Nurses usually work in reactive roles helping patients to deal with the sequelae of imbalance. What might be the consequences of nurses working to question the social values and drivers that bring about stress in this area?

Late adulthood

Mitigating the effects of physical degeneration (wear and tear, or accumulating metabolic waste) (N) (E)

In Western societies women can increasingly expect to live well into their 80s and men into their late 70s, albeit with greater levels of accrued chronic illness or physical incapacity. The physical care that nurses deliver associated with weight management, balanced diets and exercise programmes is founded upon fundamental psychological principles. Nurses need to know how to teach, motivate, support and encourage patients as they actively manage the 'side effects' of ageing

Table 5.5 *(continued)*

Sustaining intellectual function (N) (E)	In community practice, through clubs, associations, day centres, the internet and telephone advice services, in association with charities nurses are engaged in assuring older adults of the intellectual function that they can sustain using mental exercise. Where intellectual function deteriorates as in Alzheimer's disease nurses provide 'front line' support to patients and families
Sustaining independence (E)	Older people wish to retain their independence and their interdependence with their peers (community). Nurses contribute to this with home-based care, services for the blind or otherwise sense-impaired and making representations to social authorities to enable people to live in their own homes. Nurses also teach patients new skills that facilitate independence
Feeling respected, being valued (E)	Dignity and respect for patients are core objectives for nurses and government alike. Nurses establish and insist upon standards of address, dress and approach to patients by professionals
Social isolation (R)	The death of peers, the location of housing where older adults may live, physical disabilities and the costs or availability of public transport can all increase the older adult's sense of isolation and risk psychological damage. Nurses organise, facilitate and support clubs, sheltered housing and trips that enable older patients to stay in contact with each other

Answers to Exercise 5.2

1 False. Eight out of ten people who commit suicide tell someone that they're thinking about hurting themselves before actually doing it.
2 False. All types of people commit suicide.
3 False. The suicide rate among young people increased by 137 between 1960 and 1980.
4 False. Take them seriously. Listen carefully to what they are saying. Give them a chance to express their feelings. Let them know you are concerned and help them to get help.
5 False Most people who kill themselves are confused about whether they really want to die. Suicide is often a cry for help. (Bell, 1980).

References

Adams, B. N. (1983). Adolescent health care needs: needs, priorities and services. *Nursing Clinics of North America, 18,* 237–248.

Armstrong-Esther, C. A. and Browne, K. D. (1986). The influence of elderly patients' mental impairment on nurse–patient interaction. *Journal of Advanced Nursing, 11,* 379–387.

Aro, H. and Taipale, V. (1987). The impact of timing of puberty on psychosomatic symptoms among fourteen- to sixteen-year-old Finnish girls. *Child Development, 58,* 261–268.

Baltes, P. B. (1991). The many faces of human aging: toward a psychological culture of old age. *Psychological Medicine, 21,* 837–854.

Begert, L. and Jacobsson, E. (1976). Training of reality orientation with a group of patients with senile dementia. *Scandinavian Journal of Behaviour Therapy, 5,* 191–200.

Belenky, M., Clinchy, B., Goldberger, N. and Tarule, J. (1986). *Women's Ways of Knowing.* New York: Basic Books.

Bell, R. (1980). *Changing Bodies, Changing Lives: A book for teens on sex and relationships.* New York: Random House.

Berscheid, E. and Walster, E. H. (1974). A little bit about love. In Huston, T. L. (ed.) *Foundations of Interpersonal Attraction.* New York: Academic Press.

Bibring, G. L. (1959). Some considerations of the psychological processes in pregnancy. *Psychoanalytic Study of the Child, 14,* 13–121.

Birren, J. E., Butler, R. N., Greenhouse, S. W., Sokoloff, L. and Yarrow, M. R. (eds) (1963). *Human Aging: A biological and behavioral study.* Washington DC: US Government Printing Office.

Bozzi, V. (1988). Teens and condoms: an uncomfortable fit. *Psychology Today, 22,* 14.

Brody, E. M. (1990). *Women in the middle: Their parent care years.* New York: Springer.

Brooks-Gunn, J., Boyer, C. and Hein, K. (1988). Preventing HIV infection and AIDS in children and adolescents: behavioural research and intervention strategies. *American Psychologist, 43,* 958–964.

Bruch, H. (1974). *Eating Disorders: Obesity, anorexia nervosa, and the person inside.* London: Routledge.

Caplan, G. (1960). Emotional implications of pregnancy and influences on family relationships. In Stuart, H. C. and Prugh, D. G. (eds) T*he Healthy Child.* Cambridge: Harvard.

Carstensen, M. A. (1987). Age-related changes in social activity. In Carstensen, L. and Edelstein, B. (eds) *Handbook of Clinical Gerontology.* Oxford: Pergamon Press.

Cartwright, A. (1976). *How Many Children?* London: Routledge and Kegan Paul.

Chesney, M. A., Hecker, M. H. and Black, G. W. (1988). Coronary-prone components of Type A behavior in the WCGS: a new methodology. In Houston, B. K. and Snyder, C. R. (eds) *Type A Behavior: Research, theory and intervention.* New York: Wiley.

Cobliner, W. G. (1965). Some maternal attitudes towards conception. *Mental Hygiene, 49,* 4–10.

Cohen, C. I. and Sokolovsky, J. (1979). Clinical use of network analysis for psychiatric and aged populations. *Community and Mental Health Journal, 15,* 203–213.

Coleman, J. C. (1980). *The Nature of Adolescence.* London: Methuen.

Condon, R. G. (1987). *Inuit Youth.* New Brunswick NJ: Rutgers University Press.

Csikszentmihalyi, M. and Larson, R. (1984). *Being Adolescent: Conflict and growth in the teenage years.* New York: Basic Books.

Cumming, E. and Henry, W. E. (1961). *Growing Old: The process of disengagement.* New York: Basic Books.

Curtis, H. J. (1966). *Biological Mechanisms of Aging.* Springfield IL: Thomas.

Davis, K. E. and Latty-Mann, H. (1987). Love styles and relationship quality: a contribution to validation. *Journal of Social and Personal Relationships, 4,* 409–428.

Davis, R. H. (1981). The middle years. In Davis, R. H. (ed.) *Aging: Prospects and issues.* 3rd edn. Los Angeles: Andrus Gerontology Center.

Deutsch, H. (1947). *The Psychology of Women.* London: Grune Stratton.

Duck, S. (1992). *Human Relationships.* 2nd edn. London: Sage.

Engen, T. (1977). Taste and smell. In Birren, J. E. and Schaie, K. W. (eds) *Handbook of the Psychology of Aging.* New York: Van Nostrand Reinhold.

Erikson, E. H. (1968). *Identity, Youth and Crisis.* New York: Norton.

Fairburn, C. G. and Beglin, S. J. (1990). Studies of the epidemiology of *bulimia nervosa. American Journal of Psychiatry, 147,* 401–408.

Faust, M. S. (1960). Developmental maturity as a determinant of prestige in adolescent girls. *Child Development, 31,* 173–184.

Flaming, D. and Morse, J. M. (1991). Minimizing embarrassment: boys' experience of pubertal changes. *Issues in Comprehensive Pediatric Nursing, 14,* 211–230.

Friedman, M. and Rosenman, R. H. (1959). Association of specific overt behavior pattern with blood and cardiovascular findings. *Journal of the American Medical Association, 169,* 1286–1296.

Gagnon, J. H. and Simon, W. (1987). The sexual scripting of oral genital contacts. *Archives of Sexual Behavior, 16,* 1–25.

Gibbs, A. (1990). Aspects of communication with people who have attempted suicide. *Journal of Advanced Nursing, 15,* 1245–1249.

Gilligan, C. (1982). *In a Different Voice: Psychological theory and women's development.* Cambridge MA: Harvard University Press.

Goldberg, E. (2002). *The Executive Brain.* New York: Oxford University Press.

Goodman, M. J. (1982). A critique of menopausal research. In Voda, A., Dinnerstein, M. and O'Donnell, S. (eds) *Changing Perspectives on the Menopause.* Austin TX: University of Texas Press.

Gottfredson, G. (1977). Career stability and redirection in adulthood. *Journal of Applied Psychology, 62,* 329–340.

Gould, R. L. (1978). *Transformations: Growth and change in adult life.* New York: Simon and Schuster.

Granick, S. and Patterson, R. D. (eds) (1971). *Human Aging* II, *An eleven year followup biomedical behavioral study.* Washington DC: US Government Printing Office.

Greif, E. B. and Ulman, K. J. (1982). The psychological impact of the menarche on early adolescent females: a review of the literature. *Child Development, 53,* 1413–1430.

Havighurst, R. J. (1972). *Developmental Tasks and Education.* 3rd edn. New York: McKay.

Havighurst, R. J., Neugarten, B. and Tobin, S. S. (1968). Disengagement and patterns of aging. In Neugarten, B. (ed.) *Middle Age and Aging.* Chicago: University of Chicago Press.

Holden, C. (1986). Youth suicide: new research focuses on growing problem. *Science, 233,* 839–841.

Holden, U. P. and Woods, R. T. (1982). *Reality Orientation.* Edinburgh: Churchill Livingstone.

Horowitz, A. (1985). Sons and daughters as caregivers to older parents: differences in role performance and consequences. *Gerontologist, 25,* 612–617.

Jaques, E. (1965). Death and the mid-life crisis. *International Journal of Psychoanalysis, 46,* 502–514.

Johnston, L. D., Bachman, J. G. and O'Malley, P. M. (1988). *Drug Use among American High School Students, College and other Young Adults: National trends through 1987.* Rockville MD: National Institute on Drug Abuse.

Jones, H. B. (1956). A special consideration of the aging process: disease and life expectancy. In Lawrence, J. H. and Tobias, C. A. (eds) *Advances in Biological and Medical Physics* Vol IV, New York: Academic Press.

Jones, M. C. (1965). Psychological correlates of somatic development. *Child Development, 36,* 899–911.

Jones, M. C. and Bayley, N. (1950). Physical maturing among boys as related to behavior. *Journal of Educational Psychology, 49,* 129–148.

Julian, T., McKenry, P. C. and Mckelvey, M. W. (1992). Components of men's well-being at mid-life. *Issues in Mental Health Nursing, 13,* 285–299.

Kahana, B. (1982). Social behaviour and aging. In Wolman, B. B. (ed.) *Handbook of Developmental Psychology.* Englewood Cliffs NJ: Prentice Hall.

Kenrick, D. T. and Cialdini, R. B. (1977). Romantic attraction: misattribution versus reinforcement explanations. *Journal of Personality and Social Psychology, 35,* 381–391.

Kohlberg, L. (1981). *Essays on Moral Development* I, *The Philosophy of Moral Development.* New York: Harper and Row.

Lee, J. A. (1973). *The Colors of Love: An exploration of the ways of loving.* Toronto: New Press.

Levinson, D. J. (1978). *The Seasons of a Man's Life.* New York: Knopf.

Levinson, D. J. (1986). A concept of adult development. *American Psychologist, 41,* 3–13.

Levitt, M. J., Weber, R. A. and Clark, M. C. (1986). Social network relationships as sources of maternal support and well-being. *Developmental Psychology, 22,* 310–316.

Lopata, H. (1975). Support systems of the elderly: Chicago of the 1970s. *Gerontologist, 15,* 35–41.

Lowenthal, M. and Haven, C. (1968). Interaction and adaptation: intimacy as a critical variable. *American Sociological Review, 33,* 20–30.

Makinodan, T. (1977). Immunity and aging. In Finch, C. E. and Hayflick, L. (eds) *Handbook of the Biology of Aging.* New York: Van Nostrand Reinhold.

Marcia, J. E. (1966). Development and validation of ego identity status. *Journal of Personality and Social Psychology, 3,* 551–558.

Maslow, A. H. (1970). *Motivation and Personality.* New York: Harper and Row.

May, K. A. (1981). Three phases of father involvement in pregnancy. *Nursing Research, 31,* 337–342.

McCrae, R. R. and Costa, P. T., Jnr (1984). *Emerging Lives, Enduring Dispositions: Personality in adulthood.* Boston MA: Little Brown.

McElmurray, B. and Huddleston, D. (1987). The Perimenopausal Woman: Perceived threats to sexuality and self-care responses. Unpublished paper presented to the seventh Conference of the Society for Menstrual Cycle Research, Ann Arbor MI.

Mead, M. (1970). *Culture and Commitment: A study of the generation gap.* New York: Doubleday.

Meades, S. (1993). Suggested community psychiatric nursing interventions with clients suffering from *anorexia nervosa* and *bulimia nervosa. Journal of Advanced Nursing, 18,* 364–370.

Medvedev, Z. A. (1964). The nucleic acids in development and aging. In Strehler, B. L. (ed.) *Advances in Gerontological Research* I, New York: Academic Press.

Miller, B. C. and Solllie, D. C. (1986). Normal stresses in transition to parenthood. In Moos, R. H. (ed) *Coping with Life Crises.* New York: Plenum.

Milne, D. (1993). *Psychology and Mental Health Nursing.* Leicester: BPS Books (The British Psychological Society) and Macmillan.

Mitchell, J. (1972). Some psychological dimensions of adolescent sexuality. *Adolescence, 7*, 447–458.

Neugarten, B. L. (1968). The awareness of middle age. In Neugarten, B. L. (ed.) *Middle Age and Aging.* Chicago: University of Chicago Press.

Neugarten, N. (1980). *Personality in Middle and Late Life.* New York: Arno Press.

Newell, R. (1991). Body-image disturbance: cognitive behavioural formulation and intervention. *Journal of Advanced Nursing, 16*, 1400–1405.

Niven, A. N. (1977) Network Plans: Culture and Environment. Unpublished PhD thesis. University of Aberdeen.

Orem, D. (1985). *Nursing: Concepts of practice.* 2nd edn. New York: McGraw Hill.

Palmer, R. L. (1988). *Anorexia Nervosa: A guide for sufferers and their families*, 2nd edn. Harmondsworth: Penguin.

Perry, W. (1981). Cognitive and ethical growth: the making of meaning. In Chickering, A. (ed.) *The Modern American College.* San Francisco: Jossey Bass.

Powers, B. A. (1992). The roles staff play in the social networks of elderly institution-alised people. *Social Science and Medicine, 34*, 1335–1343.

Price, B. (1990). A model for body image care. *Journal of Advanced Nursing, 15*, 585–593.

Price, B. (1999) *Altered Body Image.* NT Clinical Monographs. London: EMAP Healthcare.

Roskies, E. (1988). *Stress Management for the Healthy Type A: Theory and practice.* New York: Guilford Press.

Rovee, C. K., Cohen, R. Y. and Shlapack, W. (1975). Life-span stability in olfactory sensitivity. *Development Psychology, 11*, 311–318.

Rubin, Z. (1970). Measurement of romantic love. *Journal of Personality and Social Psychology, 16*, 265–273.

Rutter, M. (1976). Maternal deprivation, 1972–1978: new findings, new concepts. new approaches. *Child Development, 50*, 283–305.

Schaie, K. W. and Willis, S. L. (1986). Can decline in intellectual functioning be reversed? *Developmental Psychology, 22*, 223–232.

Schiffman, S. (1977). Food recognition of the elderly. *Journal of Gerontology, 32*, 586–592.

Schulz, R. (1978). *The Psychology of Death, Dying and Bereavement.* Reading MA: Addison Wesley.

Schulz, R. and Ewen, R. B. (1988). *Adult Development and Aging: Myths and emerging realities.* New York: Macmillan.

Seifert, K. L. and Hoffnung, R. J. (1991). *Child Development and Adolescence.* 2nd edn. Boston MA: Houghton Mifflin.

Sheehy, G. (1976). *Passages.* New York: Dutton.

Shekelle, R., Hulley, S., Neaton, J., Billings, J. H., Borhani, N. O., Gerace, T. A., Jacobs, D. R., Lasser, N. L., Mittlemark, M. B. and Stamler, J. (1985). The MRFIT behavior pattern study: Type A behavior and incidence of heart disease. *American Journal of Epidemiology, 122*, 559–570.

Sheridan, C. L. and Radmacher, S. A. (1992). *Health Psychology: Challenging the biomedical model.* Chichester: Wiley.

Shock, N. W. (1977). Biological theories of aging. In Birren, J. E. and Schaie, K. W. (eds) *Handbook of the Psychology of Aging.* New York: Van Nostrand Reinhold.

Spence, A. (1989). *Biology of Human Aging.* Englewood Cliffs NJ: Prentice Hall.

Steiger, H., Leung, F. W., Ross, D. J. and Gulko, J. (1992). Signs of anorexia and bulimia nervosa in high-school girls reporting a combination of eating and mood symptoms. *International Journal of Eating Disorders, 12,* 383–395.

Steinbach, U. (1992). Social networks, institutionalization, and mortality among elderly people in the United States. *Journal of Gerontology, 47,* 183–190.

Stevens, J. C. and Cain, W. S. (1987). Old age deficits in the sense of smell as gauged by thresholds, magnitude matching, and odor identification. *Psychology and Aging, 2,* 36–42.

Szmukler, G. I. (1989). The psychopathology of eating disorders. In Shepherd, R. (ed.) *Handbook of the Psychophysiology of Human Eating.* Chichester: Wiley.

Toffler, A. (1970). *Future Shock.* London: Bodley Head.

Walster, E. and Walster, G. W. (1978). *A New Look at Love.* Reading MA: Addison Wesley.

Willis, S. L., Jay, G. M., Diehl, M. and Marsiske, M. (1992). Longitudinal change and prediction of everyday task performance. *Research on Aging, 14,* 68–91.

Wilson, E. O. (1978). *Sociobiology.* Cambridge: MA: Harvard University Press.

Wolkind, A. and Zajicek, E. (eds) (1981). *Pregnancy: A Psychological and Social Study.* London: Academic Press.

Worthman, C. M. and Whiting, J. W. M. (1987). Social change in adolescent sexual behaviour, mate selection, and premarital pregnancy rates in a Kikuyu community. *Ethos, 15,* 145–165.

Further reading

Price, Bob (1999) *Altered Body Image.* NT Clinical Monographs. London: EMAP Healthcare. This is probably the best first source of information on this topic. I mention here as it is particularly relevant to adolescence but it also acts as an adjunct to Bob's body image conundrum in Chapter 7.

Reed, Jan, Stanley, D. and Clarke, C. (2004) *Health, Well-being and Older People.* Oxford: Policy Press. A multidisciplinary approach to discussing some of the important basic issues facing nursing older people.

Birren, James and Schaie Warner (2001) *Handbook of the Psychology of Aging.* New York: Academic Press. Up-to-date text from two of the main international researchers in the area of adulthood and aging.

Life Events, Transitions and Crises

A practice conundrum

Your work with a case study in pain and coping associated with the last chapter may have highlighted just how differently people deal with sudden and uncomfortable change. Now we wish to develop that conundrum further and to consider the ways in which social support may serve to sustain an individual through other (potentially traumatic) life events. Your conundrum begins with a interesting activity involving a sheet of A3 paper, upon which you draw a large 'target' with three circles, one inside the other. The target represents the beginnings of a social support network map. The innermost circle represents that space within which close allies and intimate others are permitted. It is the space nearest to person at the centre of the map. The middle circle is the space where friends and close associates usually exist. This is a space of general rather than intimate support. Information shared here is not usually so revealing. The outer circle represents the space where the individual encounters passing friends, work associates or those that might be described as acquaintances. Here only the most superficial information is shared.

Develop the exercise now by asking a professional colleague to write his or her initials at the centre of the innermost circle. Next ask your colleague to add the initials of intimate friends in the innermost circle near to their own. Where such friends have close associations with each other they should be positioned in the same part of that circle. Repeat this procedure with the middle and the outer circle, adding and grouping initials of people who know each other.

Next, ask your colleague to add arrows between the initials of individuals who support each other. The direction of the arrow indicates in which direction the majority of support is provided. Of course some arrows will point in both directions because support is mutual. Encourage your colleague to ensure that arrows connect her or himself to others as well as to indicate the support provided to each other by friends. Where support is faltering or inconsistent a dotted-line arrow can be used. Having completed this part of the activity, you should have a map with web-like connections drawn upon it. Maps vary in the volume and intensity of connections represented.

It is now time to introduce an imaginary life event. Ask the nurse to imagine that she has received a sudden and pleasing promotion that offers additional salary and status but which comes with heavy responsibilities too. The nurse will have to move house, work longer hours and may have to travel/commit to unsocial hours working. The next year is going to prove very stressful but potentially rewarding long-term.

Discuss with the nurse how she would cope with this life event and how the social support network that she has might assist her or, in turn, be affected by the sudden turn of events. As you listen to her account note the importance of social support in coping with life events. What psychological adjustments seemed evident in her account and did they seem related to her stage of life?

Now examine the concepts discussed in Chapter 6 to see which were present and important in your activity. For example, did Erikson's Eight Stages of Life help you understand her situation? How did she rate the stress associated with this change? Did you witness any bargaining processes under way, similar to those discussed in association with a more fundamental change – dying? Finally, did the social support network seem to help inoculate her against the stress of change?

An almost inescapable part of modern life is change and the need to adapt to it. During the course of each individual's life many events will occur. Some of them will seem rather trivial, others will be of huge importance. Some events will be so momentous or influential that people's lives may be changed entirely. Some events will be reasonably predictable, while others will occur out of the blue. Finally, some events will be happy ones with positive outcomes whilst others will cause upset and turmoil. The role of psychology is to make some sense and meaning out of these episodes in people's lives. The first way it can do this is by attempting to provide a system for the classification of life events, crises and transitions.

Classification of life events

Kimmel (1980) distinguishes between *normative* life events – those changes that are expected according to the social norms for individuals at particular times of their lives – and *idiosyncratic* life events – those changes in life patterns that are unique to that particular individual. Normative life events would include leaving school, forming relationships, breaking relationships, and the death of parents, whereas idiosyncratic life events would include a major illness or handicap, winning a large sum of money or the death of a child.

Developmental life-span approaches endeavour to describe the normative life events that occur throughout the course of human development. One of the most well-known theories is that of Erikson (1963). In his Eight Stages of Life Erikson outlined a series of 'crises' or dilemmas that face all individuals at particular stages in their lives. These crises signal times when people face a transition or turning point in the course of their psychological development. Each developmental stage is marked by a choice between two opposing characteristics and it is necessary to resolve the crisis before being able successfully to negotiate the next in line.

Erikson's Eight Stages of Life

- *Basic trust versus basic mistrust* (birth to 1½ years old). The first crisis, or dilemma, to face the infant is whether the world is made up of safe, orderly, predictable events or irregular, unreliable occurrences. One of the most important features of the early interactions between caretaker and child is the degree of consistency, predictability and reliability of care. When infants sense that a caretaker is consistent and dependable, they develop a sense of basic trust in the parent. When they are cold, wet or hungry they know that their needs will be met. Trust, then, is the sense that others are reliable and predictable. Further, if infants develop secure attachments, they will go on to other relationships nurturing this sense with them.
- *Autonomy versus shame and doubt* (1½ to 3 years old). In this stage the child begins to exert greater control over actions and begins to explore the world by him or herself. Alongside this new-found independence comes a need for caretakers to regulate their child's behaviour, for example the little girl who has just wet her pants and is worried that others will see her in that state. Doubt stems from the realisation that one is not so powerful after all. Parents can help their children negotiate this crisis by explaining about social behaviour without crushing the child's independence. Those parents who remain insensitive to their children's needs, using shame and ridicule to confront oppositional behaviour, may produce young men and women whose shame overrides their impulses towards self-determination.
- *Initiative versus guilt* (3 to 5 years old). Building on the ability to control themselves, children now learn to make plans and set goals. They become aware that they can influence others and successfully manipulate their surroundings. The crisis comes when they realise that their most prized ambitions may be doomed to failure. When this sense of initiative results in the child 'going too far', or being made to feel incompetent, a feeling of guilt is generated. In the previous stage the child could be made to feel ashamed by other people, whereas in this stage he or she learns to make him or herself ashamed.
- *Industry versus inferiority* (5 to 12 years old). Children start to expand their horizons in this stage, and schooling provides the vehicle for the development of new skills. Play becomes more purposeful and peer-group comparison becomes an influential factor in behaviour. The danger at this stage is that children may develop an excessive feeling of

inadequacy and inferiority. Most of us can probably remember the hurts and failures of the classroom and playground. Sometimes children may have difficulty at this stage because they have not successfully resolved conflicts at earlier stages. A girl may have developed more doubt than autonomy at the second stage, hence she is unsure of herself as she tries to conquer new objectives. Good teachers, as well as good parents, can play a significant role in this crisis.

- *Identity versus role confusion* (12 to 18 years old). It was Erikson who first introduced the term *identity crisis*. This refers to confusion about one's role in the general scheme of events. Adolescents are likely to ask questions such as 'Who am I?' 'What do I believe in?' 'What am I going to do with my life?' The crisis is couched in the broad terms of culture and society, and consequently the degree of confusion is related to the clarity and consistency of each culture's norms and values. For example, in the United Kingdom at the age of 16 an adolescent can make an extremely responsible decision to get married and start a family. With the consent of parents our society condones this act. However, the same adolescent is not deemed mature enough to vote, drink alcohol, view an '18' rated film or even drive a car. It is not surprising that there is an element of role confusion when young people are treated with such inconsistency. The crisis is resolved when the young person achieves a sexual identity, an occupational identity, an ethnic identity and knows what he or she wants to do and be.

- *Intimacy versus isolation* (young adulthood). During this stage intimacy with others should develop. Erikson defines intimacy broadly as the ability to relate one's deepest hopes and fears to another person and to accept theirs reciprocally. The capacity to resolve this is again dependent on what has happened in the previous stage. If the development of intimacy is dependent on the ability to share oneself with another, it can occur only if a sense of identity has been developed. The formation of relationships gives access to individual feelings which can play a part in the development of self-confidence. If self-identity is fragile, people may try to avoid close relationships because they do not wish to expose their weaknesses.

- *Generativity versus stagnation* (middle adulthood). Generativity refers to the ability to be concerned with others, with future generations and the nature of the world and society. As Erikson puts it, 'there should be an interest in guiding and establishing the next generation'. If people fail in this task, they will tend to stagnate, become preoccupied and self-indulgent, and unable to make any contribution to the welfare of others.

- *Integrity versus despair* (late adulthood). Integrity refers to the feeling that one's life has been worth while and well spent. If, however, there is a foreboding that wrong, or no, decisions have been made and life is seen as lacking integration, then despair will be felt. Despair can also occur if it is felt that it is too late to 'make things right'. One looks back on one's life and wonders what it was all about; seeing it as unsatisfactory, yet realising that there is no time to start again. If there is a sense of having helped to create a more dignified life for oneself and everybody else, then there is a sense of wisdom as well as integrity.

Not surprisingly, Erikson's theory has its strengths and weaknesses. On the positive side, it offers a useful framework within which to view the dilemmas confronting children and adults throughout the life cycle. On the negative side the theory is a bit vague and has been described as 'fuzzy' (Bee and Boyd, 2003). Erikson recognised this criticism and said:

> I came to psychology from art, which may explain, if not justify, the fact that the reader will find me painting contexts and backgrounds where he would rather have me point to facts and concepts.

Second he seems to have rather a benign view of society as a cosy, beneficial social institution. Sometimes a healthy response to the societal ambiguities facing the adolescent would be a recognition of the difficulties involved in developing an identity.

However, the advantages of this theory for nursing practice lie in the provision of markers for those events in human development that are likely to cause people some difficulty. This enables the nurse to be aware of and understand the problems which may affect people at specific stages during their lives. What may seem an important health issue for the nurse may seem insignificant to the patient who is negotiating a personal life crisis.

Social Readjustment Rating Scale

This scale for representing normative life events was developed by Holmes and Rahe (1967). Instead of using developmental stages, they were concerned with the sorts of experiences that were likely to affect people during the course of their lives. They examined 5,000 patient records and selected forty-three events of varying severity that seemed to occur in the months preceding an illness. These events were presented to a group of 100 judges who were asked to rate them on a number of criteria:

- length of time needed to adjust to the event;
- intensity of the event;
- average amount of adaptation to the event.

They were told that marriage had a value of 500 and were asked to rate the forty-two other events, using this as a reference point. In effect, no event was found to be more than twice as stressful as marriage. The average of the numbers assigned to each event was divided by 10 and the resulting numbers became the weighting of each life event. On the basis of the results of this, the Social Readjustment Rating Scale (SRRS) evolved (see Table 6.1).

Table 6.1 *Social Readjustment Rating Scale*

Life event (*stress value*)

1   Death of spouse (*100*)
2   Divorce (*73*)
3   Marital separation (*65*)
4   Jail term (*63*)
5   Death of a close family member (*63*)
6   Personal injury or illness (*53*)
7   Marriage (*50*)
8   Fired at work (*47*)
9   Marital reconciliation (*45*)
10 Retirement (*45*)
11 Change in health of family member (*44*)
12 Pregnancy (*40*)
13 Sex difficulties (*39*)
14 Gain of new family member (*39*)
15 Business readjustment (*39*)
16 Change in financial state (*38*)
17 Death of a close friend (*37*)
18 Change to a different line of work (*36*)
19 Change in number of arguments with spouse (*35*)
20 Large mortgage repayments (*31*)
21 Foreclosure of mortgage or loan (*30*)
22 Change in responsibilities at work (*29*)
23 Son or daughter leaving home (*29*)
24 Trouble with in-laws (*29*)
25 Outstanding personal achievement (*28*)
26 Wife begins or stops work (*26*)
27 Begin or end school (*26*)
28 Change in living conditions (*25*)
29 Revision of personal habits (*24*)
30 Trouble with boss (*23*)
31 Change in work hours or conditions (*20*)
32 Change of residence (*20*)
33 Change of school (*20*)
34 Change in recreation (*19*)
35 Change in church activities (*19*)
36 Change in social activities (*18*)
37 Small mortgage repayments (*17*)
38 Change in sleeping habits (*16*)
39 Change in the number of family get-togethers (*15*)
40 Change in eating habits (*15*)
41 Vacation (*13*)
42 Christmas (*12*)
43 Minor violations of the law (*11*)

Reprinted from *Journal of Psychosomatic Research*, Vol II, Holmes & Rahe: The Social Readjustment Rating Scale, pp. 213–218, © 1967, with permission from Elsevier.

Exercise 6.1 *Coping with stress*

To obtain an indication of your own susceptibility to stress-induced illness, select those events from the SRRS which you have experienced in the past twelve months. Add together the scores for each event; Holmes and Rahe found that scoring

- 150–199 points increases your likelihood of illness by 40 per cent;
- 200–299 points increases your likelihood of illness by 50 per cent;
- 300 points and over increases your likelihood of illness by 80 per cent.

But don't worry too much if your score seems high, for, as we have seen, there are large individual differences in the way people cope with stress.

There are also some events that actually remove stress, for example a divorce may be preferable to a relationship full of conflict and friction. In addition, instead of life events causing illness, they may in fact be manifestations of an illness already present.

The main criticisms of the scale refer to the quantitative measurement (i.e. 'how much') of life stress. There is no attempt to describe or explain the qualitative features of life crises – one has to ask whether ten parking tickets are equivalent to the death of a spouse in terms of stress. While the events represented in the scale are normative, they do not necessarily depict everyday experiences.

The Hassles and Uplifts Scale

Kanner *et al.* (1981) devised the Hassles and Uplifts Scale to measure the psychological stress reflected in the occurrences of people's daily lives. The most frequently reported hassles by a sample of white middle-class adults aged 45 to 64 were:

- concern about weight;
- health of a family member;
- rising prices of common goods;
- home maintenance (inside);
- too many things to do;
- misplacing or losing things;
- yard work or outside home maintenance;
- property, investments or taxes;

- crime;
- physical appearance.

The most frequently reported uplifts by the same group were:

- relating well with your spouse or lover;
- relating well with friends;
- completing a task;
- feeling healthy;
- getting enough sleep;
- eating out;
- meeting your responsibilities;
- visiting, phoning, or writing to someone;
- spending time with family;
- home pleasing you.

A useful feature of the scale is that it measures the extent to which each event is perceived as being severe. Thus, when Young (1987) presented the scale to a sample of 448 adults aged between 20 and 60 he found that the following events were the ones that people selected as causing them some problems:

- paperwork;
- nature of work;
- work load;
- housework;
- physical appearance.

These were the events that were perceived to cause a great deal of stress:

- work load;
- free time;
- the nature of work;
- paperwork;
- money for necessities.

It can be seen that for this sample the main everyday hassles seemed to centre around work.

Therefore, in classifying life events, it is important to distinguish between everyday hassles which provide some stress and those that are likely to provide serious problems.

Models of life events

One of the main functions of research into life events has been to investigate the relationship between the events themselves and the resulting mental and physical disorders. If high levels of psychosocial stress lead to disorders, then one of the goals of nursing is to prevent the unwelcome mental and physical consequences of stressful life events in as many people as possible. This is just one of the goals of prevention, however. Equally important is encouraging competence, health and well-being. Thus primary prevention has two different goals:

- one that emphasises the prediction and understanding of physical and mental disorders as a function of the stresses and strains of everyday life;
- a knowledge of the process by which life events can lead to the development of what Maslow has described as 'psychological growth' in an individual.

The first approach focuses upon health programmes that operate before any harm has been done, thus reducing the incidence of disorder. A thorough appraisal of the types and number of life events experienced by people are important measures of the need for such programmes. Felner *et al.* (1985) in their review of the role of transitions and life events in primary prevention, concluded that:

> Identification of those conditions which consistently predispose individuals to developing physical or psychological difficulties, such as experiencing life events, may be critical to the success of efforts to justify the need for the allocation of scarce resources to preventive services. Without such evidence it may be difficult to convince those professionals trained in the more reactive, rather than proactive, human service delivery system.

But it is also clear that the adaptive impact of life events and transitions is a function of the quality as well as the quantity of experiences. Negative life events may have the potential to provide positive psychological growth. People who are experiencing a crisis are often more willing to pay attention and listen to what the nurse has to say. If the nurse can facilitate adaptation, learning and growth from the crisis, then the patient may be able to face future crises using the skills and competence that have been developed dealing with the present problem. In this sense, treatment represents the opportunity for primary prevention.

Sometimes it is better to focus on life events such as bereavement, disability, divorce, and chronic illness as a transition that involves various adaptive tasks rather than as markers of a major stress. Felner *et al.* (1985) suggest that 'A transitional framework allows us to focus on such commonalities and to develop strategies for enhancing an individual's adaptive abilities across a wide array of life changes.' Three examples of such a transitional framework or model are introduced next.

The cycle of reactions

Hopson (1981) introduces this model in the following way.

> As we began to discover other work on different transitions, a general picture increasingly began to emerge. It appeared that irrespective of the nature of the transition, an overall pattern seemed to exist.

The cycle Hopson and his associates identified consists of seven phases.

- *Immobilisation.* In the first phase the person experiences a kind of paralysis. There is a feeling of being overwhelmed by the weight of the crisis. Often people are unable to make any sense of what has happened and their powers of reasoning and understanding are disrupted. The strength of feeling in this first phase is related to the degree of unfamiliarity with the transition or crisis and expectations of positive or negative outcomes.
- *Minimisation.* A way to escape the state of immobilisation is to minimise, or even trivialise, the extent of the problem. Sometimes a person will deny that a problem exists and may even pretend to be happy. Denial can serve a useful function in giving the person time to regain composure but it will become counterproductive if allowed to be maintained over a long period of time.
- *Depression.* As the consequences of the transition become apparent, people sometimes start to feel depressed. This condition often results from a feeling of powerlessness and lack of control over the way life is going. Losing control over emotions is a particular fear in this phase and bouts of anger are often interspersed between the periods of hopelessness. Depression can occur even if individuals have created the change in life circumstances themselves, as it is a response to not knowing how to cope with the new situation. Other emotions associated with this phase are anxiety, anger and sometimes sadness.
- *Letting go.* Throughout the previous stages there has been a kind of attachment to 'life as it was'. The purpose of this stage is to become disentangled with the past and face up to the realities of the present. Letting go involves the person saying something like 'Well, here I am and I suppose the only thing to do is to face up to things as best I can. I don't know exactly what life has in store for me but I know I can survive.' This rearrangement of perspective and detachment from the past replace feelings of depression with feelings of optimism.
- *Testing.* This is a period of intense activity. In any unexplored situation there will be an experimental period when new lifestyles and new ways of coping with problems are tried out. The person may experience failures as well as successes and therefore be subject to mood swings.
- *Search for meaning.* This phase represents a more measured concern to understand the 'hows' and 'whys' of the transition. It represents an attempt not to re-establish

contact with the past but to withdraw somewhat from the furore of the testing phase and attempt to place what has happened in some kind of perspective. The search for meaning becomes a healthy form of reflective thinking.

● *Internalisation.* The product of the previous phase is access to an internalisation of feelings and meanings. During this phase these feelings and meanings are incorporated into new behaviour.

The process of the seven phases thus represents a 'cycle of experiencing disruption, gradually acknowledging its reality, testing oneself, understanding oneself, and incorporating changes in one's behaviour.' (Hopson, 1981). The level of morale during the cycle drops drastically during the third phase, only to end up in the seventh, higher than when it started.

Hopson notes that progression through the seven phases is by no means always smooth and neat. Also, each individual's progressions and regressions are unique. Some people may never get beyond the denial phase while others may become 'stuck' in the depths of depression, unable to let go. Finally, he notes that transitions are most stressful if 'they are unpredictable, involuntary, unfamiliar, of high magnitude (degree of change), and high intensity (rate of change)'.

Implications

As opposed to life event markers, this model provides an illustration of the qualitative changes that accompany life events and transitions. There is a lack of information concerning how people can be 'trained' to negotiate each of the phases so that they may reach the goal of internalisation, but in any case, this may be outside the remit of the nurse and more the responsibility of trained counsellors. If nurses have a general pattern of how patients experience life crises, they can produce a programme of care based on the general and particular needs of patients undergoing such problematic phases in their lives.

The personal competence model

Danish and D'Augelli (1982) state that 'The development of personal competence, a goal of intervention, is defined as the ability to be self-reliant and to do life planning.' Essentially this model proposes that the more resources an individual has at their disposal, the better their ability to deal with life events and crises. This model considers that there are consistent similarities between life events so that, whilst content or knowledge to confront these events may differ, the skills and attitudes necessary for a successful resolution of the problem overlap.

Danish and D'Augelli (1982) have constructed a programme designed to promote skill in dealing with life events, transitions and crises. It consists of the following six components.

- *Goal assessment.* In this part of the programme it is the individuals themselves who decide what it is important to learn, and the role of the nurse is to act in an advisory capacity and to use his or her expertise to help the patient identify goals. There are two main ways to help people identify their goals:
  - (i) to get people to concentrate on specific, positive behaviours and provide an opportunity to try them out to see if they fit in with desired needs;
  - (ii) to differentiate between those goals that are important to the individual and those that are important to others.
- *Knowledge acquisition.* One factor that may make it difficult to identify appropriate goals is lack of knowledge. Therefore it is vital that the nurse is able to provide the person with the relevant information needed to achieve his goals.
- *Decision making.* Another factor that may hinder goal attainment is a lack of decision-making skills. The approach that Janis and Mann (1977) use to help people achieve a constructive decision-making strategy is described in Chapter 7.
- *Risk assessment.* Some people will know what to do and how to do it but be prepared to take a risk. This factor is similar to the benefits/ barriers component of the Health Belief Model (see Chapter 6) and, simply stated, suggests that, if the costs outweigh the benefits, people are unlikely to take a risk.
- *Social support.* This model endorses the view that it is essential to marshal the co-operation of friends and relatives in maintaining new behaviour. Social support in this context is not just a 'buffer' but a positive resource.
- *Planning of skill development.* The last skill in the programme is being able to plan the development of skills. This is a process intended to help people design and implement their own skill programmes.

The goal of the programme is to empower people to help themselves, and so the nurse is viewed very much as a teacher using an educational approach, as well as a carer a and therapist.

The process of training in or facilitating the skills needed to confront life transitions follows a series of steps.

- The skill has to be defined in strict behavioural terms. It is no use using general terms such as 'relating better to people'. How to relate should be specified in a series of exact behaviours.
- The reasons for using a particular technique should be discussed, and the skill itself should be presented and debated.
- Some sort of yardstick or benchmark should be specified that relates to attainment criteria. People need to know when they have achieved certain levels of competence.
- It is useful to present clients with examples of effective and ineffective skills so that they can see the differences between the two.

- The skills should be practised under supervision where possible. It is not always possible for direct supervision of skills to take place, but immediate feedback on skill attainment does provide the best learning environment.
- Emphasis should be placed on continued behavioural rehearsal and practice in 'real life' contexts.
- If necessary, a behavioural checklist should be constructed for feedback. Other evaluation methods and techniques ought to be discussed.

Therefore, the format of the process of skill attainment includes an understanding of what is required, a demonstration of the skill and practice of the skill with feedback. Thus this model, or approach to life events, emphasises the role of the nurse as a teacher rather than as someone involved in clinical treatment, and there is an emphasis on prevention and 'growth' rather than treatment and cure.

A categorisation model

In contrast to the other two approaches, Moos (1986) presents a model that sets out two categories of tasks and skills that can be used to manage life transitions and crises. It is based on an analysis of a wide range of crises such as bereavement, disasters, abduction and chronic illness. The model first sets out a series of adaptive tasks which will be needed to handle the crisis; second, it describes sets of coping skills people use in a crisis; and third, it looks at factors that determine individual differences in response to crises. It will be seen that some of the features of this model are included in other models as well.

Adaptive tasks

- *Establishing meaning.* After the initial shock of the event has subsided, there is a need to understand the significance of the situation in terms of its consequences for individual adaptation. Explanations should be developed to account for the event and people should try to accept and construct a foundation for their present circumstances.
- *Confronting reality.* During any crisis or transition there are numerous tasks to be completed which are related to the event. For instance, after the death of a loved one there are funeral arrangements to be made and finances to be sorted out. People often need help in confronting these tasks so that they can deal with the main crisis.
- *Sustaining relationships.* Maintaining contact with family and friends can be a difficult task during a crisis or transition. Friends of a woman who has miscarried may not know whether or when she would like a visit. Sometimes, owing to the nature of the relationships between people and their families, communication can be difficult. Thus it is necessary to maintain adequate levels of social support within the individual's social network. Furthermore, nurses can play a significant role in creating empathic communication between family members.

- *Maintaining emotional balance.* The nature of the crisis will determine the strength and type of emotional response. However, it is important for people to try to maintain a degree of emotional balance in order to develop a positive perspective when dealing with the event. This is not to deny the individual any emotional response, as most crises involve powerful emotions, but being able to maintain a balance is the first step in developing more control over the circumstances.
- *Preserving self-image.* Many life crises involve a reduction in self-image. This is particularly evident in cases of rape. However, people who have been through a divorce may well experience difficulties in forming new relationships, owing to a low image of themselves and lack of self-confidence. It is important for the nurse to strike a balance between giving help and allowing the person to develop their own solutions and thus develop greater self-esteem.

Moos (1986) says that while all five adaptive tasks are necessary in each crisis, some will be more relevant than others depending on the specific characteristics of the event. Parents of chronically ill or disabled children will face a number of specific tasks in adapting to their child's condition (Canam, 1993). It is extremely difficult to maintain emotional balance in the case of death of a child and it may be equally difficult to regain self-esteem after rape. Thus the event, and an individual's response to it, will determine the priority of adaptive tasks.

The adaptive tasks are not easy to implement and require many coping skills to deal with them. Moos suggests that the coping skills people use in response to crises and transitions may be categorised into three groups: *appraisal-focused, problem-focused* and *emotion-focused.*

Appraisal-focused coping

This group of skills tries to modify the meaning of the situation. If a crisis is expected, such as the death of a loved one, people will often mentally prepare themselves for the event. Recalling successes in coping with past events can also prove helpful. Sometimes a crisis that seems overpowering can be better understood if it is dissected, or broken down, into manageable elements. Another appraisal-focused skill is the ability to redefine the situation in a more positive light. This may take the form of a comparison with others who are less fortunate, or it may involve constructing alternative 'worse case scenarios'. Finally, as has been stated before, denial can prove to be a positive response to a crisis in the short term if it gives a person a certain amount of 'breathing space' to come to terms with the event.

Problem-focused coping

Confronting the problem and dealing with its consequences form the main focus of this set of skills. Information skills are concerned with obtaining information about the crisis and investigating appropriate courses of action. Nurses can contribute a great deal to the development of information skills, not just by providing knowledge, but by helping the patient to develop the skill of obtaining knowledge.

A further set of skills relate to the ability to solve problems. Again, nurses can help with the development of these skills. The aim is to create an environment where people are able to cultivate a sense of competence and self-esteem. New skills go hand-in-hand with changing activities and exploring new sources of accomplishment. Thus, after a sudden death or divorce the person may experience a need to become involved in self-help groups or to seek alternative activities. Indeed, the presence of chronic illness or disability is likely to dictate a totally new perspective on life.

Emotion-focused coping

One of the adaptive tasks is emotional control, but this should not be achieved at the expense of 'bottling up' emotions. Initially it is perfectly appropriate for people who are undergoing a crisis to give vent to their feelings. This may include not only crying but anger and despair too. Sometimes laughter is involved; this does not mean that the person is uncaring, but it can reduce tension. After emotional discharge a degree of control can often be exercised and people can then start to accept the situation. Moos calls this 'resigned acceptance' and sees it as representing a conscious decision to accept things for what they are.

Variables affecting the ways in which people cope with crises and transitions

Having set out adaptive tasks and coping skills, there are three more variables that affect the ways in which people deal with life crises and transitions.

Demographic and individual differences

Age, gender, ethnicity and socio-economic status are factors known to affect the ways in which individuals manage life crises. People's cognitive and emotional maturity, their self-confidence and how they dealt with previous crises are important factors as well.

Event-related factors

These refer to the type of stressor. The specific characteristics of the events themselves will likewise effect the style of crisis management. Controllable events will command more problem-focused strategies, whereas uncontrollable events will elicit emotion-focused responses.

Environmental factors

Aspects of the social and physical environment refer to social support and cohesion, institutional community resources and voluntary services. Social cohesion can lead to the expenditure of more coping resources in tightly knit families; however, in most circumstances, social cohesion leads to more positive than negative outcomes. For example, community resources in the guise of child care facilities may prove invaluable to a person who has just become a single parent.

Nursing implications

At first sight the complexity of Moos's model may seem to make it difficult to use, with five adaptational tasks, three types of coping skill and numerous individual, event- and environmental-related factors. However, it can be used as a framework for understanding individual crises and transitions. Oleson and Shadick (1993) applied the model to the nursing care of elderly persons relocating to a nursing home. They suggest that the conceptual model depicts a process by which nurses may help elderly persons cope effectively with relocation. A nurse might think 'How on earth can I help this person? What can I do?' The models presented represent a blueprint for action. One can look at each individual situation and ask questions based on the models such as:

- What are the individual and demographic aspects of this situation? What type of event is this? What social support is available?
- What sort of adaptive tasks have priority?
- What sort of coping skills need to be defined?

And with Hopson:

- Where is this person in the cycle of transition?
- What are the characteristics of the next stage?

And with Danish and D'Augelli:

- What are the skills needed in this particular case?
- How can a programme be constructed to enable individuals to acquire the relevant skills?

Just as the person experiencing crisis or transition needs to break a seemingly overwhelming problem into potentially manageable bits, so too does the nurse.

It may prove useful to bear in mind the models of Hopson, Moos and Danish and D'Augelli when examining some specific crises/transitions such as bereavement, dying, handicap and illness.

Bereavement

Bereavement literally means 'to take away from' and is usually used when someone close has died. Grief is the emotional response to the death, while mourning is the culturally determined expression of bereavement and grief. The majority of the research into bereavement has centred on grief and has attempted to describe the common components of people's emotional response to bereavement. Most studies have attempted to describe grief as a series of stages that need to be worked through in order to achieve a healthy adjustment to loss. There seems to be considerable disagreement about the number of components to the grieving process and also whether it is necessary to proceed through all of them to reach a stage of adjustment. Lindemann (1944) originally proposed that there were three main stages:

- initial shock and emotionality;
- intermediate distress;
- a recovery phase.

Ramsay and deGroot (1977, cited in Gross, 1992) describe nine components to the grief process:

- shock and numbness;
- disorganisation;
- denial and behaving as if the deceased was still alive;
- depression, pining and despair;
- guilt, both real and imagined;
- anxiety about losing control, and the future;
- aggression and anger;
- resolution and an acceptance of the death;
- reintegration where acceptance is put into practice.

Gass and Chang (1989) analysed bereavement in terms of Lazarus's model of stress and coping. They found that both widows and widowers who had lower threat appraisal, more problem-focused and less emotion-focused coping, greater resource strength and younger age suffered less psychosocial health dysfunction.

There are distinct common themes in many of the different approaches to the grief process. Parkes (1986) has summarised these into four main stages:

- *Numbness and denial.* The initial reaction to death is usually characterised by a period of numbness, as if one's feelings have been 'turned off'. Associated with numbness is denial. This often takes the form of pretending that the deceased has in some way managed to escape death.
- *Yearning or pining.* In this stage there is a need to try to recreate the dead person. It is common for people to think that they have seen the deceased in a crowd or heard them speak. Pining, longing and a feeling of emptiness are typical characteristics of this stage.

- *Despair and depression.* Following the acknowledgement of death there is an intense feeling of despair and sometimes depression. A feeling of helplessness and hopelessness at the inability to bring back the dead person often occurs. Other emotions such as anger, guilt and anxiety may also occur in this stage.
- *Recovery and reorganisation.* Hopson (1981) would call this stage 'letting go'. At some point people realise that their lives must go on and they must attempt to break with the past. Acceptance of the death and a search for a new meaning to life are the key elements of this stage. The degree of recovery and the time span of this stage vary from person to person.

These stages should be seen as reflecting the sorts of grief reactions that occur during bereavement. Kalish (1981) has said that the stages should not be viewed as a fixed sequence of events to be followed in order to reach the final goal of recovery. There may be times when yearning and pining are felt at the same time as despair. Recovery may seem to be proceeding well when an event such as an anniversary triggers the whole grief reaction once more.

Nurses' responses to death

Wright (1991) suggests that some emotional responses to death are more difficult to manage than others. Based on his nursing experience in accident and emergency departments, he has drawn up a list of the emotional responses to sudden death that nurses find most difficult to cope with.

- *Withdrawal.* As we have seen, a period of withdrawal is a necessary part of the grieving process, since it enables the bereaved to organise themselves. However, if withdrawal leads to continued strong denial of the death, problems can arise. Under these circumstances it is appropriate to stress to the bereaved that the problem is here to stay and has to be confronted. Wright says that this period is particularly difficult for the nurse because the length varies from individual to individual and it can be hard for nurses to sit and do nothing when they are used to active care. Often the mere presence of someone is all that the bereaved person needs.
- *Denial.* Death affects nurses as well as the bereaved and sometimes going along with their need to deny the actuality of the event seems to be a caring response to their predicament. In the short term little harm will be done by denial responses, but in the long term they will prove counterproductive. Frankness and honesty communicated in a caring fashion are the hallmarks of the correct way to deal with this response.
- *Anger.* Anger often occurs in some form or another, and it can be directed at nurses, doctors, family and even the bereaved themselves. The correct way to deal with anger is not to leap to the defence of the targets of wrath but to realise that it is not a time for well thought out, logical analysis. It is important to try to empathise with the feelings

of the bereaved rather than suppress aggression. Empathy and understanding can be particularly difficult to achieve if the objects of aggression are one's colleagues.

- *Isolation.* Despite being surrounded by people, the bereaved can often feel isolated and alone. This is not the same as withdrawal but can be a response to the need to work through the loss. Nevertheless, attempting to direct attention to family and friends who can help may be counterproductive.
- *Bargaining.* This response is particularly apparent in instances of infant and child death. The parent will promise everything they have, even their own lives, in order to get their lost child back. It is seen by some as an attempt to gain control over an otherwise uncontrollable situation. Parents may get angry if nurses refuse to indulge in this bargaining process, and can start to feel discriminated against.
- *Inappropriate responses.* It may seem strange that the death of a loved one can evoke such a reaction as laughter, yet laughter may be a form of tension release or defence mechanism. Death is a huge strain on the system, and trivial, inappropriate responses may be the body's way of relieving the stress to a certain extent.
- *Guilt.* Sometimes people will test nurses with their feelings of guilt. 'It's all my fault, isn't it?' is a typical guilt response. It is important that nurses are able to reassure the bereaved person either that it is not their fault or that human nature is fallible.
- *Crying.* There are still some people who view crying as a weakness, but on the whole it is seen as a valuable reaction to death. It can break down barriers and it is a relief when it signals the end of pent-up emotion. In some cases people will want to cry but cannot. If it is at all possible they should be encouraged to cry, but sometimes crying will not occur till months, occasionally years, after the event.
- *Unfinished business.* The sudden death of a loved one leaves many things left unsaid. Nurses can help by spending some time listening to regrets about what should have been said or should have been done.

Parathian and Taylor (1993) were concerned that student nurses might be exposed to bad practice in communicating bad news to patients. They found that role modelling was successful in facilitating learning in the nursing students, irrespective of whether they were exposed to a negative instance of a poor model or a positive instance of an expert model.

Wright (1991) says that dealing with the bereaved is never an easy task, owing to the intense feelings associated with the event, and occasionally lack of information about how to deal with people who have just lost someone close to them. But if a nurse knows what to expect and is able to respond with empathy, the whole process can become somewhat less stressful for all concerned.

Bereaved children

How does death affect children? The extent to which death affects children depends on two main variables:

- the child's age;
- the child's experience of death and dying.

The first systematic study of children's conceptions of death was carried out by Nagy (1948) in Budapest. She asked over 400 children aged between 3 and 10 years to write, draw and talk about what they thought death was all about. On the basis of their responses, Nagy proposed that there were different conceptions of death at different ages.

- *Stage 1 (3–5 years old)*. In this stage children have little idea about the permanence of death. They see it as a temporary state, akin to sleeping. Indeed, one child said that the reason you had to be quiet at funerals was because you might wake the dead person up. Also, if certain requirements are met the dead person might come back to life. Therefore, according to Nagy, there is little finality to a young child's sense of death.
- *Stage 2 (5–9 years old)*. As children of this age group tend to view the world in 'concrete' terms, their conceptions of death are similar. Death now has a visual representation as the 'bogey man' or a skeleton in a black cloak. People who are clever manage to outwit death and escape. Thus one's longevity depends on how good one is at escaping death when it comes to call.
- *Stage 3 (9 years old and above)*. In this stage children develop an adult concept of death. It is viewed as inevitable, universal and irreversible.

Sometimes children confuse cause and effect and link together two unrelated events. For instance, a grandparent always said to her grandson that he should remember to brush his teeth twice a day. On the day that the grandmother died the boy forgot to brush his teeth. He thinks that not brushing his teeth led to the death of his grandmother and feels that he is to blame for her death. It may seem ridiculous to us as adults, but to the young boy it makes sense.

The second factor that affects children's concept of death is the extent of their experience of death and dying. Situations such as the death of a pet animal can promote a child's understanding of what it means to die. Bluebond-Langner (1977) found that young children suffering from terminal illnesses were able to conceive of death as being irreversible, through experiences such as the death of pets and so on. Therefore there are situations that tend to force children to view death in an adult fashion.

Schaefer and Lyons (1986) produced some guidelines on how to tell children about death. They suggest that it is no use saying things like 'Granny has just gone to sleep', as this can create false fears of sleeping. Rather, the child should be given an explanation as to why everyone is so sad (for example, 'Mummy and Daddy are sad because . . .') and be told what dead means (for example, 'The person's body has stopped working and won't go any more').

Of course children will be upset by these explanations, but Weber and Fournier (1985) say that trying to shelter children may limit their ability to learn through practical experience about this extremely important life-cycle event, and may lead them to fear death excessively.

Coping with dying

The most famous student of the process of death is undoubtedly Elizabeth Kübler-Ross (Kübler-Ross, 2000). She proposes that there are five stages to the process of dying (see Table 6.2).

Many dying patients do not always follow the trajectory predicted by Kübler-Ross and therefore the stage theory should not be accepted as a manual for dealing with dying patients. The stages of the process of dying do represent the sorts of problems the dying patient is likely to encounter, but the order and strength of the experience may

Table 6.2 *The five stages in the process of dying* (after Kübler-Ross)

I   *Shock and denial.* Denial helps prevent the patient from being overwhelmed by the initial shock of realising that they are facing death. Patients may go from doctor to doctor in the hope of obtaining a different diagnosis. Compartmentalisation, where patients hold simultaneous contradictory beliefs, may also occur. For example, they may accept that they are going to die but at the same time discuss long-term plans.

II   *Anger.* An essential stage in coming to terms with death. It is the most difficult stage to deal with because the patient's anger may come out in all directions, sometimes apparently at random. Feelings of resentment towards healthy people and 'why me?' occur at this stage.

III   *Bargaining.* In this stage the patient attempts to postpone death, often trying to 'strike a bargain with God'. This can take the form of agreeing to devote one's life to worthy causes if one is allowed to live. Bargaining involves 'faulty thought' or 'magical thinking' similar to that seen in young children's ideas about death. Depression can set in once the patient realises that no bargain can be struck.

IV   *Depression.* According to Kübler-Ross, depression occurs in approximately half the cases of people who are dying. It may be seen as a form of anticipatory grief and disengagement, but it can cause problems for the patient's family. The patient is preparing to die but friends and family are encouraging them to hold on to life a bit longer. In this stage, the patient needs permission to die so that they can let go of the people they hold dear.

V   *Acceptance.* This stage is characterised by withdrawal from others and from 'worldly concerns'. Kübler-Ross views this time as being neither happy nor sad, but a time for contemplation. This is a peaceful period, almost devoid of feeling, where the individual develops a degree of quiet expectation.

vary. Sometimes denial and acceptance alternate throughout the living–dying interval; sometimes anger is felt after bargaining and again later on. However, if patients are given the opportunity to work through the problems outlined by Kübler-Ross, they, and their families, are likely to experience fewer difficulties during the dying period.

Coping with physical handicap and illness

In 2001 the Office of Population Censuses and Surveys produced evidence that in an average health district of 250,000 about 250 people under the age of 65 years would need some form of special care owing to impairment or disability. The World Health Organisation (1980) distinguishes between impairment, disability and handicap thus:

- *Impairment* is the basic physical effect caused by illness or disease on the body or the brain.
- *Disability* is the loss of function resulting from impairment.
- *Handicap* is the social and occupational disadvantage that results from a disability.

Coping with disability

Wilkinson (1989) puts forward some factors that can influence the way people cope with becoming disabled.

- *The age of acquisition.* Congenital conditions such as spina bifida tend to have a different effect on a family than diseases that tend to be acquired later in life such as Parkinson's disease.
- *Insidious versus traumatic conditions.* Insidious diseases are diseases, such as rheumatoid arthritis, that develop gradually in people who have previously enjoyed good health. Traumatic injuries that occur suddenly, such as injuries to the spinal cord, will have a different psychological impact.
- *The stability of the condition and the prognosis.* The extent to which diseases are likely to remain stable, such as cerebral palsy, or are likely to progress, such as muscular dystrophy, will influence the individual's perception of the future.
- *The severity of disability and degree of dependence.* Different demands will be placed on carers according to the severity of the disability. The degree to which the person is restricted also affects the degree of dependence and may place further demands on carers.
- *Intellectual functioning and personality change.* Head injury and brain damage can lead to multiple disabilities affecting not only mobility, but also memory and social judgement as well. Personality changes require specific consideration.
- *Pain and other illness.* The presence or absence of pain and the frequency of periods of associated illness will affect psychological adjustment.

Research based on coping with disability is divided into two areas: an individual focus and the social context.

The individual focus attempts to view disability as a person's positive or negative reaction to their condition. In this respect one might predict that disability would invariably result in psychological distress and discomfort. Research findings are equivocal on this matter. For instance, Gardiner (1980) found greater psychological disturbances than normal in a group of rheumatoid arthritis sufferers; Motet-Grigoras and Schuckit (1986) found higher levels of depression and alcohol abuse in a group of congenitally disabled young men than in a group of similarly aged controls. However, Kostin (1973) found disabled people were not significantly different from non-disabled people with respect to overall adjustment and satisfaction with life. These differences may be explained with reference to the models of Danish and D'Augelli, Hopson and Moos presented earlier in the chapter. The degree to which people with a disability experience psychological problems will depend on various factors, including the following.

- The person's position on the 'cycle of reactions'. If a person has experienced a debilitating condition, their psychological state will mirror the degree to which they have progressed through the cycle of reactions. Thus, if a person has not managed to 'let go' of their former selves, they are liable to be depressed. If on the other hand they have managed to see themselves as a person with a disability in one area but expertise in many more, then they will have achieved a state of integration and feel more self-confident about dealing with the world.
- The extent to which the person has used adaptive tasks and developed coping skills. The ability to confront reality, establish the meaning and significance of the situation, maintain a reasonable emotional balance and develop a satisfactory self-image will determine the degree to which people with a handicap experience psychological distress.

Coping with illness

One of the first problems is finding out whether one is actually ill or not. This may seem a somewhat superficial issue, but how many of us have decided that we feel ill and have gone to see our doctor only to feel better in the waiting room? What do you do? Do you pretend that you still have the symptoms or do you say to your doctor, 'Well, I did feel ill, but do you know, I feel better now'? The perception of physical symptoms is not as 'clear-cut' as many people may think.

An illustration of the psychological, as opposed to the psychiatric, factors involved in the perception of illness is provided by the 'June Bug' incident. A textile mill in the United States was closed down because many of the workers fell ill with a mysterious illness, the 'June Bug', so called because of the month in which the 'epidemic' occurred.

It was thought that a 'bug' (insect) had infested the materials in the mill, but no evidence of its existence could be found.

Usually when no physical explanations exist for an illness, other factors are said to be involved. In this case a psychiatric explanation was put forward in the guise of a conversion reaction such as mass hysteria or hysterical contagion. A conversion reaction is the loss, or alteration, of a sensory or motor function. It is an unconscious process whereby an unacceptable reaction to a situation is converted into some sort of bodily feeling or loss of function. Such disorders are known to occur during times of stress and so it was hypothesised that the workers in the mill had converted their stress into this mysterious disease. Stress may well have been a factor in the condition, but the presumption that the disease was a case of mass hysteria is unfounded, as there is a simpler psychological explanation for this train of events at the textile mill.

The employees of the mill were all under a great deal of stress, since it was the height of the production season. The stress revealed itself in many different ways, including a number of unpleasant bodily sensations. As soon as some of the workers started to collapse, the others who were close by searched for an explanation to the events happening around them. In this case, the remaining workers formed an 'illness hypothesis' based on presumed insect infestation. The workers' 'funny feelings' now had some legitimate label – they were the result of a virus. As word got around the mill, more and more people thought that their feelings were the June Bug virus and their thoughts would be reinforced by people 'dropping like flies' all over the factory. This feature of illness behaviour is known as *mass psychogenic illness*.

Pennebaker (1984) says that symptom perception is characterised by two processes: *external* versus *internal sensory information* and *hypothesis construction*.

External versus internal sensory information

Information comes to the brain from two main sources: outside the body and from within it. At any one time, external information is competing with internal information for the individual's attention. Thus, when the external environment is relatively 'quiet', increased attention is paid to information coming from within the body. Similarly, when the external environment requires a great deal of concentration, less notice is taken of internal sensations. Therefore, people are much more likely to report internal physical symptoms and sensations when the external environment is boring or lacking in information.

Pennebaker says that if one listens to people in the cinema, there will be more coughing during the boring parts of the film than during the exciting scenes. People notice the tickling in their throats especially when someone else coughs, drawing attention to the internal sensation. Similarly, people who perceive their occupation as boring and dull report more physical symptoms and take more medication than people with interesting and absorbing jobs. Alternatively, when the external environment is particularly stimulating, or when one is concentrating on a complex task, the pain of a toothache or headache becomes less noticeable. In summary, it seems that we are more likely to notice internal sensations when the external environment is quiet, and less likely to sense these sensations when the perceptual system is engrossed in a stimulating task.

Hypothesis construction

Another aspect of symptom perception is the tendency to jump to conclusions about what is wrong, set up a hypothesis and look for details to support it. Once a framework has been established, items from the external environment are selected to fit in with it. An example of this would be a person who thinks they have a particular disease and then constructs an 'illness hypothesis' to fit the symptoms. Each internal sensation that fits the illness hypothesis is heralded as evidence of the presence of the disease; each sensation that disconfirms the illness hypothesis is ignored. Thus different people may interpret the same 'symptoms' in diverse ways because they frame their sensations differently.

Exercise 6.2 *Sensation*

This exercise is based on an experiment by Anderson and Pennebaker (1980).

Spilt your participants into three groups. Prepare some strips of reasonably rough sandpaper or emery paper. Before the experiment, tell all the participants that they have to sign a consent form as standard practice. However, there are in fact three different consent forms for the three different participant groups. These should be worded as follows.

1 I understand that I will come into contact with a stimulus that has been found to produce a mild decree of pain.
2 I understand that I will come into contact with a stimulus that has been found to produce a mild degree or pleasure.
3 I understand that I will come into contact with a stimulus that produces a sensation.

Give each participant a piece of sandpaper and ask them to place their middle fingers on the sandpaper and rub them up and down for a minute or so. It is important that each group has as little contact with the others as possible.

After touching the sandpaper, each participant has to rate the stimulus on a thirteen-point pain–pleasure scale. Provide each subject with the following scale

    –6 –5 –4 –3 –2 –1 0 1 2 3 4 5 6
    Pain   Pleasure

In the Anderson and Pennebaker (1980) experiment, participants in the pain group produced an average rating of –1.00 The participants in the pleasure group produced an average rating of +1.01, and the participants in the control group produced an average rating of +0.13.

The results you obtain may, or may not, replicate those of Anderson and Pennebaker; however it is important to remember the basic principles underlying the exercise – the relationship between a cognitive framework and the experience of emotion.

A final illustration of the interrelationship of symptom perception and different cognitive frameworks is given by Ruble (1977). The participants in the experiment were forty women who were selected because they all menstruated on the same day. They were given a simulated electroencephalic examination which they were told could locate their position in their menstrual cycle with a high degree of accuracy. On the basis of the supposed results the women were split into three groups.

- *Premenstrual group.* They were informed that they were within a day or two of beginning menstruation.
- *Intermenstrual group.* They were told not to expect the onset of menstruation for 7–10 days.
- *Control group.* They were not given any information.

All three groups completed a questionnaire about the physical and psychological symptoms associated with menstruation. The results indicated that the women in the premenstrual group rated themselves as experiencing more water retention, pain, changes in eating habits and different levels of arousal than women who believed themselves to be intermenstrual. Ruble did not deny the physical aspects of menstruation, but argued that the cognitive framework regarding the cycle location influenced the experience of symptoms.

The psychological components of illness perception have considerable significance for hypochondriasis. A common misconception of the hypochondriac is of a person who is 'putting it on'. Whilst in some cases patients who know they are healthy but wish to be sick may attempt to hoodwink the nurse into thinking that they have some ailment, the majority of hypochondriacs have a genuine although misplaced belief that they are ill. Barsky and Klerman (1983) define hypochondriasis as 'an unrealistic interpretation of one's bodily sensations as abnormal, leading to the fear and belief that one has a serious disease'. They put forward three possible reasons for the disorder.

- *Amplification of sensations.* Patients who are hypochondriacs amplify and enhance normal bodily sensations. They report increased arousal and heightened perceptual sensitivity.

- *Misinterpretation of symptoms.* Normal bodily sensations resulting from such things as indigestion and stomach flutter are misinterpreted as indications of serious illness. The incorrect diagnosis leads to an increase in emotional response which in turn can exacerbate the sensations, thus leading to a firmer conviction that they are ill.
- *Predisposition to think in physical terms.* The hypochondriac has a predisposition to view the world in physical terms. He or she is oversensitive to physical sensation and eager to substantiate feelings as indicators of dysfunction.

In summary, the primary underlying disorder of hypochondriasis is a perceptual or cognitive defect rather than the illness behaviour itself. As such, the patient will benefit from treatments that seek to identify the defect and address the irrational thoughts. The cognitive therapies mentioned in the previous chapter, such as stress inoculation training, seem ideally suited to achieve this reorientation of thought.

Once it has been established that illness is actually present, the ways in which people cope with illness will depend on several factors.

- *Severity of illness.* Although the severity of illness does not always correspond with the strength of psychological reactions, some illnesses, such as cancer and heart disease, usually produce more noticeable psychological responses than, say, asthma and arthritis, but not always. There is a range of considerable individual differences in response to illness. The person who has started to lose their hearing in one ear may construe this event as devastating, whereas the person who has been told that they have kidney disease may take it in their stride and come to terms with their circumstances.
- *Location in the body.* The site of the clinical disorder has particular significance for the patient. Clearly, people who are particularly active respond badly to illness which limits their mobility. However, disabling disorders seem to be seen as more of a threat by men than by women, while women tend to react especially badly to disfiguring diseases. Kincey (1989) says that psychological responses to surgery such as mastectomy may depend on several factors such as culture, age, personality and coping strategies. Therefore, it is important to view the disfigurement in a broad context rather than to apply only specific codes of practice.
- *Onset and duration of illness.* An unexpected and acute onset of illness may cause a number of problems in the short term, but if the illness is relatively brief, the problems will usually be resolved quite quickly. Chronic illness may have less initial impact on the patient than acute illness but often involves considerable long-term readjustment.
- *Social factors.* Experiencing illness when starting a new job is particularly troublesome, but it may seem a 'blessing in disguise' if one is looking for an excuse to escape from a difficult situation. The reactions of family and friends will also have an effect on the patient's perception of the severity of the illness and the delay between deciding that

they are ill and seeking treatment. Recovery from illness tends to be quicker in those patients who have high levels of social support from family and friends.

Models for coping with illness

Both Moos's (1986) and Hopson's (1981) models can usefully be applied to illness. Moos's approach is useful in distinguishing between the problem-focused and emotion-focused coping strategies. Thus problem-focused procedures are used to seek information, learn new skills and participate in treatment programmes. Obtaining information ranges from becoming more familiar with different forms of treatment to learning more about the causes of the illness. New skills that are associated with illness will vary in terms of their complexity. Running a home dialysis machine can seem more daunting than discovering a new way of sleeping. It is important for patients to discover, with help, their own ways of coping with the limitations imposed by illness. Specific ways of walking or sitting may minimise pain, and rearranging the home environment can often facilitate independence. Kline Leidy *et al.* (1990) propose a framework based upon nursing theory. A major premise is that individuals with limited psychosocial attributes and a preponderance of unmet basic needs will be more likely to perceive events as threatening and thus experience heightened symptoms and acute exacerbations of their illness.

Emotion-focused strategies necessarily deal with the emotional demands and consequences of illness. Moos illustrates the importance of allowing the patient time to come to terms with their condition by permitting initial denial. Helping the patient to be more objective and less overwhelmed is a useful coping strategy which at the same time permits an expression of feeling.

Hopson's model is especially relevant to those 'patients whose reaction to illness produces strong emotional feelings. When these reactions are perceived as abnormal, intervention is required. The commonest psychological response to illness is depression, which is one of the axes in Hopson's cycle of reactions. Depression is most prevalent after the initial stage of illness and it is estimated that between 20 and 30 per cent of patients suffer from depression in some form or other due to illness. When the full meaning of the situation sinks in, the person can sink to the bottom of the cycle and remain there indefinitely. The feelings of helplessness and hopelessness associated with illness result in a passive, often withdrawn response, to the situation.

If there are strong feelings of guilt, then patients may feel that the illness is justified and self-blame can occur. If, owing to self-blame, patients try to change their maladaptive behaviour so that there is less chance of the illness recurring, a small amount of self-blame can be advantageous.

Another strong emotion that tends to occur alongside depression is anxiety. This occurs as a consequence of uncertainty about the cause and outcome of the illness. It may not necessarily be related to the illness itself but may be a general response to the circumstances and conditions surrounding the patient. Coping with anxiety takes many different forms, and these have been discussed in detail elsewhere in this book. It is important to identify the type of coping strategy used by the patient and then match the treatment procedures accordingly. Thus, if a patient is using a 'vigilant' coping strategy, they will find a lack of information stressful. If, however, they are using a 'denial' coping strategy, too much detail will be counterproductive.

Nicholls (2003) makes some interesting points regarding psychological intervention in physical illness. He believes that there are three key areas of skill: *emotional care, informational care* and *counselling.*

- *Emotional care.* There is a need for care to be based on an understanding that emotional responses are part of illness. Therefore it is necessary for nurses to be able to recognise and acknowledge this part of being ill. An important skill is to be able to recognise how patients are coping and what their specific concerns about their illness are. Enabling patients to express their concerns can be difficult, but Nicholls says that this can be achieved by:
  1 making the situation non-threatening;
  2 providing the means for patients to recognise their own feelings;
  3 facilitating the expression of emotion;
  4 communicating understanding, empathy and acceptance;
  5 devoting time and support.
- *Providing information.* Since patients respond to illness and cope with it in different ways it is important to find out what they know and what they want to know. It is also necessary to realise that a patient's need for information may change over time. Therefore reluctance to discuss the details of a condition at one point does not mean that this will always be the case. Continual monitoring is required to be aware of new areas of need and evaluation of previous procedures.
- *Counselling.* This involves some of the skills examined in Chapter 1. Listening to patients and facilitating the examination of problems and fears is of primary importance in nursing care. Similarly, patients need help to explore their situation and come to an understanding of their feelings and responses. Being able to empathise with patients makes these tasks a lot easier as it is only after the predicament has been explored thoroughly that one can move on to suggesting solutions. If there is one main fault that nurses tend to make, it is jumping to conclusions too quickly. Patients need time and space to come to terms with their circumstances, and often what seems an obvious solution turns out to be inappropriate.

Summary

There are many different life crises and illnesses requiring specific forms of nursing care. Each crisis, event, transition and illness needs further analysis to understand all the issues involved. However, it is hoped that this chapter has provided the framework, or schema within which to interpret, and act on, all types of crisis and transition. The framework is not a fixed template but a process of perceiving empathically the events that patients experience.

Conundrum revisited

No matter how robust the individual proves, social support networks usually prove influential in helping individuals to cope with change. Understanding and working with social support networks can help the nurse improve care. Whilst networks are themselves disrupted by change they usually help the individual to interpret what is happening and to choose courses of action which reduce stress. Friends may, for instance, help the nurse deal with guilt about working harder and longer. They may reaffirm commitment even though contacts are now by telephone. They may help the nurse to rate the adjustment as less stressful and sustain feelings of self-competence at a time when new work requires additional learning. We hope you found that the social support network map prompted your colleague to talk about psychological concepts which are not only important regarding change but which help explain how the individual uses others to help her cope. Here, for example, is one colleague who completed this exercise talking in terms that seem very similar to those of Moos (1986) described in Chapter 11 (p. 376).

> It would be a nice surprise, wouldn't it, but my first impression is that it would mean work even to get to grips with what the change meant. I mean I would find myself trying to track all the implications of the new job. It's what my daughter would describe as a 'very grown up move' and that probably means being even more serious and professional than I am now. I would have to face how that felt, what it meant to my husband too. Then I would have to take others with me, hoping that they felt reassured by how I said I would deal with all this.

Not all social support networks work equally well, though. Some people have very thin networks with few friends in the inner or middle circle. Men tend to describe much thinner social support networks than women. Again, people who live rough on the streets are unlikely to feel well supported or to cope with life change so well. Other social support networks have relatively few connections between individuals. They are fragmented, so that the individual feels reliant upon several people to alert others to his or her situation and to secure guidance or help. Heavy reliance upon one or two friends may damage the relationships and undermine the network longer term.

As you look at the social support network did you notice where the majority of arrows pointed? Sometimes the individual draws the majority of arrows pointing inwards to the centre. Such individuals may be reporting a sense of vulnerability and/or the generosity of friends. Typically, though, a number of arrows are pointing outwards from the centre and richly between other individuals. This map suggests a considerable degree of mutual dependence and help and represents a promising network that is well equipped to help the individual manage change. You may have noted that there were some initials among the individual's friends where lots of arrows coalesced ('a star'). Such individuals are highly influential in change management. How did your colleague talk about these people as she reflected upon the change? Would you hope to meet and work with such an individual, had the nurse suffered a life-changing illness?

? Questions for further consideration

1 Distinguish between the concepts of crisis and transition.
2 What are the stages of bereavement? Do they have to occur in any specific order?
3 Discuss Erikson's Eight Stages of Life.
4 Examine the psychological components of illness perception.
5 Discuss the main issues surrounding nursing people with disabilities.
6 Compare and contrast the models of coping with life transitions, events and crises.

References

Anderson, D. B. and Pennebaker, J. W. (1980). Pain and pleasure: alternative interpretations of identical stimulation. *European Journal of Social Psychology, 10,* 207–212.

Barsky, A. J. and Klerman, G. L. (1983). Overview: hypochondriasis, bodily complaints, and somatic styles. *American Journal of Psychiatry, 140,* 273–283.

Bee, H. (1989). *The Developing Child.* 5th edn. New York: Harper and Row.

Bee, H. and Boyd, D. R. (2003). *Developing Child.* London: Allyn Bacon.

Bluebond-Langner, M. (1977). Meanings of death to children. In: Feifel, H. (ed.) *New Meanings of Death.* New York: McGraw Hill.

Canam, C. (1993). Common adaptive tasks facing parents of children with chronic conditions. *Journal of Advanced Nursing, 18,* 46–53.

Danish, S. J. and D'Augelli, A. R. (1982). *Helping Skills* II, *Life Development Intervention.* New York: Human Sciences Press.

Erikson, E. H. (1963). *Childhood and Society.* 2nd edn. New York: Norton.

Felner, R. D., Farber, S. S. and Primavera, J. (1985). Transitions and stressful life events: a model for primary prevention. In: Felner, R. D., Jason, L. A. and Moritsugu, J. N. (eds) *Preventive Psychology.* Oxford: Pergamon Press.

Gardiner, B. M. (1980). Psychological aspects of rheumatoid arthritis. *Psychological Medicine, 10,* 159–165.

Gass, K. A. and Chang, A. S. (1989). Appraisals of bereavement, coping, resources, and psychosocial health dysfunction in widows and widowers. *Nursing Research, 38,* 31–36.

Gross, R. D. (1992). *Psychology: The Science of Mind and Behaviour.* 2nd edn. London: Hodder and Stoughton.

Holmes, T. H. and Rahe, R. H. (1967). The social readjustment rating scale. *Journal of Psychosomatic Research, 11,* 213–218.

Hopson, B. (1981). Response to papers by Schlossberg, Brammer and Abrego. *Counselling Psychology, 9,* 36–39.

Janis, I. L. and Mann, L. (1977). *Decision Making: A psychological analysis of conflict, choice and commitment.* New York: Free Press.

Kalish, R. A. (1981). *Death, Grief and Caring Relationships.* Monterey CA: Brooks Cole.

Kanner, A. D., Coyne, J. C., Schaefer, C. and Lazarus, R. S. (1981). Comparison of two modes of stress measurement: daily hassles and uplifts versus major life events. *Journal of Behavioural Medicine, 4,* 1–39.

Kimmell, D. C. (1980). *Adulthood and Aging.* 2nd edn. Chichester: Wiley.

Kincey, J. (1989). Surgery. In: Broome, A. K. (ed.) *Health Psychology: Processes and Applications.* London: Chapman and Hall.

Kline Leidy, N., Ozbolt, J. G. and Swain, M. A. (1990). Psychophysiological processes of stress in chronic physical illness: a theoretical perspective. *Journal of Advanced Nursing, 15,* 478–486.

Kostin, M. (1973). The life satisfaction of non-normal persons. *Journal of Consulting and Clinical Psychology, 41,* 207–214.

Kübler-Ross, E. (2000). *On Death and Dying.* Tavistock: Routledge.

Lindemann, E. (1944). Symptomatology and management of acute grief. *American Journal of Psychiatry, 101,* 141–148.

Moos, R. H. (1986). *Coping with Life Crises: An integrated approach.* New York: Plenum.

Motet-Grigoras, C. N. and Schuckit, M. A. (1986). Depression and substance abuse in handicapped young men. *Journal of Clinical Psychiatry, 47,* 234–237.

Nagy,-M. H. (1948). The child's theories concerning death. *Journal of Genetic Psychology, 73,* 3–27.

Nicholls, K. A. (2003). *Psychological Care for Ill and Injured People: A clinical guide.* Maidenhead: Open University Press.

Oleson, M. and Shadick, K. M. (1993). Application of Moos and Schaefer's (1986) model to nursing care of elderly persons relocating in a nursing home. *Journal of Advanced Nursing, 18,* 479–485.

Parathian, A. R. and Taylor, F. (1993). Can we insulate trainee nurses from exposure to bad practice? A study of role play in communicating bad news to patients. *Journal of Advanced Nursing, 18,* 801–807.

Parkes, C. M. (1986). *Bereavement.* London: Tavistock.

Pennebaker, J. W. (1984). Accuracy of symptom perception. In: Baum, A., Taylor, S. E. and Singer, J. E. (eds) *Handbook of Psychology and Health.* Hillsdale NJ: Erlbaum.

Ruble, D. (1977). Premenstrual symptoms: a reinterpretation. *Science, 197,* 291–292.

Schaefer, D. and Lyons, C. (1986). *How do We tell the Children?* New York: Newmarket Press.

Weber, J. A. and Fournier, D. G. (1985). Family support and the child's adjustment to death. *Family Relations, 34,* 43–49.

Wilkinson, S. M. (1989). Psychological aspects of physical disability. In: Broome, A. K. (ed.) *Health Psychology: Processes and applications.* London: Chapman and Hall.

World Health Organisation, (1980). *International Classification of Impairments, Disabilities and Handicaps.* Geneva: WHO.

Wright, B. (1991). *Sudden Death: Intervention skills for the caring professions.* Edinburgh: Churchill Livingstone.

Young, V. C. (1987). Hassles, Uplifts, and Life Events as Predictors of Health. Unpublished doctoral dissertation. University of California, Berkeley.

Further reading

Bruce, N. and Carpenter, K. (eds) (1992). *Personal Coping: Theory, research, and application.* Westport CT: Praeger. Not only does this book contain a number of interesting chapters on life stress and coping, but it also contains an exposition of Moos's model of coping that is related to personal growth. The approach, which is also known as the model of Schaefer and Moos, is discussed in the context of a number of life crises.

Hopson, Barrie and Scally, Michael (1993). *Transitions: Positive Changes in your Life.* Englewood Cliffs NJ: Prentice Hall. This is a practical book designed to help people manage their own life transitions. It is based on the Hopson model discussed in this chapter and provides a good account of how to develop a response to life events.

Nichols, Keith (2003). *Psychological Care for Ill and Injured People.* Milton Keynes: Open University Press. This book investigates the psychological factors that are important in a wide range of physical illnesses. It also concentrates on the effects that hospitalisation can have on behaviour. Of particular interest is the emphasis on client-centred care.

Lutz, Tom (1999) *Crying: The Natural and Cultural History of Tears.* New York: Norton. Crying is examined from many different perspectives. We all do it, although men should, apparently, only do it once in public.

Wright, B. (1993). *Caring in Crisis.* 2nd edn. Edinburgh: Churchill Livingstone. Much of the content of the book is based on the author's extensive experience in Accident and Emergency departments. It provides a practical account of how to deal with 'crises' such as bereavement and aggression, and gives information that is specifically directed at nurses.

7

The Biopsychosocial Perspective

(1) Individual Differences

A practice conundrum

Illness or treatment may result in a wide range of psychological traumas, one of which is altered body image. A patient may be said to suffer from altered body image when his or her physical function, appearance or body sensations cause distress and significantly inhibit the ability to lead a satisfying life. Altered body image has been particularly associated with mutilating treatments, especially radical surgery associated with solid tumours (cancer) and chemotherapy to deal with widespread tumour dissemination. What is surprising though is that the nature of illness and the level of disfigurement caused are not entirely predictive of whether a patient will suffer a significant altered body image. Some patients with quite radical treatment (e.g. surgery to the head and neck) experience surprisingly modest levels of body image disruption. Other patients with more modest treatment though sometimes experience significant distress regarding their body image.

Before reading this chapter, make a list of some of the factors that may determine how patients experience alterations to their body image and why there is so much variance in the level of distress described by patients. Why is it difficult to ascertain just which patients may need more body image support?

The purpose of this chapter is to illustrate the links between different levels of explanation of behaviour: the physiological, psychological and social. Starting with psychophysiology, we can see that tumours may be responsible for aggression in the case of Charles Whitman below but do they explain why some people become aggressive on a Saturday night? In other words, in some cases there may be relatively obvious physiological explanations, in others the interplay of physiology, psychology and social factors is more subtle.

Psychophysiology

In 1966 Charles Whitman got up, shot his wife and his mother, and then went out and shot a further fourteen people. There have been many instances of such bizarre, violent acts, but what lies behind this sort of behaviour? In the case of Charles Whitman it was found that he had a huge tumour in the limbic region of his brain. Could the presence of this tumour have been in any way responsible for his behaviour? Physiological psychologists are concerned with answering these sorts of questions by examining the relationship between an individual's physiology and his behaviour.

The nervous system

The majority of psychophysiological research has centred around the human nervous system. This system is made up of a complex pattern of neural activity but has a distinct structure. The first distinction to make is between the *central nervous system* (CNS) and the *autonomic nervous system* (ANS).

The central nervous system

The central nervous system may be described as the 'executive' branch of the body; it regulates feeding and temperature, controls the movement of hands and feet, and produces imagery and thought. The CNS has two main components: the spinal cord and the brain.

The spinal cord

The spinal cord is a mass of nervous tissue occupying the vertebral canal running through the centre of the body. It is about the thickness of the little finger and is protected by bony structures organised into segments. The spinal cord has two major functions:

- It carries information from receptor sites throughout the body to the brain, and conducts information from the brain to muscles and glands;
- It plays an important role in reflexes such as the knee-jerk reaction. Reflex behaviour serves a major function in providing the body with an extremely quick response to stimulation.

The brain

The brain is divided into three parts: the *hindbrain,* the *midbrain* and the *forebrain.*

- The *hindbrain.* The lowest part of the brain, located just above the spinal cord, is the *medulla* (marrow). The medulla is responsible for basic functions such as vomiting, coughing and cardiac function, and a lesion in this area causes immediate death. Just

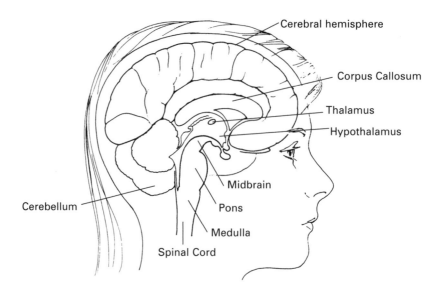

Figure 7.1 Some of the basic structures of the human brain

above the medulla lies the *pons* (bridge) which holds the 'programmes' necessary for fighting, feeding and fleeing. Damage to the pons will result in disruption of these behaviours. Behind the medulla and the pons is the *cerebellum* (little brain) which is similar in appearance to the cortex. The cerebellum is primarily concerned with the regulation of motor activities such as reaching for objects or hitting a tennis ball. Like the pons, it contains the programmes for these often 'unconscious' motor skills, and injury to this area will result in jerky, poorly co-ordinated movements.

- The *midbrain*. This is a relatively small area which forms a bridge between the hindbrain and the forebrain. Along with the pons it contains the *reticular formation* (network). Sometimes known as the *reticular activating system* (RAS), this part of the brain is concerned with maintaining levels of alertness. If an electric current is passed through a wire that has been placed in the reticular formation, an organism will immediately become alert and attentive. Thus the RAS has a significant role to play in the sleep–waking cycle. The midbrain together with the pons and medulla makes up the *brain stem*. The importance of the brain stem is signified by neurologists' use of the term *brainstem death* as an index of brain death. Indeed, the brain stem is, within limits, able to regulate the body's functions in the absence of the forebrain. In some cases of spina bifida much of the forebrain fails to develop (*anencephaly*), but as long as the brainstem is intact the body can live.
- The *forebrain*. Just above and behind the pituitary gland lies the *hypothalamus* which literally means 'under the deep chamber'. This plays an important role in the control of the body's internal functioning, maintaining a balance in the areas of eating and drinking, body temperature, motivation and sexual behaviour. The *thalamus* (deep

chamber) may be described as a large relay centre with connections between the lower portions of the brain and the cerebral cortex. Lying near the thalamus is the *limbic* system (edge or perimeter) which comprises the *amygdala, hippocampus, cingulate gyrus* and *septal area*. The limbic system structures are involved in modulating a wide range of behaviours: learning, memory, anxiety, stress and aggression. The hippocampus has been associated particularly with memory, anxiety and behavioural inhibition. However, it should not be assumed that complex processes, such as memory, are restricted to just one part of the brain; several structures are involved. The *basal ganglia* (nerve knots) are usually associated with motor structures and disorders such as Parkinson's disease and Huntington's chorea. Recently there has been a great deal of interest in the cognitive aspects of a particular part of the basal ganglia called the *caudate nucleus,* which is part of the basal ganglia (see Exercise 7.1).

Exercise 7.1 *The Necker cube*

Look at the cube in Figure 7.2. The cube can be viewed in two ways and if you look at it for a while the second image should become visible. Once you can see them both, the two images will swop around quite regularly. After a while, try to hold one of the images. You will probably find that you can't; the images will continue to swop around. Flowers (1993) found that people suffering from Parkinson's disease take more time than non-sufferers to see the other dimension of the figure and once the two images have begun to interchange find it difficult to hold one for any length of time. It has been suggested that damage caused to the caudate nucleus may be responsible for this particular dysfunction. People suffering from Parkinson's disease often have difficulty in changing from one train of thought to another, but seem to have normal cognitive functioning in other areas of thought processes.

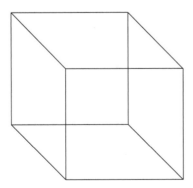

Figure 7.2 The Necker cube

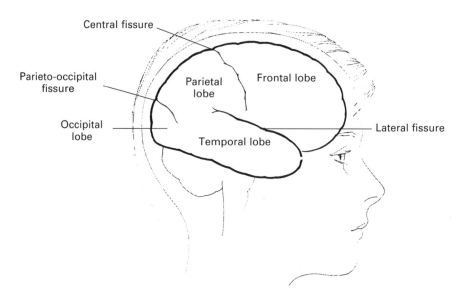

Figure 7.3 The lobes of the human brain

Lying over the parts of the forebrain mentioned so far are the *cerebral hemispheres*. The top layer of the hemispheres is called the *cerebral cortex* and is made up of a large series of grooves or convolutions, necessary to pack the 30 cm of surface area into such a small space. The cortex is divided by a number of fissures into four regions or lobes: *frontal, parietal, occipital* and *temporal* (see Figure 7.3).

The frontal lobe contains the *motor cortex* which is concerned with the control of movement in various parts of the body. More cortex is taken up with those parts of the body which require sensitivity or large amounts of precise motor control, such as the fingers, whereas less cortex is taken up with the trunk. Damage to the motor cortex does not necessarily result in total paralysis; sometimes it can lead to lack of fine control over movements, as other regions of the brain can often provide a 'back-up service'. The parietal lobe contains the *somatosensory cortex* which receives information from skin senses such as touch, temperature and pressure. Again, more area is assigned to the more sensitive parts of the body such as the lips. The occipital and temporal lobes are concerned with vision and hearing. About two-thirds of the cortex do not have a specific function and are known as the *association cortex*. Higher-order mental functions such as thinking and learning are thought to be the responsibility of the association cortex but have so far largely defied attempts at localisation. The cortex is of special interest to physiological psychologists because it is the last part of the brain to stop growing and undergoes more change after birth than any other area of the brain.

The autonomic nervous system

The *autonomic nervous system* (ANS) is concerned with regulating functions of the body such as heart rate and blood pressure in response to physical demands, or to ensure the smooth running of the digestive system and body temperature control. The system has two parts: the *sympathetic* and the *parasympathetic*. If an organism is faced with an emergency the sympathetic branch of the ANS will increase the heart rate and blood flow to the skeletal muscles, open the respiratory passages and stimulate the adrenal gland. The parasympathetic branch of the ANS tends to have the opposite effect, slowing, calming and generally conserving energy. A balance is normally maintained between the two systems with one or the other being called into action to respond to specific circumstances.

The autonomic nervous system uses the hypothalamus to orchestrate its effects in two ways: by direct neural excitation and by stimulating the endocrine glands to release hormones. Basically, the hypothalamus influences the endocrine system via the *pituitary gland* which in turn secretes hormones to influence other endocrine glands.

Emotion

The physiological structures most often associated with emotion are the hypothalamus and the limbic system. It seems that electrical stimulation of the hypothalamus produces emotional reactions such as fighting or running away (MacPhail and Miller, 1968). Some parts of the limbic system excite or arouse the organism, whilst others inhibit the organism; damage to such areas can result in the loss of all emotion or loss of all inhibition. Hence certain structures of the brain regulate emotional responses, and strong feelings are accompanied by physiological reactions. When a person is angry they are often aware of their heart beating faster and their face becoming flushed.

There has been considerable interest in the relationship between specific feelings and their associated physiology for a long time. One of the earliest theories of emotion was proposed by William James who said that we do not hit out because we are angry but vice versa:

> We feel sorry because we cry, angry because we strike, afraid because we tremble, and not that we cry, strike, or tremble because we are sorry, angry, or fearful, as the case may be.

A Danish physiologist called Lange, working independently of James, produced a similar theory. The two were combined to form the James–Lange theory of emotion which states that it is the perception of bodily states that results in emotion – 'I'm trembling, so I must be afraid.' This theory was later contested by Walter Cannon (1927) who pointed out that many non-emotional stressors, such as high fever, produce a peripheral arousal state similar to that of rage. Injections of adrenaline produce arousal but do not result in the experience of specific emotions. This conflict of opinion was resolved by Schachter and Singer's (1962) famous experiment. They postulated that the experience of emotion could not be explained solely in terms of physiological processes; people experiencing arousal of some kind will look for an explanation in their immediate surroundings.

Schachter and Singer injected male participants with either adrenaline or a placebo. The participants were told that they were being given a vitamin supplement, 'Suproxin', in order to examine its effects on vision. There were four groups of participants:

- One group was informed of expected physiological consequences, such as increased heart-rate and palpitations.
- One group was misinformed of the physiological consequences to expect.
- One group was left ignorant of the physiological consequences to expect.
- One group was given saline injections.

Whilst the participants (one at a time) were waiting for what they thought was the real experiment, their environment was varied in two ways:

- *Euphoria*. A confederate of the experimenter entered the room and behaved in a 'happy' way, making paper planes, laughing out loud, and so on.
- *Anger*. The participant and the experimenter's confederate were asked to fill in a questionnaire while the stooge became increasingly angry and violent and eventually ripped up the questionnaire.

The experimenters predicted that those participants who were left in ignorance of the source of their arousal would use their immediate environment as a source of information. Thus those participants in the third condition would interpret the effects of the drug differently according to whether they were in the 'euphoric' or the 'angry' condition. The experimenters found that those participants who had been given no explanation for their arousal did indeed feel and act more emotionally than those given an explanation or a placebo. Thus the adrenaline caused anger in one situation and euphoria in another. This led the experimenters to propose that emotional state is determined by an interaction between physiological state and the cognitive environment.

Implications for nurses

A woman is admitted to an Accident and Emergency department having been knocked off her bicycle. Early clinical observations show markedly raised cystolic blood pressure, pulse rate and respiration. The patient says she is short of breath and experiencing palpitations which she is convinced are due to the anger she feels towards the motorist who caused the accident and to fear and panic about the accident itself. She thinks everyone is making too much fuss and wants to go home.

There are a number of ways in which these clinical observations could be interpreted. It is important not only to understand how the patient may explain them within the context of his or her cognitive environment, taking into account the possibility of erroneous attribution, but also to be aware that nurses may be making clinical assessments and looking for explanations using similar potentially incorrect strategies.

Most of us have had physiological sensations as a result of emotional arousal. Think about the last time you were really anxious, perhaps waiting to take an exam. You may well have had sweaty hands, a rapid thumping heartbeat and needed to go to the toilet frequently. When the exam was over the physical symptoms disappeared.

Physical symptoms can occur because a patient is anxious about being in hospital – this is a healthy response to a stressful situation. However, they can also occur as a more serious mental health problem. Imagine having these sensations without knowing the cause and consequently not knowing when they will end. Imagine these sensations lasting day after day. You would probably have difficulty in coping with everyday activities and need some form of help. This experience is often described as an *acute anxiety state*.

Transmitting messages

Messages are carried to and from different parts of the brain by neurons or nerve cells. There are four main parts to a cell:

- the *cell body*: the body of the nerve cell and the control centre;
- the *dendrites*: tree-like growths attached to the cell body whose main function is to receive messages from other neurons;
- the *axon*: carries messages to other nerve cells;
- the *terminal buttons*: found at the end of the axons.

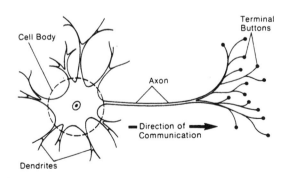

Figure 7.4 The main parts of a cell

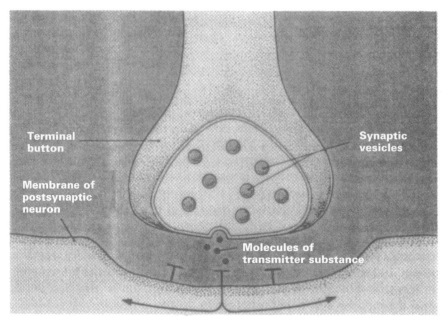

Activation of receptor site excites or
inhibits postsynaptic neuron

Figure 7.5 Transmitting messages

The messages carried by the axon involve electrical current, but this current is unlike electricity travelling down a wire. Electricity travels at about 200 million metres per second; the axon transmits information at less than 200 metres per second. When an axon is triggered at one end it sends an action potential down to the other end rather like a 'Mexican wave' travels around a sports ground. When the action potential reaches the terminal buttons, a chemical called a *transmitter substance is* secreted. This chemical substance is then picked up by the receptor sites of the next neuron. The transmitter substance is then 'put out of commission' by the terminal buttons, taking them back (re-uptake) or deactivating them with enzymes. The conjunction between one neuron's terminal buttons and another's dendrites is called the *synapse,* of which there are basically two types – *excitatory* and *inhibitory.* Excitatory synapses increase the probability that the axon of the next neuron will fire, whereas inhibitory synapses will cause the next neuron to fire at a low rate or not at all. The synapse is one of the most important features of the nerve cell, since many drugs produce their effects by stimulating or blocking the receptor sites.

Drugs can exert an important influence on the complex biochemical events that take place when one neuron communicates with another. There are two main ways that drugs operate:

- They can take the place of natural transmitter substances acting in their place. For example, Curare replaces the transmitter substance acetycholine, producing paralysis;
- By stimulating or preventing the release of transmitter substances. The drug Reserpine prevents synaptic vesicles from storing norepinephrine (another common transmitter substance) leading to a lowering of blood pressure.

It might be interesting to look at how some other drugs achieve their effects (Table 7.1). Psychophysiological approaches to the explanation of behaviour provide a useful

Table 7.1 *Some drugs and their effects*

Drug: amphetamines
- *Physiological mechanism*: stimulate release of norepinephrine and receptor sites
- *Behavioural effect*: increases levels of mental and physical activity

Drug: Imipramine
- *Physiological mechanism*: inhibits re-uptake of norepinephrine by terminal buttons
- *Behavioural effect*: reduces depression

Drug: Botulinum
- *Physiological mechanism*: prevents release of acetylcholine
- *Behavioural effect*: leads to food poisoning

Drug: Chloropromazine
- *Physiological mechanism*: binds to dopamine receptor sites preventing dopamine from reaching them
- *Behavioural effect*: reduction in schizophrenic and psychotic symptoms

Drug: LSD and Psilocybin
- *Physiological mechanism*: influences transmission at synapses in the brain where serotonin is the transmitter substance
- *Behavioural effect*: produce major changes in perception

Drug: barbiturates
- *Physiological mechanism*: inhibit all neural activity
- *Behavioural effect*: reduce anxiety and levels of activity

Drug: nicotine
- *Physiological mechanism*: attaches itself to receptors normally sensitive to acetylcholine and stimulates neurons
- *Behavioural effect*: acts as a stimulant

insight into the interaction between basic physiology and psychological functioning. This also illustrates the ways in which psychology has become integrated with other basic sciences.

Sleep

About one-third of our lives is spent sleeping. Sleep is so important to us that as early as 1970 Dunlop estimated that in Britain one night's sleep in ten is induced by hypnotic drugs. Or, put another way, on any night in Britain 3.5 million people will take a sleeping pill. More recently, about 10 million prescriptions were written for sleeping pills in the United Kingdom in 2004 (*Drug and Therapeutics Bulletin*, DTB).

Perceptions of our sleeping habits are not always correct. Rachman and Phillips (1975) investigated a group of 'good sleepers' and a group of 'poor sleepers'. The good sleepers estimated that it took them about seven minutes to fall asleep, whereas the poor sleepers thought that it took them at least an hour. When both groups were studied, the poor sleepers only took eight minutes longer than the good sleepers to fall asleep. Misperceptions of sleep patterns are important because hypnotic drugs are often prescribed in response to complaints based on the patients' own perceptions. A more recent study by Stepanski *et al.* (1989) found that insomniacs slept an average of 364 minutes per night and the control group 419 minutes per night. Daytime sleepiness did not differ between groups; in fact, there was a trend for daytime alertness in the insomniacs. The subjective element of sleep has been highlighted by Rogers and Aldrich (1993) with respect to the opposite of insomniacs – people who suffer from narcolepsy (sleep attacks). They found that 'nap therapy' improved alertness and reduced the frequency of sleep attacks.

The main reason for the comparative delay in sleep research in the twentieth century is that sleep behaviour is not open to direct observation (Jensen and Herr, 1993). It was not until the early 1940s that the electroencephalograph (EEG) started to be used extensively in sleep research. The EEG measures changes in the electrical activity of the brain. During the course of each night's sleep the brain produces different types of electrical activity and these can be measured by the EEG.

In order to understand these patterns of electrical activity, it is necessary to map the changes occurring during a typical night's sleep. Sleep is thought by many to be a time when the body can rest and recuperate. While the body may be relaxed, the brain is far from inactive. When a person is relaxed but awake, the EEG measures alpha waves. These are fast, low-voltage waves which have an unsynchronised pattern of firing. As the individual falls asleep, *hypnagogic imagery* – very vivid, distinct images – precedes the true onset of sleep. *State 1 sleep* is represented by a slowing down of the heart rate, and the presence of theta wave forms on the EEG. The sleeper can still be woken easily at this stage. *Stage 2 sleep* shows clear signs of 'sleep spindles' (periods when a large number

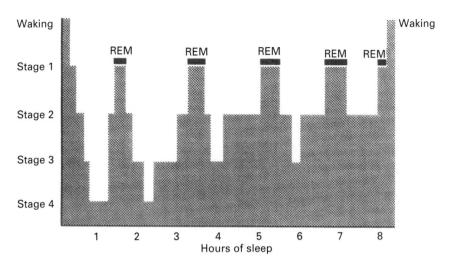

Figure 7.6 The stages of sleep

of neurons become synchronised, firing in unison) but it is still easy to wake someone. *Stage 3 sleep* is marked by the presence of 'delta' wave activity for at least 20 per cent of the time. Delta waves are slow, high-voltage waves which indicate deep sleep. *Stage 4 sleep* is the deepest stage and delta wave activity accounts for 50 per cent of the time. It is extremely difficult to wake a person in this stage, and often the most fearful nightmares occur during this stage.

It takes about sixty minutes to achieve Stage 4 sleep and people normally spend up to twenty-five minutes in this stage. The process is then reversed, moving back to stage 3 and then to stage 2. After about ninety minutes a different form of sleep occurs. This is called *rapid eye movement* (REM) sleep. This form of sleep is characterised by the return of fast, low-voltage activity and rapid movement of the eyes. Sometimes this type of sleep is referred to as 'paradoxical', since the EEG readings indicate wakefulness, but the individual is clearly fast asleep. If woken during this stage, people usually report dreaming, and most dreams do occur during REM sleep. The stages are repeated, with the periods of REM sleep increasing and the depth of sleep decreasing. The individual differences in patterns of sleep have implications for nursing care. In hospitals it is often inappropriate to have standardised times for sleeping and giving medication; information about individual sleep patterns needs to be included in any nursing assessment.

There are individual differences in the amount of sleep needed. It seems as if some people are able to function perfectly well on very little sleep, whereas others need their eight hours. Webb and Cartwright (1978) said that 6 per cent of men and 14 per cent of women suffer from insomnia. Insomnia was found to be attributable to several causes, the most common of these being anxiety and depression.

Sleep deprivation

There are therefore two types of sleep: *slow wave sleep* (SWS) and *rapid eye movement Sleep* (REM). There have been a number of investigations into the extent to which people need both types of sleep, conducted either by depriving subjects of all sleep or depriving them only of REM sleep by waking them up as soon as it occurs. Wilkinson (1968) suggested that the main consequences of total sleep deprivation are progressive deterioration in the performance of various tasks and an associated change in mood. However, the extent of the deterioration depends on the nature of the task and on the motivation of the person. Broadbent (1963) said:

> a sleep-deprived man is not like a child's mechanical toy which goes slower as it runs down, nor is he like a car engine which continues until its fuel is exhausted and stops dead. He is like a motor which after much use misfires, runs normally for a while, then falters again, and so on.

The world record for sleep deprivation is held by Randy Gardner, who stayed awake for 264 hours. On his first night asleep he slept for fifteen hours, but by the second night had returned to his normal eight-hour cycle and showed no psychological or physical deterioration. Williams *et al.* (1964) found that in the first recovery sleep following total deprivation, the amount of Stage 4 sleep increases much more than other stages, including REM. This indicates the body's particular need for this stage of sleep.

Studies of partial sleep deprivation have concentrated on depriving subjects of REM sleep. Cartwright *et al.* (1967) have concluded that:

- there is a progressive increase in the number of awakenings required to maintain REM sleep deprivation;
- there is an REM sleep 'rebound' effect. Recovery sleep after REM deprivation contains many more incidents of REM sleep.

They did not find evidence of even minor psychological changes following REM sleep deprivation.

The evidence suggests that the body can function without substantial periods of sleep but may 'misfire' occasionally. The two most important types of sleep are Stage 4 SWS and REM sleep, and it is also interesting to note that the majority of dreaming occurs in these two types of sleep. Hodgson (1991) has related the need for sleep to nursing practice. It is suggested that importance should be given to individualised patient care and that the nurse is in a unique position to facilitate patient needs.

The need to dream?

There have been numerous theories which have attempted to explain the need to sleep and dream. *Freudian theory* views dreams as an expression of repressed, sexual desires, whereas *evolutionary theory* examines the role of sleep in the survival of the species, noting that sleeping animals are often less conspicuous to would-be predators. However, the *psychophysiological perspective* attempts to explain sleeping and dreaming in terms of the functions and processes of the body.

Hobson (1990) put forward two main explanations for the need to sleep and dream.

The neuronal rest hypothesis

The small neurons with large synaptic gaps are more likely to lose transmitter cells than large neurons with little distance between the gap. It is the small neurons (aminergic neurons) that work frequently and continuously during the waking state. This may lead to a greater amount of transmitter cells becoming depleted. Hobson suggests that it is the small aminergic neurons which show the most dramatic decreases in firing rate during SWS sleep, falling to their lowest levels during REM sleep. Thus the periods of SWS and REM sleep enable these neurons to 'stock up' on their neurotransmitter supplies. An analogy might be to view the brain as a supermarket where certain sections produce greater turnover than others, having to be replenished during the night for the following day.

The reconstructive hypothesis

Although the aminergic neurons are resting, the rest of the system is a hive of activity. Another function of REM sleep is to maintain the basic circuits of the brain. Much of our daytime behaviour is insufficient to activate a large proportion of neural activity, therefore many areas of the brain need to be exercised to ensure that they do not suffer from disuse. It is rather like a car that is kept in a garage all the time – it needs to be started up once a day to keep it in functional order. The high level of 'redundant' firing during REM sleep thus serves a maintenance or reconstructive role. Hobson also suggests that as REM sleep is overrepresented during early intra-uterine life, peaking at about thirty weeks of gestational age, there is further evidence of its reconstruct ional role. If these propositions are correct, then we need SWS and REM sleep to service and replenish the systems of, the brain.

The spandrels of sleep

A proposition put forward by Flanagan (2000) is that dreams are the 'spandrels' of sleep. Spandrels is an architectural term for the triangular bits in between the arches of a bridge and say a road going along the top. They serve no function but are a by-product of the arches which have an important function supporting the bridge. Thus Flanagan (2000) says that dreams are a by-product of sleep whose function is tangential to the importance of sleep. This does not mean that dreams are useless, they result from our need to find, or even create, meaning from our lives even when we are asleep. In this explanation he differs from Hobson (1990) by proposing that dreams do not really have a *function* at all and that the important cognitive functions are best served by sleep not by dreams. He accepts Hobson's point about the developmental importance of REM sleep but says that once it has served its function in completing the visual system, it no longer has any use.

Hopefully, Flanagan would accept that even if dreams do not have a significant physiological function, if they have a role in creating meaning in our lives, then they have an important psychological function.

Personality

The term 'personality' is used by many people in the course of everyday conversation, yet if you were to ask them to define what they mean by it, they would struggle to reply. The popularity of the expression is matched only by the wealth of attempts to classify it as a concept. Thus the first endeavour must be to represent the different theories, definitions and descriptions of the personality construct before investigating its usefulness in the context of nursing care. Broadly speaking, one can divide personality theories into three main groups: *psychodynamic, psychometric* and *humanistic*.

Psychodynamic theories

As the name suggests, these theories involve elements of action and change. Personality is not simply something with which one is born; it develops through a dynamic interaction between the individual and the environment. There is no doubt that the most famous of the psychodynamic theories comes from Sigmund Freud (1856–1939). Freud called his theory *psychoanalysis* and spent the best part of thirty years developing it. It is impossible to do justice to the wealth and breadth of his writings in just a few lines, but it is important that nurses become familiar with some of the basic concepts of his theory, as many of the terms used in psychiatry are derived from his work.

Psychoanalytic theory

Freud's theory is more than a personality theory, for it includes a theory of motivation and a range of psychotherapies. However, with regard to personality, it is often useful to divide this theory into two main components: the *structure of personality* and the *development of personality*.

Personality structure

According to Freud, personality is made up of three parts: the *id*, the *ego* and the *superego*.

- The *id* is largely concerned with our instincts and basic needs. It resides in our unconscious and thus we are not aware of the exact status of this need or desire.

Impulses arising from the body's needs build up into a tension requiring release, and it is the job of the id to make this happen. This results in pleasure if it succeeds and frustration if it does not.

- The *ego* tries to maintain a balance between the id and external reality. It is the 'executive' branch of the personality, and directs the ways in which unconscious needs may be realised.
- The *superego* represents the 'moral' branch of personality. It occurs later in Freud's theory and is concerned with whether the actions determined by the ego are allowed. It personifies the influence of culture and society on the behaviour of the individual. Whenever id impulses arise and are given direction by the ego, the superego acts to decide whether they conform to the norms of society.

> The ego's relation to the id might be compared with that of a rider to his horse. The horse supplies the locomotive energy, while the rider has the privilege of deciding on the goal and of guiding the powerful animal's movement. But only too often there arises between the ego and the id the not precisely ideal situation of the rider being obliged to guide the horse along the path by which it itself wants to go.
>
> (Freud, 1964)

The structural components of personality, together with external factors, interact in such a way as to be in continual conflict. These conflicts require resolution if a person is to function normally. The id is always governed by the *pleasure principle* which makes continual demands upon the ego for satisfaction of its needs. The ego has to consider the needs of the id in terms of the possibilities presented by external reality. This is called the *reality principle*. The result of these conflicts is anxiety. A separate form of anxiety is associated with each of the ego's 'three tyrannical masters'. Thus, *reality anxiety* (such as fear of snakes, the dark, and physical harm) is related to the ego, *neurotic anxiety* (such as fear of uncontrollable urges) is related to the id, and *moral anxiety* (such as fear of being punished for doing something wrong) is related to the superego. If the ego has difficulty resolving a conflict, it will call upon a strategy to defend itself from harm. These strategies are called *defence mechanisms*, of which there are five main ones.

- *Repression.* The principle of this defence mechanism is 'what we don't know can't hurt us'. Threatening thoughts are prevented from emerging into awareness; to prevent anxiety we may 'forget' the name of someone who has hurt us or 'forget' to pay a bill that would put intense strain on the household budget.
- *Reaction formation.* The ego disguises an undesirable emotion by focusing on its opposite. A child's jealousy for a newborn brother or sister may be manifested as love and affection; outward chastity may hide sexual desire.
- *Projection.* It is easier for the ego to handle external threats than internal dangers. Therefore, anxiety-arousing thoughts and feelings are accredited to others rather than

to the self. 'I want to hurt her' becomes 'She wants to hurt me.' Violence is made legitimate because it is done in self-defence.

- *Regression.* This occurs when a person reverts to an earlier stage of development. When life becomes 'too much', people retreat to times when life was much simpler. The sorts of behaviour associated with this defence mechanism are childish and often infantile.
- *Fixation.* A part of the personality becomes 'stuck' and remains secured to an earlier period of development. The person is not permitted to proceed entirely to the next stage of development.

For example, the pleasures of sucking experienced by a baby during breast or bottle feeding may lead to a reluctance to give it up, and the infant will resist being weaned.

Developmental structure

Freud believed that the foundations of personality lay in the child's progression through a series of developmental stages.

- *The oral stage: birth to one year.* The experience of sucking introduces the infant to both the pleasures and pains of the world. Pleasure stems from sucking and chewing, pain from frustration and anxiety. Parents influence the way drives are satisfied by the way in which they respond to the child at this point.
- *The anal stage: one to three years.* During this stage children go through toilet training. If toilet training is particularly harsh, defecation can become a source of great anxiety for the child, as the child's immediate need for gratification is frustrated by the parents' demands for voluntary expulsion to be delayed. The *anal retentive personality* is characterised by excessive tidiness and orderliness; a compulsion for everything and everyone to be placed in perfect order. The *anal expulsive personality* is characterised by messiness and a tendency to be slipshod. Sometimes uncontrollable expulsion is manifest in temper tantrums or excessive physical behaviour. The aim of parents at this stage is to allow enough, but not too much, gratification, and to help the child develop enough, but not too much, self-control. However, parents who are strict about toilet training may also be strict about tidiness, so the significance of the anal content of the stage may be overestimated.
- *The phallic stage: three to five years.* During this stage, pleasures and problems focus on the genital area. In boys, conflict centres around the sexual desire for their mother and the consequent fear of their father. This is known as the *Oedipus complex* from the Greek myth of Oedipus who unwittingly killed his father and married his mother. As a result of the boy's desire, he is afraid that his father may take retribution by castrating him (the *castration complex*). The resolution of this dilemma occurs by the boy identifying with his father and striving to be like him. For girls, this stage represents a similar desire for the opposite sex-parent. The successful or unsuccessful resolution of the Oedipus complex was thought by Freud to be the determining

factor in all later neuroses. The ability to restrain the impulse for ego gratification results in the development of the superego or conscience. It should be remembered that Freud based his initial observations on a small sample of largely Austrian middle-class women at the beginning of the century and therefore the extrapolation of his analyses to women in present-day society is limited.

- *The period of latency: five years to puberty.* During this period the child experiences a period of relative 'sexual' calm and concentrates on interacting with children of the same sex. Sexual energy continues to flow but is channelled into social concerns such as interaction with peers and teachers, and into clubs and sport. Development continues but is not accompanied by the storms and stresses of earlier stages.

- *The genital stage: adolescence.* The physiological changes of puberty result in mature, adult sexuality with the biological aim of propagating the species. The choice of companion is not entirely independent of the experiences of the earlier stages. A young woman may choose a 'father figure', depending on the attitudes and patterns that have developed in the earlier years. Freud says that some internal conflict will be inevitable throughout the life span, but by the genital stage the individual has achieved a relatively stable personality.

To many people Freud's theory of personality seems somewhat far-fetched. However, it must be said that when anyone mentions the word psychology the first name that comes to mind for most people is Freud's. But let us take an objective view of this theory and assess its strengths and weaknesses.

- *Strengths.* Freud may not have discovered the unconscious but he certainly popularised it. Freud illustrated that we may not always be aware of the reasons for our behaviour but that they do have an explainable cause. Through the use of *hypnosis, dream analysis* and *free association* it was thought to be possible to gain access to the true motives behind behaviour. Whether access to the unconscious in this manner is possible is uncertain; however, most people would accept that we as individuals are not always the best judge of our own designs and motives. Another strength of the theory is its emphasis upon the importance of childhood in shaping the adult personality. Whether an emphasis on the sexual nature of personality development is a strength of the theory can be questioned, but certainly it is this aspect of the theory that often causes the most controversy.

- *Weaknesses.* There is no doubt that the theory is not scientific. Indeed, Freud never intended it to be so. However, in seeking to explain everything it could be said that he explains nothing. Let's take the following example. Suppose a child is observed during infancy to undergo extremely strict toilet training. What could we predict about the child's later personality? According to the central argument of the theory, the child should become compulsively neat, tidy and over-controlled. But the defence mechanism of reaction formation (see p. 231) would predict that the child would react against the strict toilet training by becoming messy, dirty and irresponsible. Whether the child becomes messy or neat, Freudian theory has an explanation and therefore becomes inherently untestable.

The emphasis on sex in childhood strains many people's credulity. Over the past twenty to thirty years, developmental psychologists have found children to be curious, self-motivated, social beings who seek excitement and thrills. They are not anxiety-ridden creatures trying to reduce tension created by sexual dilemmas. They are curious about sex, but then they are curious about many things in the world.

In summary, Freud provided a rich source of hypotheses for developmental research and founded a dynasty of psychoanalysts such as Carl Jung, Karen Horney, Harry Stack Sullivan and Eric Erikson. Unfortunately, its usefulness as a psychological theory of personality depends on whether one believes it or not, and has nothing to do with scientific validity.

Psychometric theories

Exercise 7.2 *Personality inventory*

Choose as participants for this experiment some friends who have never studied psychology. Ask them if they would mind spending some time doing a three-part test that will give them an indication of their personality. Tell them that all scores will be entirely anonymous and the results conveyed via coded numbers. You can either give them the test in print form or read the questions out loud.

The GU11 (BL version) Personality Inventory

I   Indicate whether you think the following are true or false:

		True	False
1	Happiness is more important than success	☐	☐
2	Men and women can be both sympathetic and assertive	☐	☐
3	Our lives are largely controlled by fate	☐	☐
4	I like to be liked by other people	☐	☐
5	I am usually quite positive about life	☐	☐
6	The clothes one wears reflects one's personality	☐	☐
7	Sometimes I feel shy when I meet people for the first time	☐	☐
8	I like to watch sport on television	☐	☐
9	Occasionally I have dreams I don't quite understand	☐	☐
10	I sometimes boast a little	☐	☐

II Look at (listen to) the following words and give the first word that comes into your mind. Please try to respond as quickly as possible.

Tape	Mouse
Pencil	Car
Mother	Exam
Blood	Food
Yellow	Friend
House	Water
Useful	Man

III Which of the following do you prefer?

1 (a) Watching television
   (b) Having a conversation
2 (a) Going walking
   (b) Watching movies
3 (a) A noisy party
   (b) Art galleries
4 (a) People who work hard
   (b) People with flair
5 (a) A holiday on a farm
   (b) A holiday by the sea
6 (a) Spicy food
   (b) Plain food
7 (a) Going for a ride on a bike
   (b) Riding an exercise bicycle
8 (a) Lots of acquaintances
   (b) A few special friends
9 (a) Classical music
   (b) Rock music
10 (a) New clothes
    (b) Eating out at a good restaurant

A day, or at least a few hours, after giving your friends the test, read them the following description:

This person has several interesting personality characteristics. For most of the time he/she is quite friendly and sociable. However, sometimes he/she can feel a bit shy, and somewhat inhibited. A major personality characteristic of this person is that he/she is not easily influenced by other people. Instead, he/she usually needs to have reasonable evidence before making up his/her mind and doesn't jump to conclusions. This person can be quite down-to-earth and businesslike if the situation requires. But he/she also has a colourful imagination, and can be quite creative. Overall he/she seems to be somewhat above average in maturity and thoughtfulness.

After carrying out this test and reading this analysis to your friend ask them whether they think that this personality assessment is at all accurate. In most cases the answer will be in the affirmative and some may even go further and say that the results are quite surprisingly appropriate.

There are two main reasons for your friends' reactions:

- The 'personality assessment' is couched in terms so general that they can apply to almost anyone. Some astrologers make use of the same principle and word their predictions so broadly that they will fit a wide range of events.
- The results are achieved because many people place great faith in tests, especially if they seem to be measuring personality in a comprehensive fashion. Therefore, it is crucial that you explain to your friend that this was not a real psychological test and that the results were made up. You should also explain to your friend that only qualified people are allowed to administer psychological tests. They are usually Chartered Psychologists but if not, they must possess a certificate from the British Psychological Society to show that they are qualified to administer psychological tests. Therefore you and your friend should make sure that any person testing you has the necessary qualifications. You should also try to ensure that the test you are taking has been standardised; that is, it is both *valid* (measures what it claims to measure) and *reliable* (measures what it claims to measure consistently). If you are unsure about any of these conditions you should decline to take the test.

'Trait' versus 'type'

Psychometrics is an approach to personality which focuses on psychological measurement. Measurement in this context involves the assigning of numerical values to psychological variables. There are two main approaches to the measurement of personality characteristics: by *trait* or by *type*.

It has been estimated that there are at least 18,000 words that have been used to describe personality differences (for example, shrewd, lazy, shy, aggressive, stupid). These words do not attempt to describe the whole person but one aspect of their personality, a person's *personality traits*. On the other hand, descriptions such as 'he's a bit of an extrovert' or 'she's an argumentative sort' refer to the person as belonging to a class of individual, thus categorising them as a particular *type*.

Cattell's trait theory

We have seen that there are a vast number of personality traits, far too many to put in a questionnaire. Raymond Cattell (1946) identified what he called twelve *primary factors,* or *source traits,* that were basic to each individual's personality. Essentially, Cattell was able to group the thousands of what he called *surface traits* into these twelve basic categories of source traits. Subsequent work led to the number being revised to sixteen and it became known as the Sixteen Personality Factor Questionnaire (16PF).

The sixteen factors are *bipolar;* that is, they represent two extremes of a particular dimension. For example, submissiveness (submissive, mild, accommodating, comforting) versus dominance (dominant, aggressive, stubborn, competitive). Most people's scores do not lie at the extremes of the scale but somewhere in the middle.

The test has been very successfully used in personnel selection. A company may give the 16PF to its best salespeople and put all the personality profiles together to produce a 'best salesperson profile'. Prospective employees are then given the 16PF and their profile is compared with the 'best salesperson profile' to see how similar they are. If there is quite a close relationship between the two profiles it is assumed that the person has the personality qualities of a good salesperson. Those companies with a thorough selection process will not base their whole selection procedures on the 16PF, but will use a variety of techniques including interviews and the following up of references as well. However, this method will work only if it is feasible to select the 'best' individuals. The best salespeople may be the ones who sell the most goods, but how one selects a group of the 'best nurses' may be a much more difficult task.

Big five models

There are two models that have been referred to as 'big five' models. The first was developed by Costa and McCrae (2005) and consists of five factors: Openness, Conscientiousness, Extroversion, Agreeableness and Neuroticism (OCEAN). The traits associated with each of the factors are:

- *Openness*: generating ideas, use of fantasy, aesthetic perspective, feeling dominant.
- *Conscientiousness*: self-discipline, sense of duty, order, competence, deliberation.
- *Extroversion*: excitement-seeking, assertiveness, activity, positive emotions, warmth.
- *Agreeableness*: altruism, modesty, tender-minded, straightforward, trust.
- *Neuroticism*: anxiety, self-consciousness, vulnerability, hostility, depression.

The model was developed by observing that five similar factors were present in many personality studies over a period of several decades. Costa and McCrae (1992) then set about designing a questionnaire based on these five factors called the NEO-PI. This has been used in many contexts since its construction and the authors present evidence for the stability of the five factors, particularly over the age of 30 (Costa and McCrae, 2005).

However, a major criticism of this five-factor approach is its ethnocentric bias. Although the authors document the test's usefulness in Western society, it is not clear whether the five factors would stand up in non-Western cultures.

Goldberg (1981) also produced a personality inventory containing five factors: Extroversion, Agreeableness, Conscientiousness, Emotional stability and Intellect. At first sight it seems that this model is the same as that of Costa and McCrae (1992), with intellect substituted for openness, but there is a much more important difference between the two and this is that Goldberg pays attention to the social and cultural aspects of personality. Somer and Goldberg (1999) looked at the use of their inventory in Turkey. They found that the Turkish 'intellect' factor was closer to the 'openness' of Costa and McCrae. Because traditionalism versus modernism seemed to be an important aspect of Turkish life, this element was much more prominent in the Turkish responses to the inventory. However, despite their attempts to address cultural aspects of personality it is hard to see how, say, the Mundoogumoor of New Guinea would fare when confronted with the inventory. It can be argued that concepts such as extroversion have been socially constructed in the West and as such have meaning only in a Western context.

Is personality determined by our genes?

The answer is that it depends on what is meant by determined. Certainly there is evidence of a strong heritability factor (Loehlin, 1992), but this still leaves genetic factors accounting for approximately less than half the variability in personality. However, bear in mind when looking at the evidence from twin studies that 'reared apart' can sometimes mean the twins were separated at less than 1 year old to between 1 and5 years old. Also, children brought up in the same family do not always share a similar environment, especially as they grow older and the impact of life outside the family gains importance. Thus the evidence from these studies may not be as robust as one might think. Some even question the usefulness of the term 'personality', preferring to use 'a disposition to act in a particular way in specific circumstances' instead, but we will keep with the term for the moment.

Eysenck's type theory

At about the same time that Cattell was busy developing his measures of personality, Hans Eysenck was conducting his own investigations into the structure of personality. He noted that introversion and neuroticism seemed to be identical when measured by the personality tests of the time. This was consistent with Freudian theory, but inconsistent with his findings that there were two factors: a dimension of introversion–extroversion and a dimension of neuroticism–stability. Eysenck (1970) proposed that people can be categorised into four general types according to their position on these two dimensions (see Figure 7.7).

Eysenck tried to relate his personality types to neurophysiological processes. He

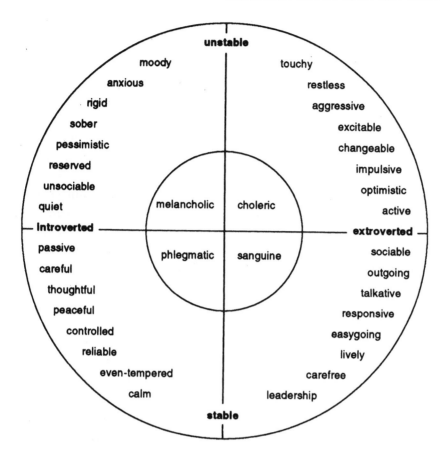

Figure 7.7 Eysenck's four general types

© H. J. Eysenck, 1965, from *Fact and Fiction in Psychology*. Reproduced by permission of Personality Investigations.

suggested that introverts are neurologically chronically over-aroused and seek to reduce this excitation by avoiding extra stimulation from the outside world. Extroverts are chronically under-aroused and have to pursue extra stimulation and new experiences. According to the theory, extroverts will more easily become bored than introverts but are less likely to feel guilty and anxious. (Note that the four personality types correspond to the four humours of pre-scientific medicine: *melancholic* (too much black bile), *choleric* (too much yellow bile), *phlegmatic* (too much phlegm) and *sanguine* (too much blood).)

A question that is often asked about both personality tests is 'How do you know people aren't lying or manipulating the answers to portray whatever personality they want?' Each test deals in different ways with people who are 'economical with the truth'. The 16PF has 236 items on the scale. Cattell solves the problem of people lying by placing similar items at, say, Nos 14 and 173, 63 and 126, 91 and 208, and so on. By the time most people have reached No. 42 they cannot remember their response to No. 24.

If people respond in a contradictory fashion to similar components of the test the responses are disregarded.

Eysenck deals with the problem in a different way. In his questionnaire he has a number of 'lie detector' questions like 'Do you sometimes get cross?' or 'As a child, did you always do as you were told immediately and without grumbling?' The questions refer to situations that most people have experienced – most of us have at some time been cross or hesitated to do what we were told. Therefore, if someone gets a high lie score, they may not be truly representative of the general population and the scores are rejected.

Eysenck and Cattell have a certain amount in common but they disagree on basic issues such as whether traits or types are the fundamental variables of personality. For Cattell, there are many traits, which develop in different ways. Some are inherited, while others are the result of early experiences. Eysenck believes that his basic dimensions of personality have their roots in neurophysiology and are largely genetically determined.

Jung's Psychological Types

In 1921 Jung had finished his massive work on Psychological Types. He had moved even further away from Freudian theory and was now more convinced by the work of William James, in particular James's distinction between 'tough-minded' and 'tender-minded' personality types. The tough-minded person tended to be governed by 'stubborn irreducible facts', whereas the tender-minded person approached life with an organising set of principles and ideas. Thus the characteristics of tough-mindedness were: materialistic, pessimistic, sceptical, sensationalistic and pluralistic; the tender-minded person was: idealistic, intellectual, optimistic and believers in free will. Already in his mind was the dichotomy between extroversion and introversion (Jung in fact used the spelling 'extravert', but 'extrovert' is normally preferred these days.) The third main contribution to the development of his theory of types came from his interest in the Gnostics. They used a typology containing the functions of thinking, feeling and sensation. Seeking to 'balance or complete' the system, Jung added the function of intuition so that there were now four categories of extroversion and four categories of introversion comprising eight psychological types:

- *Extrovert–thinking*. Loves facts and loves building them into theories. Often intolerant of other's ideas.
- *Extrovert–feeling*. According to Jung, usually a woman and 'tends to exhaust emotions in external relations'. Readily suggestible and identifies with others in a conventional way. The 'show-business' type.
- *Extrovert–sensation*. Usually men. Consists of the practical, imaginative, hard-headed type of person. They are hungry for external stimulation and hate boredom. Hedonists.

- *Extrovert–intuition*. Intensity of judgement is emphasised here. Can be unstable and impulsive. Relationships are often unstable. Adventurers and explorers would be in this group.
- *Introvert–thinking*. Scholars and philosophers would be placed here. The emphasis is upon concepts rather than facts. Intellectually arrogant and somewhat lacking in feeling.
- *Introvert–feeling*. These people have strong likes and dislikes but often are incapable of expressing them. Sometimes this group is described as mysterious and enigmatic. Jung places nuns, poets and musicians here.
- *Introvert–sensation*. The characteristics include irrationality, sensuality and difficulty communicating. They 'feed' on sense impressions. Jung mentioned Van Gogh here.
- *Introvert–intuition*. He placed himself in this category. People in this group have little concern for what other people think of them. They pursue their own thoughts and often see themselves as misunderstood. Mystics and even simple daydreamers would be included here.

These are the eight main types Also within the typology are eight 'inferior functions' attached to each type. They serve to augment the interpretation of the type by taking some of the characteristics from the polar opposites.

It is probably this latter feature of Jung's theory that led to critics becoming somewhat confused by the exact criteria by which one type was different from another. Hence the theory was increasingly ignored by mainstream psychology, particularly since Jung attempted to assuage his critics by adding on more and more cavils so that the usefulness of the theory became severely compromised.

Just after the Second World War, Isobel Myers and her mother Katherine Briggs resurrected, if you like, Jung's typology and added a further element, that of judging versus perceiving, to become the Myers–Briggs Type Indicator (MBTI). This has sixteen types (Table 7.2) made up of four dimensions:

- Extroversion versus introversion.
- Sensing versus intuition.
- Thinking versus feeling.
- Judging versus perceiving.

Table 7.2 The sixteen types of Myers and Briggs

ISTJ	ISFJ	INFJ	INTJ
ISTP	ISFP	INFP	INTP
ESTP	ESFP	ENFP	ENTP
ESTJ	ESFJ	ENFJ	ENTJ

One of the main aims of the MBTI is to help people determine their own personality preferences, but it has been used extensively in job selection and personnel training to match employees and prospective employees to the most appropriate position within an institution.

In that there is a degree of self-selection inherent in the test used to determine types, it has had some success, but others have been critical of its use as a model of personality owing to the vagueness of many of the terms, most people being able to find something that fits with their ideas of themselves.

Both type and trait approaches are useful attempts to represent personality, but their limitations lie in the view that much of our personality is in some ways prescribed and stable. This need not be the case, as we shall see in the next approach to individual temperament.

Humanistic theories

Kelly's personal construct theory

Kelly's theory differs totally from the theories of Eysenck and Cattell. He sees personality as a process of change rather than stability. According to Kelly (1955) people construct models of the world in terms of pairs of opposing concepts called *personal constructs*. People are continually striving to make sense of the world and anticipate possible events, and so we tend to see people in terms of being either pleasant or unpleasant, intelligent or stupid, kind or nasty. Kelly says that we all have a fixed number of constructs which are essentially basic discriminations, sometimes not having labels. Constructs can be relatively tight (the opposing concepts deciduous–evergreen are restricted largely to trees) or relatively open (friendly–aloof can be used in a number of different contexts). The constituents of constructs such as events, objects and people are termed *elements*.

The most important feature of Kelly's theory is its emphasis on the process of change in personality development. When one sets up a construct it acts as a working hypothesis which can be either confirmed or refuted by experience. Thus, as you read this, you may consider me to be a person who knows quite a bit about personality theories; however, on meeting me, you might decide that my knowledge is largely superficial. In this instance I have gone from one end of your construct to the other. You may decide that this construct is not really relevant, and you would rather formulate a hypothesis of me as a good or bad writer. In this instance you would have discarded your former construct as being not really applicable and substituted a new one that seems more relevant. (You may like to think of some circumstances where your construct changed in relation to a particular individual and note that it was not just a change in your opinion but a difference in the way you viewed that person.) A good way to examine Kelly's personal construct theory is to complete a Kelly grid for yourself.

Exercise 7.3 *Kelly grid*

Figure 7.9 shows a partially completed Kelly grid. Along the top are elements, that is, descriptions of types of people you might know. There are three circles in each row of the grid. These can be placed where they are by you or someone else. In this example I have provided the selection but you may wish to provide your own. The constructs on the right of the grid are arrived at by thinking of some way in which two of the encircled elements are the same and different from the third. In this example I have decided that I know a successful person (Jim) and a happy person (Mary), who are quite carefree and happy-go-lucky, and an ethical person (Joan) who is the opposite – very principled. Two crosses are placed in the two common elements and all the other elements in the row are examined to determine whether they are either more carefree (they get a cross) or more principled (they get a blank). Look at Figure 7.8 and see how I have developed the constructs. If I were to complete the exercise properly, I would continue till I had run out of constructs.

The next stage is to measure the similarity between my constructs. To do this I make a copy of the crosses and blanks in row 1 on a piece of paper. I place the paper under row 2 and count the number of times that a cross in row 1 matches a cross in row 2 and a blank matches a blank. A circle without a cross counts as a blank. Next, I place the paper under row 3 and repeat the procedure for all the rest of the rows. Now I copy row 2 on to a piece of paper and compare it with the remaining rows, repeating the procedure until I have a set of matching scores, as in Table 7.3.

If constructs are identical they will have a score of 20. If they have a score of 0, they are still identical but expressed the other way round. Thus scores tending toward 0 and 20 express similarity and scores that tend toward 10 express less relationship. I now have a measure of

Table 7.3 *Similarity between constructs*

Row	No. of matching scores
1 and 2	10
1 and 3	7
1 and 4	11
2 and 3	8
2 and 4	11
3 and 4	7

those constructs which relate well to each other. Try this exercise for yourself (Figure 7.9 provides a blank grid for you to use) and you will provide yourself with an outline of your personality that consists of the constructs you use to describe the world and their similarity. (For a more detailed journey through constructing and using Kelly grids see Stevens (1996: 162) – it is well worth the effort.)

Personality assessment is another way of trying to find out what lies behind our behaviour. Although it bears little resemblance to psycho-physiological techniques, the information which studies of personality can provide adds another dimension to our overall explanations of behaviour.

Summary

In the first part of this chapter the structures and functions of the central nervous system (CNS) and the autonomic nervous system (ANS) have been described. The CNS can be described as the executive branch of the body, regulating feeding and temperature, controlling movement and producing thought. The brain and spinal chord are the main components of the CNS. The ANS is divided into the sympathetic and parasympathetic and is responsible for regulating heart rate and blood pressure in response to physical demands, digestion and temperature control.

The physiological reactions associated with emotion have been discussed with particular reference to the work of Schacter and Singer, who concluded that emotional state is determined by the interaction of physical state with cognitive environment. Attention has also been paid to the role of the CNS in sleep and the individual nature of sleep patterns. Insomnia and sleep deprivation and the function of sleep and dreaming have been discussed in relation to health maintenance and nursing care. The process by which messages are transmitted through nerve cells has been described along with the physiological and behavioural impact of various commonly used drugs on neuro-transmission.

In the second part of the chapter, three broad theories of personality were described. I looked at Freud's contribution to psychodynamic theory in terms of its strengths and weaknesses. Psychometric theories depend on an assumption that personality is stable and can be measured; the two main approaches to personality measurement are those which focus on traits and those which focus on type. These were discussed and examined in relation to their contribution to personality theory and limitations. Lastly, humanistic theories have been discussed, focusing in particular on Kelly's personal construct theory. This theory views personality as a process of change through continually trying to make sense of the world.

Constructs

1 Carefree – principled
2 Kind – cruel
3 Confident – anxious
4 Understanding – self-centred
5
6
7
8
9
10
11
12

Construct	1 Me	2 Father	3 Mother	4 Sister	5 Brother	6 Best friend	7 Partner	8 Ex-friend	9 Rejecting person	10 Attractive person	11 Boss	12 Happy person	13 Pitied person	14 Neighbour	15 Successful person	16 Ethical person	17	18	19	20
1 Carefree – principled	×	×	×			×				×		⊗		×	⊗	O				
2 Kind – cruel		⊗	⊗		×	×	×		O			×		×	×	×				
3 Confident – anxious	O	×		×	×	⊗	⊗			×	×				×	×				
4 Understanding – self-centred			×			×	⊗			×	O	×		⊗	×					

Figure 7.8 A Kelly grid

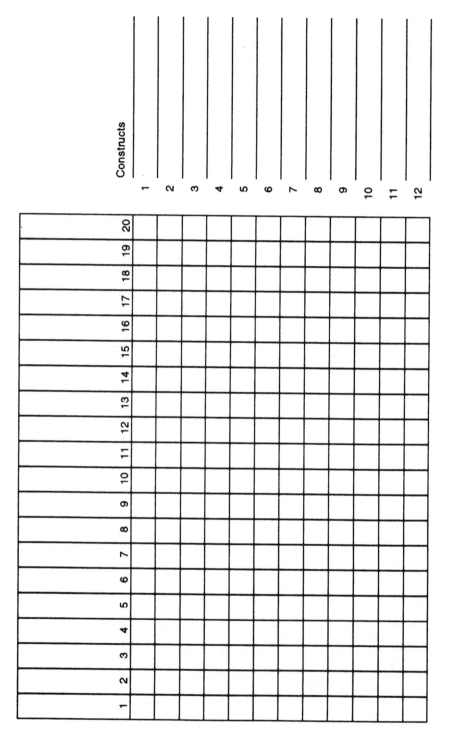

Figure 7.9 A blank Kelly grid

Conundrum revisited

As you read through this chapter a number of interesting points may have emerged regarding how patients might experience altered body image. The first of these is that we know our body (its dimensions, capacity, weight, strength and many other things) through neurological sensations entering the brain. Neurological sensations will tell us where our limbs are positioned, even if we closed our eyes and were not able to verify this matter visually (proprioception). There are a number of things that may now happen to distort the sensations that tell us about the body. Pain may affect our estimation of the size or the importance of the organ affected. If you have suffered from a dental abscess, for instance, it is likely that you will have estimated that a large part of your mouth was affected, even though the abscess lay beneath just one tooth. Sleep and stress also influence the ability of individuals to make sense in changes to body function or appearance. When individuals are tired they are less co-ordinated and may report that the body feels 'heavy' or 'slow'. The individual's perception of body function has changed. Equally, the use of drugs can significantly alter the individual's body image. Amphetamines, for instance, increase the patient's sense of power and control, the availability of energy to live 'life in the fast lane'. Whilst some physical changes may be associated with drug taking drugs also distort perceptions of the body.

Altered body image has its origins in more than altered sensations or perceptions of the body, however. Individuals ascribe meanings to their body, describing it in terms of satisfaction (cathexis) and often using analogies (as a tool or house, as something trustworthy or untrustworthy, vibrant or worn out). We form mental images of the body and are more or less satisfied with each of these.

A number of theories in Chapter 7 may be brought to bear, suggesting why some patients develop greater degrees of altered body image. They discuss the ways in which we form images of the body and of the self. If you support Freud's analysis, individuals develop their personality, their sense of self, based in large part upon psychological work associated with the body and its functions. Patients who were at a less secure stage of personal development may be less well placed to deal with the challenges associated with rapid changes in body function or appearance. The argument might run that individuals have insufficiently developed egos to deal with the sudden discrepancies (between reality) and the body as it *should* be.

Alternatively altered body image may be understood in terms of personality and, in particular, personality traits. Imagine that you were given £100,000 to be split up, insuring different parts and functions of your body against dysfunction or disfigurement. Some individuals might consistently spend more of their allocated money upon physical appearance over function. They might value such elements consistently highly (a trait) and therefore suffer a greater deal of loss when illness or treatment impairs them. Folk wisdom reminds us that 'beauty is only skin-deep', but in practice many individuals spend a significant amount of time, money and energy on sustaining their appearance.

Eysenck's work on personality types is also relevant. For instance, patients who display an extrovert personality may be able to draw upon a wider social circle to help them deal with body image threats. Extroverts make friends easily, they are gregarious. Extroverts, though, are also more dependent upon the opinion of others, seeking approval for their appearance, behaviour and identity. If the patient's social network is not supportive, the extrovert patient could be ill placed to deal with sudden changes in body image.

Lastly, Kelly's account of personal constructs can be applied too to body image and coping in the face of adversity. His theory points out that personal constructs are developed more or less subconsciously to help individuals antic- ipate and cope with day-to-day living. Some personal constructs are relatively superficial and are freely discussed and happily updated or even abandoned. Other personal constructs are deeper-seated and closer to the person's iden- tity. They are rarely talked about, confronted or adjusted – at least, not with- out difficulty. Given this description it is arguable that patients who have deeply seated personal constructs linking physical function or appearance with self-worth (I am attractive and desirable) may suffer badly in the face of disfig- urement. Equally, those patients with personal constructs concerning their abil- ity to change and adapt (I am resilient and nothing gets me down) may draw upon this when confronting body image adversity. The patient believes that he is able to cope and recalls past successes to address the current challenge.

Altered body image, then, is a good example of where neurophysiology meets neuropsychology. Individuals' experience the body using neurological transmissions but they make sense of such sensations by deciding what this means concerning the self. Is the pain permanent, will the treatment leave me scarred and will I be able to rise about such misfortune? Patients may habitu- ally deal with changes in a familiar fashion (behaving according to trait). They may be more or less equipped to suffer insult to body function or appearance, or try to deal with the situation using personal constructs that have seemed useful in the past. All of these psychological theories could contribute to a debate regarding why patients vary in the degree of distress they suffer after body image insult.

? Questions for further consideration

1 Examine explanations of dreaming.
2 What are the psychophysiological correlates of emotion?
3 How are messages transmitted to the brain?

4 Compare and contrast *type* and *trait* theories of personality.

5 What is meant by a personal construct? How is it measured?

6 Discuss the problems associated with assessing the validity of psychodynamic theories of personality.

References

Broadbent, D. E. (1963). Differences and interactions between stresses. *Quarterly Journal of Experimental Psychology, 15,* 205–211.

Cannon, W. B. (1927). The James–Lange theory of emotions: a critical examination and alternative. *American Journal of Psychology, 39,* 106–124.

Cartwright, R., Monroe, L. and Palmer, C. (1967). Individual differences in response to REM deprivation. *Archives of General Psychiatry, 16,* 297–303.

Cattell, R. B. (1946). *Description and Measurement of Personality.* New York: World Book Company.

Costa, P. T. and McCrae, R. R. (1994) 'Set like plaster'? Evidence for the stability of adult personality. In Heatherton, T. F and Weinberger, J.L. (eds) *Can Personality Change?* New York: American Psychological Association.

Costa, T. P. and McCrae, R. P. (2005). *Personality in Adulthood.* New York: Guilford Press.

Dunlop, D. (1970). Abuse of drugs by the public and by doctors. *British Medical Bulletin, 26,* 236–239.

Eysenck, H. J. (1970). *The Structure of Human Personality.* 2nd edn. London: Methuen.

Flanagan, O. (2000). *Dreaming Souls.* New York: Oxford University Press.

Flowers, K. (1993). Unpublished personal communication.

Freud, S. (1964). New introductory lectures on psychoanalysis. In Strachey, J. (ed.) *The Standard Edition of the Complete Works of Sigmund Freud.* London: Hogarth Press.

Goldberg, L. R. (1981) Language and individual differences: the search for universals in human lexicons. In Wheeler, L. (ed.) *Review of Personality and Social Psychology* II, London: Sage.

Hobson, J. A. (1990). *The Dreaming Brain.* London: Penguin.

Hodgson, L. A. (1991). Why do we need sleep? Relating theory to nursing practice. *Journal of Advanced Nursing, 16,* 1503–1510.

Horne, J. (1992). Stay awake, stay alive. *New Scientist, 133,* 20–24.

Jensen, D. P. and Herr, K. A. (1993). Sleeplessness. *Nursing Clinics of North America, 28,* 385–405.

Kelly, G. A. (1955). *The Psychology of Personal Constructs* I–II. New York: Norton.

Loehlin, J. C. (1992) *Genes and Environment in Personality Development,* Newbury Park CA: Sage.

MacPhail, E. M. and Miller, N. E. (1968). Cholinergic brain stimulation in cats: failure to obtain sleep. *Journal of Comparative and Physiological Psychology, 65,* 499–503.

Rachman, S. J. and Phillips, C. (1975). *Psychology and Medicine.* London: Temple Smith.

Rogers, A. E. and Aldrich, M. S. (1993). The effect of regularly scheduled naps on sleep attacks and excessive daytime sleepiness associated with narcolepsy. *Nursing Research, 42,* 111–117.

Schacter, S. and Singer, J. F. (1962). Cognitive, social, and physiological determinants of emotional state. *Psychological Review, 69,* 379–399.

Somer, O. and Goldberg, L. R. (1999) The structure of Turkish trait-descriptive adjectives. *Journal of Personality and Social Psychology, 76,* 431–450

Stepanski, E., Koshorek, G., Zorick, F., Glinn, M., Roehrs, T. and Roth, T. (1989). Characteristics of individuals who do, or do not, seek treatment for chronic insomnia. *Psychosomatics, 30,* 421–427.

Webb, W. B. and Cartwright, R. D. (1978). Sleep and dreams. *Annual Review of Psychology, 29,* 223–252.

Wilkinson, R. T. (1968). Sleep deprivation: performance tests for partial and selective sleep deprivation. In Abt, L. E. and Reiss, B. F. (eds) *Progress in Clinical Psychology* VII. London: Grune and Stratton.

Williams, H. L., Agnew, H. W. and Webb, W. B. (1964). Sleep patterns in young adults. *Electroencephalograph in Clinical Neurophysiology, 17,* 376–381.

Further reading

Flanagan, Owen (2000) *Dreaming Souls.* Oxford: Oxford University Press. I have always found dreams fascinating. Something we all apparently do, or have, and yet we know so little about them. This book goes quite a way to making the picture a bit clearer.

Goldberg, Elkhonon (2001) *The Executive Brain.* New York: Oxford University Press. An interesting journey through the frontal lobes of the brain. With a particularly important chapter 11 on cognitive rehabilitation.

Kiersey, David and Bates, Marilyn (1984) *Please Understand Me.* Del Mar CA: Prometheus Nemesis. Essentially a type of Myers-Briggs approach. But it does contain a wealth of detail on the 'four types' and also an opportunity for you to assess yourself using their own scale.

The Biopsychosocial Perspective

(2) Pain and Stress

Whilst psychophysiology and personality are two *areas* that illustrate a biopsychosocial perspective, two important *topics* in health also serve a similar function: pain and stress. This means that one cannot investigate the psychology of pain and stress in isolation from biological and social factors. Pain and stress are neither physiological, psychological nor social, but a combination of all three. Therefore, it is important to examine the ways in which the components of pain and stress interact to produce two of the major topics in nursing practice. Karoly and Jensen (1993) have said that pain is one of the most pervasive symptoms in medical practice, the most frequently stated cause of disability, and the single most compelling force underlying an individual's decision to seek or avoid medical care.

A practice conundrum

In our conundrums to date we have encouraged you to use the contents of a chapter to verify or modify your understanding of problems that you have confronted in practice. In this chapter we are reversing that process and encourage you to read the contents of Chapter 8 as part of preparation to investigate the meaning of pain, coping and support for one patient that you assist. In conducting your case study it is important to follow three key principles:

- To place patient needs first. Whilst you seek to understand and reflect upon pain and coping, your responsibilities to help the patient tackle pain remain uppermost.
- As you engage in helping the patient to cope with pain make notes on whether your support appeared to modify the patient's perception of pain and coping as well as whether pain was relieved. Perceptions of circumstance and ability to deal with pain influence patient coping.

● Balance the need to understand and learn with the need to respect privacy. Ask the patient's permission to explore this case study in more depth and be prepared to listen and observe as well as to ask questions.

To help you organise your case study use the following headings and date your entries so as to reflect the changing circumstances of the patient:

● Patient history.
● Pain dimensions (e.g. physical, emotional, acute on chronic).
● Contexts or origins of pain. (What does the patient think causes or exacerbates his or her pain?)
● Description of pain. (How is pain described? What words, symbols or analogies are used?)
● How is coping described/conceived by the patient?
● How does the patient see nursing support/intervention (e.g. heading off pain or sustaining personal coping)?
● What seems most helpful to the patient?

Once your case study is complete, discuss with colleagues the extent to which psychological concepts and patient insights have helped you to deepen or diversify your appreciation of pain, coping and what is supportive regarding nursing care.

Pain

Imagine, for a moment, that you are a patient on the burns ward of a hospital. A recent accident has left half your body covered with deep burns. Pain has become your constant companion; pain-relieving medications have been minimised or withheld altogether, as they may result in prolonged periods of sleep, and resultant inability to comply with the high levels of fluid intake required. The isolation necessary to avoid infection allows you time to recall all aspects of your present condition: the original trauma, the personal and financial ramifications, the possibility of incapacitation and disfigurement, and the excruciatingly painful medical treatments you must undergo.

Your treatment, referred to as 'open treatment', requires the bandages which cover (and may cling to) your wounds to be removed. Hydrotherapy (or 'tubbing') follows, exposing your temperature-hypersensitive skin first to air, then to a whirlpool bath of water, in rapid succession. Debridement (the removal of devitalised tissue) is then accomplished by means of cutting tissue away, pulling it away with forceps or rubbing wet gauze across the surface of the wound. In addition to experiencing the pain of this treatment, you can see with your own eyes the extent of the tissue damage inflicted by the burns. Application of an antibacterial compound and redressing the wound complete the procedure: a regimen that will be repeated twice daily for a period of several weeks. What can be done for a person who has to experience such excruciating pain?

We will all experience pain at some time during our lives although maybe not as much as in the example given; indeed, it often serves as an indication that something is wrong. However, not all people experience pain. There are some people who have a congenital insensitivity to pain. Melzack (1973) cites the case of a young Canadian woman who seemed perfectly normal except for the fact that she never appeared to experience pain. As a child she had bitten off part of her tongue whilst chewing and had burnt her legs when she kneeled on a hot radiator to peer out of a window. According to Melzack, she not only felt no pain in response to scalding water, electric shock and icy water, but showed no changes in blood pressure, heart rate or respiration either. Fortunately this condition is rare, for whilst the absence of pain may seem desirable, this woman died at the age of 29 because her body was unable to use pain as a sign of danger. Pain, it seems, is not a simple sensory phenomenon but a rather complex entity. Therefore, the first stage in any analysis of pain is to determine precisely what we are talking about.

Sanders (1985) defines pain as 'the sensory and emotional experience of discomfort, which is usually associated with actual or threatened tissue damage or irritation'. However, explanations of pain fall into two categories – types and theories.

Types of pain

The first distinction to make is between *sensory* pain and *reaction* to pain. Sensory pain relates to the pain threshold – the point at which stimulation becomes painful. If stimulation increases the pain can become unbearable. The points at which pain is felt and at which it becomes unbearable differ from person to person; some individuals will feel pain when others will not because they have a different pain threshold. Reaction to pain is the observable component, as it is possible to estimate degrees of pain only by observing an individual's reactions to it – we cannot feel another's pain. There are large individual and cultural differences in the ways people react to pain, however, and one must be careful not to fall into the trap of stereotyping a patient's pain responses on the basis of their cultural origin. Davitz and Davitz (1985) presented nurses from the United States with the following brief description of an adult patient:

Michael O'Hara, aged 37, Irish, was struck by an automobile. He was admitted to hospital with a fractured femur and facial injuries. Currently in traction, he is to remain hospitalised for an indefinite period.

The nurses were asked for their ratings of the patient's physical pain and psychological distress. The experimenters then varied the ethnic background of the individual while keeping the other details constant (Oriental, Mediterranean, Black, Spanish, Anglo-Saxon/Germanic and Jewish). For both physical pain and psychological distress, the American nurses believed that Jewish and Spanish patients suffered most, while Oriental and Anglo-Saxon/Germanic patients suffered the least. Davitz and Davitz (1985) state that:

> in discussing our research with nurses, we have found that some nurses react defensively to our findings. They strenuously insist that they never generalise, that they treat all patients as individuals. That may indeed be the case for particular nurses, but our data do indicate that in general, American nurses in fact tend to share certain generalised beliefs about patients.

A second distinction that has been made is between *organic* and *psychogenic* pain. When discomfort is caused by tissue damage such as a serious burn, it is described as organic pain. When there is pain, but no apparent tissue damage, psychological factors are deemed to be responsible and this is called psychogenic pain. Many researchers now recognise that nearly all pain has physiological and psychological components and different pain experiences involve different mixtures of organic and psychogenic causes. Thus the distinction between organic and psychogenic pain is not particularly useful, and leads to some health care professionals thinking that pain with no obvious physical cause exists only in the patient's mind. There are several types of pain with no apparent physical basis.

- *Phantom limb pain.* According to Bakal (1992), about 5–10 per cent of patients who have had a limb amputated will experience phantom limb pain. This is pain which is experienced in a limb that is no longer there or has no functioning nerves. Patients can feel either recurrent or continuous pain which has been described as burning, shooting or cramping. People who have had their hand amputated have been known to report feelings as if their fingernails are digging into the palm of their phantom hand. This may happen if the amputation stump is stimulated, as it contains severed nerves which would have carried messages to the missing limb.
- *Neuralgia.* This type of pain involves recurrent episodes of intense shooting or stabbing pain along a nerve. Attacks of neuralgia can occur very suddenly and without any evident cause. Sometimes very minor stimuli can trigger an attack – a ball of cotton gently drawn across the skin will often produce an attack, whereas a stronger stimulus such as a pinprick will not.
- *Causalgia.* This is usually experienced as recurrent episodes of severe burning pain, and occurs in a part of the body that has been injured but now has healed. Thus a person previously wounded in the arm may feel as if the arm is being pressed against a hot pipe even though the wound has healed and the nerves have been regenerated. Like neuralgia, minor stimulation can set it off.

Acute and chronic pain

Loeser and Fordyce (1983) state that acute pain and chronic pain have nothing in common save for the four-letter word *pain*. Acute pain involves short-term and usually reversible discomfort, whereas chronic pain often has no identifiable cause, is not temporary, and involves psychological adjustment. Unfortunately, most research has been concerned with the analysis of acute pain, often under laboratory conditions, and thus does not necessarily relate to most chronic pain sufferers. Turk *et al.* (1983) say that a person's psychological adjustment to pain will depend on whether the underlying condition is benign or malignant and worsening. They propose three types of chronic pain. (The distinctions between different types of pain will become increasingly important when we consider ways of controlling pain later in the chapter.)

- *Recurrent pain:* originating from benign causes and characterised by intense pain episodes followed by periods of relief (for example, migraine headaches, tension headaches, myofacial pain).
- *Intractable/benign pain:* present most of the time with varying levels of intensity (for example, chronic lower back pain).
- *Progressive pain:* characterised by continuous discomfort, associated with malignancy, and a worsening condition (such as rheumatoid arthritis or cancer).

Theories of pain

There are three major theories of pain: *specificity theory, pattern theory* and *gate control theory.*

Specificity theory

This theory proposed that there are specific pathways responsible for transmitting pain messages to a pain centre in the brain. The theory is usually accredited to Von Frey in 1894, but in fact it had its roots in the much earlier work of the French philosopher Descartes. Von Frey suggested that the quality of skin sensations such as cold, warmth, pain and touch depends on the type of nerve endings that are stimulated. Different structures of nerve endings made some of them responsive to one kind of stimulus and unresponsive to others. Pain was thought to be associated with stimulation of the free nerve endings. However, this explanation has proved to be simplistic, since stimulation of the outer ear (which has only free nerve endings) can produce a wide range of sensations such as warmth, cold, touch, itch and pain.

Pain signals are thought to be carried by two types of fibres, A-delta and C fibres, which follow different paths when they reach the brain. A myelin sheath around the fibres facilitates the transmission of signals. Lyn (1984) suggests that the myelinated A-delta fibres represent immediate or sharp pain, whereas unmyelinated C fibres produce dull or aching pain. The thoracic and abdominal organs have a different nerve supply from the skin and injuries to the thoracic and abdominal organs usually have to be extensive before severe pain is experienced. (However, minimal tissue damage caused by the passage of renal stones can cause extreme pain.) Localisation of pain from these areas may be difficult, and pains originating from internal organs can sometimes feel as if they are coming from other parts of the body such as the skin. This is known as *referred pain* and occurs when the sensory impulses from the internal organ and the sensory impulses from the skin use the same pathway to the brain (Francis, 1987). Thus, although the appendix is located lower down on the right side of the body, pain from appendicitis is felt in the upper abdomen. Similarly, pain in the ear may be the result of toothache.

However, there is no evidence of a pain centre in the brain as postulated by Von Frey, and whilst specificity theory can help to explain why some injuries are perceived as painful, it cannot explain congenital insensitivity to pain or even why sometimes environmental factors can distract an individual to the extent that no pain at all is experienced.

Pattern theory

This theory tries to relate the experience of pain to particular patterns of impulses in the nervous system. It proposes that pain may occur as a result of any kind of stimulus, as long as that stimulation is intense. The receptors for pain are shared with those of touch, so that differences in *quantity*, rather than *quality*, of nerve fibre discharge produce differences in quality of sensation. A small degree of stimulation will be classified as touch, whereas strong stimulation will be classified as pain. Exactly the same kind of nerve fibres are discharging, but the difference in sensation is due to the amount of discharge.

One problem with pattern theory is that sometimes mild stimuli can trigger intense pain, as in the case of causalgia or neuralgia. However, more serious problems for both pattern and specificity theories are that they do not consider psychological factors, such as the meaning of the situation, personality and culture, in the perception of pain. One attempt to integrate both psychological and physiological perspectives into a theory of pain is the *gate control theory* of Melzack and Wall (1965).

Gate control theory

This, is based on the principle that neural mechanisms can control a 'gate' in the spinal cord to prevent pain messages from reaching the brain. The theory states that there are certain neurons, called *interneurons*, which are located in the spinal cord. These interneurons receive inputs from nerve fibres which carry pain messages, and information, such as pressure and temperature, from the skin senses.

When the interneurons are stimulated (mainly by fibres from the skin senses), the gate is closed and the pain messages are barred. There may therefore be some validity in the saying 'rubbing it makes it better'. In contrast, when the interneurons are stimulated by fibres carrying pain messages inhibition takes place, the gate remains open and an unobstructed route exists to the brain. Melzack and Wall (1965, 1982) suggest that information descending from the brain can also open and close the gate. Therefore psychological factors such as a person's emotional state and the context of the situation would be important determinants in the perception of pain.

The experience of pain

The experience of pain is governed by three components: *sensory/physical, emotional* and *cognitive.*

- *Sensory/physical.* The sensory/physical component of the pain system transmits primary sensory information, such as the location of the pain and whether it is a pricking, burning or aching pain.
- *Emotional.* This component has two parts: (1) the degree to which we want to escape pain; and (2) our emotional response to it.
- *Cognitive.* Pain after a serious accident may indicate the need for rest and relaxation, whereas the pain caused by terminal disease may include factors such as anger and frustration, making the pain more difficult to tolerate.

These three components of pain also affect the opening and closing of the gate in gate control theory. Some conditions that may affect the opening and closing of the gate are given in Table 8.1.

Since its conception nearly thirty years ago, gate control theory has been the source of considerable debate. In its original 1965 formulation, most discussion centred on determining the exact nature of the anatomical and neurophysiological mechanisms responsible for the perception of pain. Melzack and Wall (1965) thought that a part of the spinal cord called the substantia gelatinosa was of prime importance for the gating process, but research has so far failed to establish its exact function in the gate control

Table 8.1 *Conditions affecting gate opening and closure*

	Sensory/physical	*Emotional*	*Cognitive*
Opening the gate	Nature of injury	Anxiety	Attending to the pain
Closing the gate	Massage	Relaxation	Distraction

theory. Accordingly, Melzack and Wall (1982) revised their model in the following three main ways.

- They attempted to state the multiple functions of substantia gelatinosa in the process.
- They proposed a descending inhibitory input to the gate from the brain, i.e. the brain was able to control the function of the gate.
- They established the involvement of endorphins (morphine-like substances) in the experience of pain.

There is still doubt concerning the nature and location of some components of gate control theory; nevertheless, it represents a major step forward in the integration of psychological and physiological components of pain and has stimulated a multidisciplinary view of pain research and treatment.

What influences the perception of pain?

Many people think that the more the body is harmed or injured the more pain will be experienced. This is not necessarily correct, as the degree of injury does not always correlate with the amount of pain. Thus it is appropriate to examine some of the factors that have been thought to influence pain in order to establish the true nature of any association. At this point we should distinguish between pain *tolerance* and pain *threshold*. The majority of research has investigated people's ability to tolerate pain as opposed to their capacity to distinguish pain from sensation. Some factors that have been thought to influence pain tolerance are: *the degree of injury, the placebo effect, culture, emotion, personality* and *memory.*

Degree of injury

In a famous study comparing American soldiers injured on the battlefield with civilians hospitalised for major surgery, Beecher (1959) found that 80 per cent of the hospitalised patients requested morphine, compared with 33 per cent of the soldiers. As the differences were not due to shock or trauma-induced analgesia, Beecher proposed that the context in which the hospitalisation took place was an important factor in the differential experience of pain. For the soldiers, the fact that they had escaped death on the battlefield countered the pain being felt, while the civilians undergoing major surgery did not have such positive connotations. Beecher concluded that the degree of injury to an individual is not necessarily proportional to the amount of pain experienced.

The placebo effect

McCaffery (1983) defined a placebo as 'any medical treatment that produces an effect in a patient because of its implicit or explicit therapeutic intent and not because of its specific nature'. Some research has shown that placebos seem to produce substantial relief in about half as many patients as does a real drug (Melzack and Wall, 1982). Unfortunately, the effectiveness of placebos tends to decrease with recurrent use.

There are a number of hypotheses about why placebos can reduce pain. A popular explanation is that the patient's belief that a treatment will work activates the release of substances in the body called *endogenous opoids* (from *endogenous,* meaning 'developing from within' and *oid* meaning 'resembling') which inhibit the transmission of pain signals (Fields and Levine, 1984). But why a belief that having taken something to make the pain better should stimulate the body to produce more pain-relieving substances is still unclear. Another explanation is that the placebo effect acts at a 'higher' level in the brain. One of the main functions of pain is to signal to the brain that something is wrong; if a person takes a placebo and believes it to work then the brain does not need to monitor the pain anymore since the treatment is in place. Thus the brain sends messages to inhibit the transmission of pain signals, and the individual experiences a reduction or extinction of the pain.

Culture

There are cultural differences in both the response to pain and the behavioural expression of pain. Melzack (1973) presents striking evidence of the way in which in some cultures under certain circumstances respond to apparently excruciating pain with no visible reaction. In some remote Indian villages a hook swinging ceremony takes place, in which a young man has two hooks inserted into his back, is hoisted on to a pole and is paraded from village to village. Melzack (1973) says that during the whole of this procedure the young man seems to display no pain. It is impossible to measure the exact amount of pain experienced by the young man, but by most people's standards the hook-swinging ceremony would be judged to be unbearably painful. This response to pain is further evidence that the meaning of the situation, for example, its religious significance, is important in the experience of pain.

There are also cultural differences in the behavioural response to pain. Zborowski (1969) found that expressions of pain differed among ethnic groups in medical settings and suggested that the differences were due to the attitudes and values of the ethnic groups. Third-generation Americans were found to respond to pain in a 'matter of fact' way and as if they should be good, uncomplaining patients. A sample of Irish patients was found to be similar in the expression of pain, but they chose to communicate their suffering to observers. More overt responses were observed in Italian and Jewish samples. The Italians felt that pain should be avoided at all costs, whereas the Jewish sample was much more concerned with the memory of the pain.

While culture does seem to affect the expression of, and response to, pain, nurses should beware of falling into the 'stereotype trap'. Davitz and Davitz (1985) found that although their sample of American nurses strenuously insisted that they weren't influenced by stereotypes, and treated all patients as individuals, it was found that they did tend to share generalised beliefs about patients.

Emotion

Kleinknecht and Bernstein (1978) posted anxiety questionnaires to a sample of patients before they came for dental treatment. They measured attendance, split the patients into high and low-anxiety groups and asked the patients to indicate how much pain they had experienced during their appointment. The high and low-anxiety groups were compared and it was found that the high-anxiety patients reported more pain than the low-anxiety patients. This difference was not due to the type of treatment, since similar procedures were adopted for all patients. Therefore it seems that there is a connection between anxiety and pain. Walding (1991) reviewed the relationship between pain and anxiety for patients undergoing surgery. The conclusions were that there was a relationship between pain, anxiety and perceived powerlessness. Decreasing perceived powerlessness reduced anxiety, and thus helped to reduce pain.

Cooper *et al.* (1987) found an association between levels of stress in children and migraine headaches. Children who suffered from migraine were asked to keep diaries of their headaches over a four-month period. It was found that migraine sufferers with high levels of anxiety had more frequent and severe headaches than those with lower anxiety. The relationship between pain and anxiety can therefore be seen to be circular. The fear of pain or the anticipation of high pain levels will increase anxiety, which in turn will lead to a self-fulfilling prophecy, because an increase in anxiety will lead to an increase in pain sensitivity.

Personality

One of the tests that has been used extensively in the analysis of pain is a personality test called the Minnesota Multiphasic Personality Inventory (MMPI). Connolly *et al.* (1978) gave a sample of eighty women the MMPI and then monitored their pain and anxiety levels during childbirth. They found that women who scored high on the 'anxious–depressive' scale of the MMPI displayed higher levels of pain and anxiety. Further, Rappaport *et al.* (1987) highlighted the differential personality characteristics associated with chronic and acute pain. Individuals who suffered from chronic back pain showed an MMPI profile characterised by high levels of neuroticism, while individuals with acute pain recovering from injury showed slightly elevated neuroticism scores but scores which were nevertheless well within the normal range. These findings also indicate the different psychological effects which can result from conditions that are expected to end soon compared with those that may never cease.

Memory of pain

Lander *et al.* (1991) examined 138 children aged between 5 and 17 years who were attending an out-patient lab for venipuncture. The children reported their anxiety and expected pain levels before venipuncture, immediately after their visit and two months later. Four patterns of response were identified when prediction, recall and accuracy were examined (see Figure 8.1). The largest group (*n* = 74) was labelled *realistic*, since experienced and recalled pain scores were comparable. Many children in this group also had expected pain that was equivalent to their experienced and recalled pain. A second group (*n* = 23) was identified for whom the experience seemed irrelevant – recalled and expected pain were the same no matter whether the experienced pain was high or low. A third group (*n* = 23) was designated *overreactors* because more pain was recalled than had been experienced or expected. Finally, the fourth group was labelled the *denial* group, as they recalled having very little pain despite expecting and experiencing mid to high levels of pain. These findings indicate that memory of pain is not always accurate, and that children possess different types of coping strategy to deal with painful experiences. With respect to older people aged between 55 to 87 years, Walmsley *et al.* (1992) found that memories of prior pain experience had a significant effect on expectations about post-operative pain. Ratings of past pain experience correlated significantly with pain expected post-operatively. Finally, Niven and Murphy-Black (2000), in a review of pain during childbirth, found that women do not completely forget the pain and that recall was often vivid but not always entirely accurate. They also found that memories of labour pain could produce intense negative reactions in a few women, but were more likely to give rise to positive consequences related to coping, self-efficacy and self-esteem.

Assessment of pain

A study by Camp and O'Sullivan (1987) found that nurses were not very good at finding out about patients' experiences of pain. Nurses were observed to document less than 50 per cent of what the patient reported as pain, and these findings show that some nurses do not give sufficient importance to patients' reports of pain. Harrison (1991) also points out that nurses often provide inaccurate and biased estimates of their patients' pain. There are several methods of assessing pain, and they may be grouped under the following headings: *self-report methods, psychophysiological measures* and *behavioural assessment*.

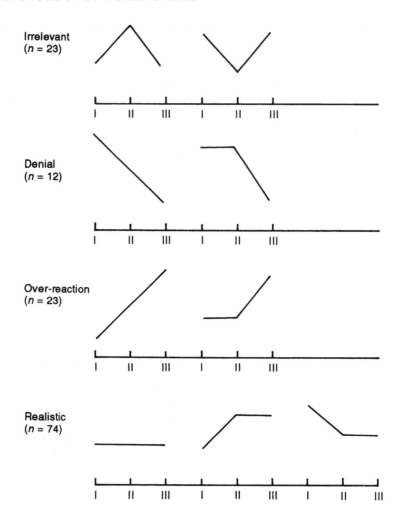

Figure 8.1 Four patterns of response among 5–17 year old venipuncture subjects, including variations in each category. *Key*: I expected pain, II experienced pain, III recalled pain

Reprinted from *Behaviour Research and Therapy*, Vol 30, Lander 'Children's Pain Predictions and Memories', pp 117–124, 1991, with permission from Elsevier.

Self-report measures

One of the easiest and most direct methods of assessing pain is to ask the patient to indicate the degree of discomfort on a rating scale. *Visual analog scales* use a 10 cm long line with 'I have no pain' at one end and 'My pain is as bad as I can imagine' at the other. The patient marks a point on the line equivalent to the pain's intensity.

A second type of scale, the *category scale,* uses a line but has the following categories of pain interspersed along it: No pain; Mild; Discomforting; Distressing; Horrible;

Excruciating. La Montagne *et al.* (1991) found that when children rated their pain using a visual analogue scale, there was a significant correlation between the nurses and physicians' ratings of the childrens' pain and their own ratings of pain.

Pain questionnaires are another type of self-report procedure. The most famous is the McGill Pain Questionnaire (MPQ) which consists of a list of words categorised into dimensions that include twenty subclasses which describe pain. The sensory dimension includes the temperature subclass hot; burning; scalding; searing; while the affective dimension includes the fear subclass fearful; frightful; terrifying. This questionnaire has proved useful in both the research and the clinical domains and has helped to distinguish different patterns of pain. For example, people suffering from toothache will choose different patterns of words in the MPQ from people suffering from arthritis.

Psychophysiological measures

Another range of techniques involved in measuring pain uses psychophysiological indices. As pain tolerance is associated with heightened autonomic activity, measures such as heart rate and skin conductance have been employed to indicate levels of pain. Further, muscle tension has also been linked with pain, hence the use of the electromyograph (EMG), which measures electrical activity in muscles, to assess various pain states. Finally, the electroencephalograph (EEG) is used to measure evoked potentials, the sharp surges or peaks of electrical activity in the brain. Chapman *et al.* (1985) found that the amplitude of these evoked potentials increased with the presence of pain and decreased when analgesics were administered to the patient.

The advantages of psychophysiological measurements over self-report methods are that they do not suffer from response bias. When asked about their pain, people may not tell the truth, but it is very difficult to fake psychophysiological measures. However, changes in autonomic functioning, muscle activity and evoked potentials also happen in response to other stimuli besides pain, and therefore can give an inaccurate picture of purely pain experience.

Behavioural assessment

The University of Alabama in Birmingham (UAB) Pain and Behaviour Scale was developed for use by nurses in the course of their everyday ward routines (Richards *et al.,* 1982). The nurse has the patient perform several activities and rates their behaviours in such areas as patient mobility and use of medication on a three-point scale labelled 'none', 'occasional' and 'frequent'. The ratings are added up to provide a total pain score. The authors suggest that the scale is easy to use and acts as a valid and reliable behavioural measure of pain. It is also useful in training nurses to become more aware of the nature of their patients' pain.

Management of pain

The majority of methods used to reduce or alleviate pain involve some kind of pharmacological treatment. However, a number of psychological approaches have been devised to moderate the experience of pain.

Acupuncture

Acupuncture is the process of inserting fine needles under the skin at selected points and vibrating them. The Chinese have been practising acupuncture for over 2,000 years, and the ancient Chinese thought that life energy flowed through pathways in the body, called *meridians*. Pain could be relieved by inserting a needle at specific points in the body, reducing the life energy passing through the meridians. Unfortunately there is no evidence of these meridians but there is evidence of the effectiveness of acupuncture in reducing pain. So how good is it? Melzack and Wall (1982) reviewed the evidence for the efficiency of acupuncture in relieving, and in some cases removing, pain. They came to several conclusions

- Only a small proportion of the population are likely to benefit from acupuncture. Even in China, physicians perform less than 10 per cent of their operations using acupuncture analgesia.
- Acupuncture is rarely effective for surgery in Western cultures and may produce only mild analgesia.
- Patients who benefit most from acupuncture have shown themselves to be open to suggestion and easily hypnotised.
- Acupuncture does not appear to be a success in ameliorating long-term, chronic pain.

Hypnosis

Barber (1986) tells of a surgeon in the latter part of the nineteenth century who removed a cancerous tumour from a woman's breast using hypnotism to control the pain. During the procedure, the woman was able to engage the surgeon in conversation and showed no signs of feeling pain. This situation contrasts with the widely held picture of a hypnotist seated in front of a person swinging a gold watch on a chain saying, 'You are going to sleep, you are going to sleep.'

In fact the hypnotic procedure varies enormously, from altering a patient's negative perception of pain to developing deep feelings of relaxation that are incompatible with pain. The main question, as with acupuncture, is 'Does it work?' The short answer is 'Yes, it does, but only with a limited number of the population.' For some individuals hypnosis can produce pain relief very quickly and dramatically. For others it may produce only temporary unawareness of what is going on around and about the person.

Indeed, Barber (1982) has likened the process of becoming hypnotised to becoming involved in a good book, and suggested that there was a link between suggestibility and hypnotism. He proposed (1986) that:

- People often show as much pain relief when given suggestions about how they are feeling as when they have been hypnotised;
- those people who are highly suggestive receive the most pain relief;
- distraction is often used in association with suggestion to reduce pain.

This last point fits in well with the view of Pennebaker (1984) who regards distraction as evidence of the role cognitive components play in diverting attention away from the internal sensations of the body. Thus an individual is likely to feel more pain when the external environment is boring than when it provides distractions to absorb the attention.

Hilgard and Hilgard (1975) take an opposing viewpoint with regard to the mechanisms of hypnotism. Suggestions may *modify* the emotional response to pain, but hypnosis actually *blocks* a large amount of pain from awareness and therefore being under hypnosis is an altered state of consciousness. As evidence for their claim, they report an experiment on the *hidden observer phenomenon*. The participant was hypnotised to feel no pain in one arm and then asked to immerse that arm in a bucket of ice-cold water. The activity of the other arm was to be kept out of awareness. The person was required to rate how much pain they experienced in the immersed arm on a scale from 0 (no pain) to 10 (unbearable pain). The participants in the experiment invariably reported 0. They were also asked to use the same numerical scale for the hand that was out of awareness, but they would not be aware of what the hand was writing. While the subjects were overtly describing a 0 degree of pain, the hand out of awareness was writing 2, 5, 7 and 9 degrees of pain. Hilgard and Hilgard say that the hidden observer in the participant's brain was reporting normal pain while the hypnotised part of the brain was facilitating no pain at all. Thus the experimenters suggest that the mind is capable of blocking and monitoring pain at the same time. Hypnotic procedures can prove a useful source of pain relief to some people in some circumstances; however, their widespread use by large numbers of individuals is unlikely.

Cognitive restructuring

There has been considerable interest in the relationship between people's thoughts and their experience of pain. The term *cognitive restructuring* refers to the ways in which people are able to manipulate the way they think about pain in order to reduce the harmful effects of the experience. Essential to the concept of cognitive restructuring is the idea of control. There are two forms of cognitive control: *informational* and *strategic*.

Informational control

Informational control may be defined as 'the provision of information which enables people to predict accurately what is about to happen to them'. An experiment illustrating the use of informational control in the alleviation of pain was conducted by Johnson (1975). In a laboratory setting he exposed three groups of male participants to pain. One group was given information about the types of physical sensations they might be expected to experience as a result of the procedure; a second group was given information about the procedure, but no details about the sorts of sensations to expect; and a third group was not given any instructions at all. Johnson found that information about the nature of physical sensations likely to be experienced significantly reduced discomfort. Providing the second group with details of the procedure itself produced levels of discomfort no different from those of the control group who had received no instructions at all. The intensity of the sensations was similar for all groups, but more accurate expectations were associated with a significant reduction in distress.

Comparable findings have been found in the context of patients' preparation for surgery. However, when preparation involves a number of additional components, such as reassurance, emotional support and coping techniques, information about sensations alone is not enough in itself to reduce discomfort. Information needs to operate in conjunction with reassurance, emotional support and coping techniques to prove effective (Johnson and Wallace, 1990).

Strategic control

Cognitive strategies can be classified into three types: *distraction, imagery* and *reinterpretation.*

Distraction

Many people suffering from headaches or toothache have found that becoming engrossed in a task often negates the awareness of pain. Thus, actively engaging a distraction strategy can reduce pain. Sometimes the strategy may be passive (looking at a picture, listening to a tape) or active (singing a song, solving problems).

Beales (1979) performed a study on twelve children attending an Accident and Emergency department. The children, who were aged between five and thirteen years old, were observed whilst a nurse sutured a wound. The nurse tried to distract the children by talking to them whilst hiding the first suture from the child's sight. Beales noted that whenever the nurse said something like 'There, that didn't hurt, did it?' the children reported pain on subsequent sutures. Further, they found that children experienced more pain if comments were made on the unpleasantness of the wound, such as saying 'Ugh! That looks a bit of a mess, doesn't it?' Beales summarises the findings of the study as follows.

- Sometimes nurses feel they have to justify giving information about pain in order not to deceive patients. This practice may amplify the pain experience.
- Pain may be increased by the non-verbal behaviour of parents suggesting the procedure is painful.
- When their cases were being discussed, the children would sometimes misunderstand and exaggerate what was being said, thus leading to more pain and distress.

McCaul and Malott (1984) reviewed studies on the effectiveness of distraction in reducing pain and concluded that it is a useful technique as long as the painful stimulus is not too severe (for example, sutures, injections, dental drilling, early stages of childbirth). As pain increases, the ability to use distraction techniques becomes harder and harder. Also, the distractive task must attract a relatively high degree of attention and involvement on the patient's part to maintain the diversion. McCaffery (1990) says that research supports some of the older methods of pain control such as distraction (especially humour) and cutaneous stimulation.

Imagery

Guided imagery is a strategy that asks the patient to imagine a mental scene incompatible with the pain. Usually the scenes are pleasant ones of beaches or meadows, but not always (see Exercise 8.1).

Exercise 8.1 *Use of guided imagery*

The following is an example of a visualisation strategy to deal with pain resulting from a cut hand.

- *Stage 1.* Sit down in a comfortable chair in a quiet room. Take some time to relax your body, using a relaxation exercise that suits you. In your mind's eye, try to picture yourself sitting in the chair Allow *your* body to merge with the visualised figure so that you feel you are the figure sitting in the chair in your mind. Try to think of your body and your image as identical twins, fitting perfectly together.
- *Stage 2.* In your mind's eye, look at your hand. See it slip like a glove from the body. As it moves away from you, it grows larger and larger, until it becomes as big as a house standing just twenty yards away from you sitting on its base at the wrist.
- *Stage 3.* Stand up in your mind body and walk towards the hand. When you are about half-way there, turn round and see your other body, sitting in the chair. Say to it, 'Cross your legs,' and it does so. If it doesn't return to the chair and try again. When you see your

● *Stage 4.* When you reach the hand, you notice a door which you open and walk through. The hand is 'hollow, and a ladder is against the wall of the hand on the side of the palm and alongside the wound. On the floor are some patching materials, some tape and glue. You place these materials in the bucket and start to climb up the ladder to begin your repair to the cut.

● *Stage 5.* You repair the cut in whatever way seems best to you. You might want to place glue on the edges of the cut, position the patching material, and secure it with tape. After you have patched it up, quietly watch it for a few moments to make sure it is firm. When you are sure, climb down the ladder. However, if the patch starts to slip, start your repair again and continue till you have a patch that will hold.

● *Stage 6.* When you have achieved your desired result descend the ladder, put the materials back on the floor, go out of the door, walk back to your body, turn round and sit down.

● *Stage 7.* You look at your huge mind-hand and notice there is no wound. The hand gradually shrinks as it slowly moves towards you. Finally, when it is the right size, it slips back into place just like a glove.

● *Stage 8.* Relax for a while, then open your eyes, feeling good. Ignore your hand initially, allowing time for the body to integrate the visualisation without interference.

(This exercise may also prove useful for people who are anxious about dental care. In that case, a tooth should be substituted for the hand.)

The imagery technique is in many ways similar to distraction. The main difference is that imagery is based on imagined rather than real stimuli and thus does not have to depend on the environment to furnish distracting situations.

Reinterpretation

This is where the patient substitutes constructive thoughts for ones that arouse harm and pain. Fernandez (1986) says that the pain experience can be redefined by using reinterpretative self-statements. These self-statements may try to reduce the unpleasantness of the situation by containing messages such as 'It's not the worst thing that could happen to me, and just think of the benefits later on', or they could redefine the context completely. An example of the latter process would be asking a person who has her hand in icy water to think of herself as the hero of an Eskimo settlement which has become dangerously short of food. In order to feed her family she has cut a hole in the ice to get fish. She knows that if she holds a small piece of bread under the water as bait it will attract fish. It is only a matter of time, she has to hold her hand under for a few more minutes and she will have saved her family.

McCaul and Malott (1984) suggest that both distraction and imagery are particularly useful for mild pain, and cognitive reinterpretation is beneficial for higher levels of pain. Cognitive restructuring techniques can be used in conjunction to provide a multimodal treatment programme. Turk *et al.* (1983) encouraged participants to increase their resistance to pain and stress by giving them a general instruction about the nature of pain; training participants to relax; providing a selection of restructuring strategies; asking participants to imagine the painful situation and their reactions to it; and getting them to play the role of a teacher instructing someone else in the procedure.

The experimenters provide evidence of the effectiveness of this treatment programme in the alleviation of chronic pain in particular. However, it is not always possible to spend the appropriate amount of time needed to develop suitable pain management skills.

CBT and chronic pain

Pain behaviour

The behavioural approach to pain concentrates on the observable features of pain behaviour. The three learning mechanisms that characterise pain behaviour are: *operant conditioning*; *classical conditioning*; *modelling*.

Operant conditioning

Operant conditioning is underpinned by two key concepts: *reward* and *punishment*. Pain behaviour is frequently related to some form of reward. If something desirable occurs whenever a person displays pain behaviour, such as attention from a spouse or parent, that behaviour will be reinforced and is thus likely to be prolonged or repeated. Sometimes pain behaviour involves negative reinforcement, such as avoiding something undesirable like a stressful job or avoiding contact with a threatening person. It might seem proper to respond to someone in pain in a supportive and attentive fashion, but according to the operant approach to pain this will only result in rewarding the pain behaviour.

Giving a person attention every time they report pain will increase the pain behaviour because attention acts as a reward. Varni and Thompson (1986) describe how the rehabilitation of a 3-year-old girl with severe burns was hampered by rewarding pain behaviour. On trying to walk the girl cried, 'Ow! My leg hurts.' The nurse replied quickly, 'I'm sorry it hurts so much – can you show me where? Maybe we had better do some exercise some other time.' This resulted in the physical therapy essentially being terminated because of the patient's interfering pain behaviours. Pain behaviours such as crying, complaining of the pain and resisting the nurse's efforts to put her splints on were maintained by the hospital staff's attention to those behaviours, thus allowing her to avoid unpleasant activities such as physical therapy. Varni and Thompson decided to change the situation by instructing the hospital staff to ignore the pain behaviours instead of paying them attention, give rewards for suitable behaviour – 'If you don't cry while I'm doing this, you can have some chocolate cake after' – and commend her every time she engaged in adaptive activities. These changes had a startling effect in decreasing the child's pain behaviours. She started to comply with the nurse's requests for exercise, and to assist the nurses in her physical care.

Classical conditioning of pain

Classical conditioning can explain how features of the environment which were previously unconnected with pain can take on huge significance. If a person with chronic back pain goes for a walk and at the end of 100 ft always experiences intense pain, then the distance of 100 ft gradually becomes associated with back pain. The person has become conditioned to respond to the distance of 100 ft rather than to the actual amount of walking. Furthermore, when the critical distance is about to be reached, increased anxiety about the imminent pain will occur.

Another example of the process of classical conditioning in pain is the case of a patient with chronic lumbar pain. This patient used to report increased pain and muscle spasm around about the time he was going to sleep on the ward. Thus he began to associate going to sleep with the muscle spasm and experienced considerable anxiety in the evening when the time to go to sleep approached. This anxiety, in turn, enhanced the pain and pain behaviour. Another person may have experienced pain when given an injection in the past, so that injections have become associated with pain. The traumatic experience may not have initially occurred in hospital, but it has become generalised to all needles in all settings.

Modelling

One of the best illustrations of the way in which a 'model' can influence the experience of pain is provided by Craig and Prkachin (1978). In this experiment, volunteers were exposed to a series of electric shocks. The shocks ranged in intensity on a scale of 1 to 5 and participants were required to rate them for painfulness. Physiological measures of skin conductance and heart rate were taken. The electric shocks were given to the volunteers in the presence of a confederate of the experimenters who also was thought to be receiving shocks but actually did not receive any. In the experimental condition, the confederate always rated the shock after the volunteer and on each occasion her ratings were 25 per cent lower. In the control condition, the volunteer was unaware of the confederate's perception of shock. The results of the study showed that those participants exposed to the 'pain-tolerant' model reported less discomfort than the participants in the control condition. More important, the physiological data indicated that heart rate and skin conductance were significantly lower for those subjects who were exposed to the pain-tolerant models. The experimenters propose that exposure to someone who seems to be experiencing less pain results in the patient not only reporting less pain but actually seeming to experience less pain.

Cognitive Behaviour Therapy

Sometimes called 'multimodal therapy' (see 'Stress', p. 288), this approach amalgamates the emotional, cognitive and behavioural correlates of pain into one therapeutic approach. Starting with a physiological perspective, it is important to use techniques such as relaxation, visualisation and distraction to reduce anxiety and other emotional aspects of pain. Alongside the physiological, cognitive components need to be addressed. Thus patients are encouraged to confront their thoughts about pain such as 'It will never end and if anything just get worse', replacing them with a more adaptive version such as ' I know it may be bad at the moment, but there is an end and if I can just get through this bit by concentrating on what I have to do tomorrow . . .' Finally, certain behaviours may be antagonistic to the experience of pain. The idea is to identify these behaviours and replace them with behaviours which may in fact reduce pain. Sometimes when people are concentrating very hard on completing a particular task well they 'forget' all about any pain. In a review of behavioural treatments for pain, Van Tulder *et al.* (2000) found evidence of reduced pain intensity and increased functional status such as return to work. Also, Eccleston *et al.* (2002) found evidence for the effectiveness of psychological treatments such as relaxation and CBT in reducing the pain of chronic or recurrent headache in children. and adolescents.

Nursing implications

The type of pain management procedure chosen will depend in part on the nursing context. Thus, procedures used in Accident and Emergency departments will not necessarily be applicable to patients being prepared for surgery or patients with chronic pain. The following represent some general guidelines relating to the context-specific nature of pain management.

- As anxiety is related to pain, nurses should try to reassure the patient by talking and developing a therapeutic relationship. The mere fact that a nurse is there and talking to a patient often reduces anxiety. Patients arriving in Accident and Emergency departments are often anxious because they do not know how long they will have to wait, so explanations about estimated waiting time along with explanations of how the department functions can reduce a patient's anxiety.
- One of the main problems for patients going into hospital is their perceived lack of control. Ways in which nurses can give patients a greater sense of control are to

provide information as above, but also to try to involve the patient in their own care by asking them to hold the end of a bandage or move a limb in a particular way.

● The nurse should possess a repertoire of pain management techniques and try to match them to the specific situation and to the specific patient. This is not always easy but can be achieved if the nurse is able to talk to the patient about their normal patterns of coping with pain and determine the ways in which the patient explains the cause of events.

● Finally, it is important to consider the relatives of the patient. Often it is easy to become wrapped up in the care of the sufferer without realising what the consequences are for relatives or friends. Seeing someone whom you love and care for in pain can be an extremely distressing experience, and therefore attention to the needs of relatives is important as well as care of the patient.

Whilst some studies have indicated that nurses' knowledge of pain is not what it might be (Ferrell *et al.*, 1992), they also indicate that this lack of knowledge can easily be reversed given appropriate training (Hamilton and Edgar, 1992).

Conundrum revisited

It would be trite to try and second-guess what your case study may have taught you, but there are a number of assertions that you may like to compare with your own findings. You may discover that your case study enables you to either support or refute these. What is important is that you are engaged in understanding pain, coping and support using psychological concepts introduced within your reading.

● *Assertion 1*. Even when pain has a physical origin (for instance a burn) it is still fundamentally a psychological experience. The physical sensation of pain forces the patient to focus upon the experience, to interpret what it means and the threat that it poses to future health or well-being. As one patient observed, 'For most of your life your body does what you expect it to. It obeys you and doesn't cause problems. It is sort of silent. When you get pain like I have, there is no more silence.'

● *Assertion 2*. Patients redefine their self-worth, who they are and how they think others probably see them through their efforts to cope with pain. Successful coping enables the patient to sustain dignity, whilst chaotic coping (where strategies are rapidly adjusted or abandoned) leaves the patient feeling that the locus of control is with the pain or the professionals assisting.

● *Assertion 3*. Patients assisted to develop coping strategies that seem meaningful to them are more successful and feel more independent. Whilst tackling the origins of pain (e.g. combating infection) and altering the receipt

of sensation (e.g. analgesia) are important, measures associated with the development of coping are key to patient well being.
● *Assertion 4*. An understanding of pain and coping concepts may usefully be used by the nurse to enable the patient to understand his situation, how he feels and what might seem acceptable solutions.

Stress and coping

There is no doubt that stress has become a very fashionable concept for explaining a wide variety of conditions. It has been used to designate psychological symptoms preceding an illness, feelings of anxiety, discomfort, arousal, and many other conditions. Attempts to define stress are hampered by this broad collection of concepts and contexts in which the term is used. We can, however, look at different models of stress: physiological and psychological, the different types of cognitive appraisal techniques that are used to cope with stress and the various methods of stress management.

The nature of stress

Stress can be conceptualised in three ways.

● *Stress as a stimulus*. This view sees stress as something that happens to us, perhaps arising from having a highly stressful job, or being put under pressure by not having time to complete tasks. Events and circumstances conspire to cause feelings of tension that can be interpreted as stress.
● *Stress as a response*. Sometimes stress refers to how we respond to situations. The expression 'being wound up' is a perfect description of how stress can occur as a product of the ways in which we react to people and to circumstances. A person's response to stressors is usually termed *strain*.
● *Stress as a transaction*. Stress can be both a stimulus and a response. Often, people become so tired that they worry about whether they can do their job properly. On the other hand, having to perform a particularly demanding task can cause tiredness. There is a transaction between people and their environments, resulting in each affecting, and being affected by, each other.

A physiological model of stress

Selye (1956) proposed that the body's response to stressful stimuli occurs in three stages. He called these stages the General Adaptation Syndrome (GAS).

- *Stage 1 – the alarm reaction.* Blood pressure initially drops below normal, then rises quickly. The pituitary gland produces adrenocorticotropic hormone (ACTH), which stimulates the adrenal glands to secrete adrenaline into the bloodstream. This reaction is sometimes known as the 'fight or flight' response because it enables the organism either to face up to the stress or run away from it. The high level of arousal cannot be maintained for very long and if the initial stress is too severe and persists, then the organism may die in this stage.

- *Stage 2 – the resistance stage.* If the stress continues but is not strong enough to cause death, the body goes into a stage of resistance. The pituitary still produces ACTH and the adrenal cortex continues to produce glucocorticoids which stimulate the conversion of fats and proteins to sugars, thus producing energy. Arousal decreases somewhat and the body starts to replace the hormones released by the adrenal glands. Often there are few outward signs of stress but the ability to resist new stressors is reduced. Many stress-related diseases occur in this stage. The glucocorticoid hormones inhibit the formation of antibodies and decrease the formation of white blood cells. In males, sperm production drops and in females the menstrual cycle is disrupted.

- *Stage 3 – the exhaustion stage.* If the stress continues, the body's ability to maintain its resistance ultimately collapses. Disease and physiological damage are likely to occur, resulting in breakdown.

According to Seyle (1956), this physiological response pattern occurs regardless of the nature of the stimulus. Cold, electric shock, illness and emotional conflict will all produce the same response pattern. However, the model cannot explain why in some cases one person will experience stress while another will not, as exactly the same situation can produce GAS in one individual and not in another. It is not whether the event is stressful or not, but whether a person *thinks* it is stressful. This may be termed *cognitive appraisal,* and according to Bakal (1992) the psychological perception of threat is far more important than a simple analysis of the physiological effects of heat, shock and trauma on the body reserves.

A psychological model of stress

The psychological perspective emphasises the importance of how stressors are interpreted by individuals. In what has become a famous experiment, Richard Lazarus illustrated how presenting participants with different instructions altered their stressful experiences. Lazarus *et al.* (1965) showed participants a thirteen-minute black-and-white film about industrial accidents entitled *It didn't have to happen.* The film depicted three accidents: a man running the tips of his fingers through a ripsaw; a man losing his finger; and a worker being impaled by a plank of wood that had flown out of a machine. Participants were assigned to one of three conditions.

- *Control.* These participants were given no explanation of the events that they were about to see in the film. They were told to pay close attention to what was happening in the action sequences.
- *Intellectualisation.* This group of participants were told to analyse the film from an academic viewpoint. They had to view the film whilst assessing the internal dynamics of various situations. They were required to determine the effectiveness of the techniques used by the foreman to influence safety procedures and thus they had to try and view the film in a detached, analytical manner.
- *Denial.* The third group of participants were told that the events were all staged by actors using special effects and that nobody really got hurt in the film despite the vivid scenes.

Lazarus and his colleagues found that both the intellectual and the denial instructions reduced the participants' emotional responses to the film. Participants in the control condition had significantly higher heartbeat rates and showed more skin conductance than the participants in the other two groups. Therefore, the experimenters concluded that varying the instructions reduced the emotional response to stressful sequences in the film by allowing the participants to appraise the stimuli in a less threatening manner. They had 'devalued the threat'.

One of the outcomes of this research programme was the development of a cognitive model of stress (Lazarus, 1966). The initial component of the model relates to the perception of threat. Any potential stressful stimulus is appraised in terms of the effects it may have on an individual and the consequences of their actions. Whenever a stressful situation occurs the first reaction is 'How much am I in danger from this situation?' This is called *primary appraisal.* Following the primary appraisal of threat comes a *secondary appraisal.* Here the individual asks, 'What am I going to do and what are the likely consequences of my action?' Thus a nurse might find him or herself in a situation where the initial response is to worry about how he or she is going to be affected by the stress, then to be concerned about what he or she is going to do about it and how that is going to affect his or her life. Factors which influence the appraisal process are *social* and *cultural background* and *previous experience of similar situations.*

The next stage in the model is the use of coping mechanisms to deal with the stress. These are also classified into two categories: *problem-focused* and *emotion-focused.* Problem-focused strategies involve taking direct action with the stressful stimulus itself, and the individual tries to remove or reduce the threat. Emotion-focused strategies concentrate on altering one's reaction to the event.

Mary has some exams coming up in the next few days. These are important exams, and not surprisingly they are causing her a certain amount of stress because she is not sure if she will be able to pass them. A problem-focused coping strategy would be to either revise harder or decide not to take the exams. In each case the stress is confronted; in the first instance the stressful stimulus is reduced, and in the second it is removed.

However, Mary feels that she can't just run away from her exams and has revised until she thinks her brains are going to burst. She decides to adopt an emotion-focused coping strategy. After her usual time revising in the library, she resolves to go home and have a nice relaxing bath, followed by reading a good book on the sofa. Tomorrow she thinks she might ask around to see if anyone is interested in going out in the evening to enjoy themselves. The stressful stimulus is still there but she has altered her response to it and now no longer feels quite so worried about passing her exams.

Nursing intervention techniques can be enhanced when they are consistent with the patient's preferred coping style. Martelli *et al.* (1987) found that patients with problem-focused, emotion-focused or mixed-focused coping styles were able to cope more effectively when these styles were matched with appropriate interventions. They also noted that the mixed focus intervention was the most effective strategy, indicating that it is important to tackle stress from both problem- and emotion-focused viewpoints.

A central concern in nursing practice is the use of denial and intellectualisation coping mechanisms to deal with stressful situations. Bakal (1992) suggests that one of the reasons why some nurses are good at hiding their emotions is that they are in fact not feeling any emotion. Continual exposure to particularly stressful stimuli may result in an increased use of intellectualisation as a coping strategy. This may serve to distance the nurse from the stressful stimulus. However, if this stimulus is a patient or colleague, then the quality of interpersonal interaction could be affected.

Steptoe and Vogele (1986) attempted to replicate the Lazarus *et al.* experiment, using the same film about industrial accidents but changing one of the conditions. Medical students were allocated to one of three conditions: *control, intellectualisation* or *sensation focusing* (which replaced Lazarus's denial condition). Participants allocated to the third condition were given instructions to concentrate on their emotional feelings and note their physical sensations while watching the film. Psychophysiological measures of heart rate and skin conductance were taken, as were subjective emotional responses to the film. The latter were measured using a symptom–emotion checklist based on one developed by Pennebaker (1982).

The results indicated no significant differences between any of the conditions on any of the measures except for the sensation-focusing condition which produced significantly lower levels of heart rate and skin conductance than the other two. It seems that, in this instance, intellectualisation did not work, whereas concentrating on one's sensations did. How may this finding be explained? One explanation is that the participants spent so much time concentrating on their sensations that it distracted them from the film. Leventhal (1990) put forward another theory that concentrating on finding labels for one's emotions serves to objectify the experience. It may be that sensation-focusing is a form of forced intellectualisation whereby the subjects have no choice but to try to interpret the sensory inputs in a nonemotional manner.

As with pain, involving patients in their own care can serve to intellectualise or objectify the experience, which may for some prove a useful strategy to reduce anxiety and stress. For others it may not work at all because they are adopting a counterproductive coping strategy.

Coping strategies

Another dimension to coping strategies is the emphasis on the distinction between those people (*blunters*) who tend to deny the stressful elements of a situation and those (*monitors*) who prefer to examine what is going on around them (Miller, 1987). (Other words that have been used by experimenters to describe blunters are *repressors, deniers, avoiders* and *information avoiders*, and for monitors *sensitisers, vigilants* and *information seekers* (Murray and Niven, 1992).) Miller developed a technique to measure people's preferred coping styles. She presented people with a series of scenarios such as imagining they were afraid of the dentist and had to have some dental work done, or being held hostage by a group of armed terrorists in a public building.

After each scenario the person is presented with eight statements, half of which are of the monitoring variety (for example, in the hostage situation: 'If there was access to a radio, I would stay near it and listen to the bulletins about what the police were doing') and half would be of the blunting variety (for example, in the dental situation 'I would do mental puzzles in my head').

Participants are asked to select the statements that reflect how they would react to the situations portrayed in the scenarios, and are categorised as either blunters or monitors on the basis of their responses. Clearly, the type of coping strategy that is usually adopted by a patient will have a significant effect on the effectiveness of nursing interventions. As has been suggested above, 'tailoring' interventions to match coping styles may lead to a greater reduction in patients' stress and anxiety.

A final dimension of coping processes is the cognitive/behavioural distinction. This is not so much a dimension as two distinct classifications. Curry and Russ (1985) reviewed the literature on the types of coping strategies used by children in stressful circumstances (see Table 8.2).

More research is needed on the extent to which anxious people are more likely than non-anxious people to use specific strategies, whether young children use different coping strategies to older children and the developmental factors that influence the different choices of coping strategy.

Stress and illness

Stress can be both a direct and an indirect factor in illness. For instance, stress causes direct changes in the production of adrenalin and noradrenalin that can result in blood clotting, an increase in blood pressure and heart rate, fat deposits and immuno

Table 8.2 Coping strategies used by children

Behavioural coping strategies

- *Information seeking.* An attempt is made to gain information by asking questions and watching what is going on. Any medical instruments are inspected and their functions explored.
- *Support seeking.* The child attempts to develop a supportive relationship with the nurse, involving physical and verbal interaction.
- *Direct efforts to maintain control.* The child tries to participate in the treatment process or establishes limits and conditions.

Cognitive coping strategies

- *Reality-orientated working through.* The child has specific, correct thoughts about procedures before, during and after treatment: 'The cut looked quite big, so I thought I would probably have to have stitches for it to mend properly.'
- *Positive cognitive restructuring.* The child attends to positive factors of the treatment programme: 'I tried to think good thoughts and that I would be getting a present at the end of it.'
- *Defensive reappraisal.* Superstitious thoughts and an attempt to deny the stressful elements of the situation: 'I thought the needle was really made of rubber and just squirts water. It wasn't really going into my arm.'
- *Emotion-regulating cognitions.* Self-statements to allay fear and anxiety: 'I said to myself, God is with you, so don't worry.'
- *Behaviour-regulating cognitions.* Self-statements aimed at controlling and regulating behaviour during treatment: 'I told myself to try and keep still.'
- *Diversionary thinking.* Diverting thoughts away from the situation: 'I tried to concentrate on the Garfield poster on the wall.'

suppression. Cortisol can lead to a decrease in the immune function, leading to greater susceptibility to infection, with chronic stress being more likely to increase cortisol secretion. Also cortisol decreases the number of active T cells which could influence tumour development (Kiecolt-Glaser and Glaser, 1992). However, it can also affect health indirectly by causing us to eat more, drink more, smoke more, etc. One interesting recent development is the area of psychoneuroimmunology (PIN). This simply states that a person's psychological state can influence the functioning of their immune system via their nervous system. At first it was thought that the immune system was independent of other bodily systems but it seems it is not (Ader and Cohen, 1993). Factors such as mood, beliefs (pessimism versus optimism) and emotional expression/suppression have all been associated with health outcomes (Daruna, 2004).

Stress and work

Burnout may be defined as 'the process where professional attitudes and behaviour change in negative ways in response to some form of job stress'. There have been many articles on burnout in a wide range of health care journals, from the stress symptoms and burnout of comparative groups of UK and Australian podiatrists (Mandy and Tinley, 2004) to the coping strategies used by mental health nurses to deal with job stress (Taylor and Barling, 2004). This illustrates the concern of health professionals about the problem and also provides us with a number of different interpretations of the phenomena. Some of the characteristics that have been put forward to describe the burnout syndrome are:

- labelling patients;
- Feeling unappreciated and guilty;
- a sense of failure;
- intolerance of colleagues and patients;
- hating going to work every day cynicism and dislike of patients;
- illness and absenteeism;
- clock-watching;
- exhaustion;
- isolation and withdrawal;
- 'going by the book' all the time;
- lack of concentration;
- boredom;
- sleep difficulties;
- depersonalisation.

Dewe (1989) examined a sample of 1,801 general nurses for evidence and frequency of tension tiredness at work. There were five main sources of stress:

- *Work overload.* Problems of staff shortage and dealing with too many patients were the most stressful experiences, allied to trying to maintain high standards at the same time.
- *Difficulties in relating to other staff.* Arguments conflict with colleagues were found to be the next stressful events.
- Problems with nursing critically ill patients.
- Anxiety and concern over patient treatment.
- Patients' condition.

This study is interesting because it was conducted over fifteen years ago many of the findings would not be out of place today.

Stress management

> Every time someone tells me to 'just relax' I know something nasty is going to happen to me.
>
> (Comment from a patient)

Over the years, people develop a variety of techniques to manage stressful circumstances. Unfortunately some of them, whilst successful in the short term, may prove counter-productive in the long term. A few drinks after work may lead to a dependence on alcohol and actually increase stress over a period of time. Sometimes people find themselves in novel stressful situations where their previous coping strategies seem inappropriate. Thus there is a need to give people help in learning new and successful ways of managing stress. I will now examine some of these techniques.

Relaxation

Relaxation is a skill. The ability to relax can be developed in much the same ways as interpersonal skills can be developed – with practice. There are a number of techniques that have been constructed to help people relax, the most common being progressive muscular relaxation. Edmund Jacobson (1929) thought that all forms of tension, including mental tension, were based on the contraction of the muscles. Thus, if people could be taught to relax their muscles, their minds would become relaxed too. The technique is based upon the fact that every time a muscle contracts it creates a series of neural impulses that are sent to the brain. If many muscles are activated, tension is created. Progressive muscular relaxation aims to teach individuals to recognise when excessive muscle contraction occurs and provides training in how to relax these muscles.

Lohaus *et al.* (2001) looked at two types of relaxation training on children aged between 10 and 12 years. They used progressive muscular relaxation and imagery-based relaxation techniques to see if they could affect physiological measures such as heart rate, galvanic skin response, skin temperature and self-reports. They found that although the children reported that both relaxation techniques increased their feeling of well-being and mood, these did not always correspond to the physiological measures and a decrease in heart rate was not always associated with a decrease in skin temperature. These findings indicate that one must be careful when using different indices of stress reduction but, perhaps more important, that perceptions of stress are not always indicative of the 'physiological experience' of stress.

Another relaxation technique concentrates on breathing and is known as deep diaphragmatic breathing. This can function as a relatively brief relaxation exercise, and after practice can be reduced to just a few minutes. As the exercise is relatively unobtrusive and also, with practice, short, it can be used in all sorts of stressful situations. The diaphragm is a large sheet of muscle extending across the lower edge of the rib cage under the lungs and attached to the back. If we use it to facilitate our breathing, it can help us to breathe more deeply and to relax more fully. Most people tend to breathe using the muscles around the chest. To use the diaphragm correctly the abdomen should move outwards when you inhale and pull inwards when you exhale. When achieved, this technique will fill the lungs more fully and the body will receive more oxygen.

Exercise 8.2 *Relaxation*

- If you are able, assume a comfortable position and close your eyes.
- Become aware of your breathing.
- Notice whether you are breathing through your nose or your mouth
- Notice the pace of your breathing.
- Notice all the muscle groups in your body. Which are tense and which are relaxed? (Those who have practised progressive muscular relaxation have an advantage here.)
- Become aware of your breathing again
- Begin breathing through your nose, exhaling through your mouth.
- Continue, and try to breathe more deeply. To assist you with this you can now use your diaphragm. As you inhale, push your abdomen outwards so as to draw your diaphragm downwards and fill your lungs more fully. As you exhale pull your abdomen inwards so as to expel air. Try this for a couple of minutes. (You may wish to use your hand to monitor the movement of your abdomen.)
- As you continue to breathe try to hold your breath for a few seconds. Inhale to a count of four: 1 . . . 2 . . . 3 . . . 4. Hold it for a count of four: 1 . . . 2 . . . 3 . . . 4. Exhale slowly to a count of eight: 1 . . . 2 . . . 3 . . . 4 . . . 5 . . . 6 . . . 7 . . . 8. (Repeat a couple of times.)
- As you continue, monitor the sensations within your body, particularly when you exhale, and notice the relaxing effect of breathing out slowly and rhythmically.

The evidence for the effectiveness of relaxation techniques in reducing stress tends to be ambivalent. In a review of the literature, Borkovec and Sides (1979) found some studies had suggested very little difference between relaxation groups and control groups. One of the reasons for these findings is that many of the studies used different measures of stress and this may account for the discrepancies. Another explanation is that relaxation reduces stress not so much by reducing muscle tension, but by arousing pleasant thoughts in people while they are completing the exercise (Peveler and Johnson, 1986). More simply, relaxation may not be effective in reducing stress because people are not prepared to spend the time in practising the technique properly and therefore do not reap the benefits. However, Wynd (1992) used relaxation training to reduce the stress associated with relapse rates in smoking cessation. As the relaxation was learned by the patients, the perceived stress was reduced and smoking abstinence was maintained.

Biofeedback

Biofeedback is a technique which monitors the status of a person's physiological processes (such as heart rate or muscle tension), amplifies them and feeds the information back to the individual. Budzynski (1973) said that biofeedback training has three objectives:

- to develop an increased awareness of internal physiological states;
- to establish control over these states;
- to be able to transfer this control from the clinic to everyday situations.

The last objective is particularly important, for if the patient cannot use the technique in a context other than the laboratory or clinic then the usefulness of the method is limited, to say the least. Miller (1978) found that whilst patients were able to reduce their blood pressure using biofeedback training in the laboratory, when they returned to their natural environment the changes were not always maintained. However, when biofeedback was combined with other techniques such as breathing and relaxing self-statements, Blanchard *et al.* (1988) found it to be an effective treatment for hypertension. Furthermore, patients were able to obtain these results in their own homes.

A number of years ago Meichenbaum (1976) argued that when biofeedback works, it does so by creating the conditions for people to change their behaviour and their thinking from encouraging sickness to discouraging it. People's ability to control their muscles is generalised to an overall ability to be more in control of their lives. They may also pick up health-supporting attitudes from their therapists. Meichenbaum is supported in his view by a case cited in Bakal (1992). A patient was an outstanding success in a biofeedback training programme designed to reduce her terrible headaches. After twelve biofeedback sessions she reported a near total disappearance of headaches. However, the physiological data indicated that she had gained little or no control over the muscle activity of her forehead. Scientifically, it seems that the function of biofeedback is quite complex and more research is needed to pinpoint exactly what is happening during the treatment programme. In the meantime, if it works for some patients, it doesn't really matter why.

The cognitive behavioural approach

The cognitive/behavioural approach to stress management emphasises the role of faulty cognition and irrational beliefs in the perception of stressful stimuli. Meichenbaum (1977) and Meichenbaum and Cameron (1983) have produced a stress management programme based on cognitive, behavioural principles which they have called *stress inoculation*. This technique begins with a phase designed to provide the patient with a conceptual framework for understanding the problem. The main goal of the initial phase is to change self-talk from negative to positive statements, in order to get patients to think differently about themselves. Patients are encouraged to react more objectively to stressful situations and to try to pay less heed to their emotional reactions. Thus a person who is prone to severe attacks of anxiety would be urged to first of all determine the circumstances that produce the anxiety. It is helpful if the patient keeps a diary of daily events and notes the behaviours and thoughts which accompany the anxiety attacks. This information can be used to inform the patient that anxiety involves physiological responses such as sweaty hands, increased heart rate, tense muscles, and so on. If patients can detect the physiological signs of anxiety, these may be used as cues to employ suitable coping mechanisms.

Cognitive coping may take the form of using strategies such as relaxation and deep diaphragmatic breathing to reduce physiological arousal, or it may take the form of focusing attention on the task in hand and not on feelings of fear. Details of the intensity and prospective duration of emotions are useful, as is an evaluation of patients' coping strategies. Thus there are three main phases to stress inoculation programmes.

- *The conceptualisation phase.* Here the person learns about the nature of stress and how people react to it.
- *The skills acquisition phase.* The person learns behavioural and cognitive skills to use in emotion-focused and problem-focused coping.
- *Application and follow-through.* The last phase involves making the transition to using the coping skills in the real world.

An example of stress inoculation to deal with the management of anger is given by Novaco (1975). The importance of redefining or changing the structure of maladaptive thoughts is emphasised, along with conducting a situational analysis and using relaxation skills. Novaco recommends the stress coping thoughts listed in Table 8.3 to deal with anger.

Table 8.3 *Stress coping thoughts* (adapted from Novaco, 1975)

1 Preparing for provocation
This may upset me, but I think I know how to deal with it.
What is it that I have to do?
I can work out a plan to deal with this.
I can manage the situation, I know how to regulate my anger.
If I find myself getting upset, I'll know what to do.
There won't be any need for an argument.
Try not to take this too seriously.
This could be a testy situation, but I believe in myself.

Table 8.3 *(continued)*

2 Impact and confrontation
Stay calm. Just continue to relax.
Just as long as I keep my cool, I'm in control.
Just roll with the punches.
You don't need to prove yourself.
There is no point in getting mad.
Don't make more out of this than you have to.
I'm not going to let this person get to me.
It's really a shame that this person has to act like this.
For someone to be that irritable, they must be awfully unhappy.
If I start to get mad, I'll just be banging my head against a wall. So I might as well
    just relax.
I can't change this person with anger, I'll just upset myself.

3 Coping with arousal
My muscles are starting to get tight. Time to relax and slow things down.
Getting upset won't help.
It's not worth it to get so angry.
Let them make a fool of themselves.
I have a right to get annoyed, but let's keep the lid on.
Time to take some deep breaths.
My anger is a sign of what I need to do. Time to cope.
Try to reason it out.
Let's try a co-operative approach. Maybe we are both right. They'd probably like me
    to get angry. Well, I'm going to disappoint them.
I can't expect people to act the way I want them to.
Take it easy, don't get pushy.

4 Reflecting on the provocation
(a) When the problem is unresolved:
     Forget about the aggravation. Thinking about it is only doing me harm.
     Try to shake it off and think about something more important.
     Relaxation is much better than anger.
     These feelings will go away sooner or later. Let's make it sooner.
     What about laughing at it? Is it really so serious?
     Don't take it personally. Take a deep breath.
(b) When the conflict is resolved and the coping successful:
     I handled that one pretty well. It worked.
     That wasn't as hard as I thought.
     It could have gotten a lot worse.
     I actually got through that without getting too angry.
     I guess I've been getting upset for too long when it wasn't even necessary.
     I think I'm getting better at this.

The importance of managing anger/hostility is illustrated by Barefoot *et al.* (1983). They examined the records of 255 physicians who had taken a psychological test that included a scale for hostility when they were in medical school twenty-five years earlier. Those with high scores for hostility were found to have rates for both coronary heart disease and overall mortality which were several times higher than those with low hostility scores. Maybe a further cognitive coping self-statement should be included: 'I'm not going to let this person kill me'.

Control

Research has found that people who feel that they have little, or no, control over events in their lives experience high levels of stress and anxiety. One factor that has been found to increase people's sense of control is predictability. Weiss (1972) gave three rats a combination of electric shock and tones. Two of the rats received small electric shocks to their tails, the third did not. The first rat heard a tone ten seconds before the shock. The second rat was presented with a series of random tones totally unconnected with the shocks. Thus, the first rat was able to predict when the shocks would occur, the second rat could not. The third rat heard randomly presented tones but was given no shock. When autopsies were performed on the three rats it was found that there were significant differences in the amount of ulceration found in the stomach. The third rat which had received no shocks was found to have little ulceration of the stomach. The second rat, which was unable to predict the onset of shock had extensive ulceration. The first rat, which was able to predict the shock, had levels of ulceration similar to the rat which had received no shock at all. Both the first and second rats had received exactly the same stimulus but the degree of perceived control had determined its physiological effects.

One must always be wary of extrapolating results from animal studies to human behaviour; however, Rodin *et al.* (1979) have found similar results concerning perceived control using human subjects. In a densely packed lift, people who were standing close to the control panel felt less crowded and actually thought the lift was larger than those people who were standing some distance from the panel. Brown (1990) investigated the anxiety experienced by patients undergoing surgery for renal calculus disease. It was found that pre-operatively fear of general anaesthetic was a main factor, and post-operatively pain was the most commonly identified stressor. Careful pre-operative explanation was found to reduce stress.

In the hospital environment perceived control has been found to influence stress factors. Volicer *et al.* (1977) asked medical and surgical patients to rate hospital practices in terms of their perceived stressfulness. Events that were rated as very stressful included: people thinking they might have cancer; losing their sight; and knowing they had a serious illness. Most people would not be too surprised at these findings. However, other events that were rated as very stressful included patients not being told what is wrong with them; not knowing the results or reasons for treatment; or having questions ignored. Collectively these events may be construed as a lack of perceived control or the feeling of not knowing what is going on. It may not be possible to cure people with serious illnesses but the stress that occurs from patients not knowing what is happening to them can be reduced by using many of the interpersonal skills discussed in Chapter 1.

Control can be an important factor in preparing parents for their children's ICU experience. Miles and Mathes (1991) found that parents found the child's behaviour, the child's emotional response, and parental role alterations the most stressful events in the ICU. When parents were given adequate information they responded with lower levels of stress.

In many circumstances where patients are facing some kind of stress, the knowledge that they have some element of control will often help to dilute anxious feelings. Note that patients do not have to have *actual* control, but they do have to feel or think that they have some control or else stress and anxiety will usually follow. Thus nurses should try to improve predictability and create an atmosphere of control and mastery when dealing with patients who find themselves feeling anxious.

Social support

Can the presence of friends or relations reduce stress? The answer to this question is that social support *normally* has a beneficial effect in reducing stress, but not always (Callaghan and Morrissey, 1993). Social support may be defined as the help that a group of people such as family and friends provide, or are thought to provide, in stressful situations. Duck (1998) says that there are three important sorts of social support.

- *Emotional support.* This refers to the knowledge that one is loved and cared for. It can be achieved by giving presents and compliments, expressing concern, taking an interest in other people's well-being, arranging to spend time together, remembering special events and being prepared to listen without jumping in with solutions.
- *Esteem support.* This type of support is concerned with providing people with the knowledge that they are valued and held in high esteem. Treating other's opinions as important, asking advice and allowing them to take the lead all contribute to a sense of self-esteem.
- *Network support.* Knowing that one belongs to a network of mutual support.

These three types of support are developed through the exchanges of everyday life. They do not just exist when stress occurs, but are part of the results of dealing with friends during the course of daily life. One feature of social support is that it can provide a 'buffering' effect to stressful events. However, Cohen and McKay (1984) say that this buffering effect will work only under the following certain conditions.

- *Appropriate tangible support.* Tangible support, such as the offer of money or care, will be effective only if it is viewed as warranted. Offers of inappropriate tangible support can result in feelings of inadequacy and indebtedness, which will inevitably compound a patient's problem.
- *Social acceptability.* One way that social support acts as a buffer against stress is to help people redefine the situation as less stressful by turning to others who have experienced comparable circumstances for advice and help. This action will be of use only if the source of the stress is socially acceptable. Wortman and Dunkel-Schetter (1979) found that patients suffering from cancer were reluctant to discuss their condition and failed to seek out other cancer patients owing to the stigma attached to their condition. Many cancer patients often avoided publicly stating that they had cancer. However, on the positive side, social support can enhance coping strategies by suggesting alternative coping strategies based on other's previous experience and getting people to focus on the more positive aspects of the predicament.
- *Loss of self-esteem.* Social support can play a significant role in elevating low self-opinion. Yet it will be effective only if a person's interpersonal relationships allow others to play a part in developing emotional support. If stressful events weaken one's feelings of belonging or being loved, emotional support can sometimes replace or strengthen these feelings.

When social support acts as a negative buffer to stress, it is usually due to the sorts of factors just mentioned. Help is not always offered in effective ways and when it is offered and not wanted it becomes intrusive and excessive. Finally, it is important to distinguish between the actual supportive behaviour of friends and kin and the way a person feels about the support that is an offer. A person may feel secure in the knowledge that he has a fully functioning support network ready to help whenever the need arises when in actual fact such may not necessarily be the case. An important factor is the actual behaviour of people who constitute the support network. Gottlieb (1985) says that successful coping depends on the belief that others will provide help if asked and the actual manifestation of support in a crisis. Aaronson (1989) investigated perceived and received support during pregnancy. It was found that received support was just as important as perceived support in facilitating positive health behaviours such as abstinence from alcohol, cigarettes and caffeine.

In his book on the psychology of happiness Argyle (1987) concedes that negative buffering can occur and sometimes people leave a support group feeling worse than when they went in. This often happens when the sole purpose of the group is to grouch about each individual's particular problems. What constitutes happiness, according to Argyle (1987), is having a good time and being able to share it with one's friends and relations. Thus, the effectiveness of social support in ameliorating the effects of stress will depend to a large extent on the nature of the support and the context in which it is applied.

Multimodal stress management programmes

A number of people have suggested that stress management cannot be achieved through one procedure alone and that a multimodal approach is needed. Suinn (1980) developed a stress management programme consisting of two phases. First, people are taught to reduce their exposure to situations which cause stress, for example deadlines, rapid paced activities and confrontations. Second, anxiety is reduced by the use of relaxation training techniques. This approach mirrors the coping theories of Lazarus and Launier (1978) by emphasising a need to 'attack' the source of stress (*problem* or *active coping*) and then to try to deal with the impact of the stressor on the individual (*emotional* or *palliative coping*).

An advantage of multimodal stress programmes is highlighted by Pearlin and Schooler (1978) who say that having a particular weapon is one's arsenal is less important than having a variety of weapons. Thus Roskies (1987) advocates the use of a variety of techniques under three main headings: *physiological, behavioural* and *cognitive*. In her stress management programmes for healthy Type A individuals she starts by getting her subjects to recognise their own personal tension signs and the situations that provoke them. Subjects are required to complete a diary during the day, starting from when they wake up in the morning till they go to bed at night. They have to list the events as they occur, for example:

Woke up – Argued with son – Started work on a new project – Finished first draft – Had lunch – Late for meeting – Meeting exceedingly boring – More work on new project – Drove home – Had tea – Spoke to son about argument – Spoke to wife about son – Watched TV – Went to bed.

Each event is monitored for low, medium and high tension levels. Finally, tension signs are divided into their physical and emotional components. Thus some of the events would appear like this:

		Tension signs	
Event	*Tension level*	*Physical*	*Emotional*
Arguing with son Anger/Frustration	High	Knot in stomach	
Boring meeting	Low	Sleepy	Boredom
Project work	Med	Concentration	Resignation
Talk with wife	High	Tense shoulders	Anger/Guilt

The purpose of this stage of the programme is to: make people more aware of the situations that create tension in their lives; enable people to recognise their own personal tension signs; and determine the emotions associated with the tension signs.

Having developed skills in recognising tension, the next stage is concerned with developing skills to manage the tension. This is achieved by learning to discriminate between relaxed and tense muscles, being able to relax muscle groups using progressive muscular relaxation and eventually, learning to use a simple command to relax the whole body. Once these new skills have been acquired they can be used to monitor and regulate tension during the day, prepare for potentially stressful situations such as interviews and meetings, and maintain self-control during a crisis.

The second stage in the programme involves behavioural stress awareness. Again, a diary is constructed of the day's events.

Travelling to college – Lectures – Lunch – Game of squash – Library – Going home – Tea – Work on essay – Read book – Go to bed

Low, medium and high tension levels are assigned to each event. Tension signs now include a behavioural component. Table 8.4 gives examples of behavioural stress awareness.

Two good reasons for managing behavioural tension are the acknowledgement that: the act of raising one's voice and getting angry increases unpleasantness for you as well the other person/people; behaving angrily towards others leads them to respond in kind.

Having developed the ability to recognise the situational and interpersonal 'triggers' likely to arouse tense behaviour, the next stage is to substitute behaviours that will cause less psychological harm. This may be achieved in a number of ways.

- *Time out.* Placing a delay before any action, such as counting to ten, can reduce the 'size of the response'.

Table 8.4 *Behavioural stress awareness*

- *Event 1* Travelling to college, the bus is too slow
  Tension level: Medium
  Tension signs: (a) Emotional/physical – impatience
                 (b) Behavioural – keep looking at watch
- *Event 2* Eating lunch
  Tension level: Low
  Tension signs: (a) Emotional/physical – quite relaxed
                 (b) Behavioural – tend to gobble food
- *Event 3* Work on essay
  Tension level: Medium
  Tension signs: (a) Emotional/physical – concentration
                 (b) Behavioural – tap pencil

Table 8.5 *Linking emotions and self-talk*

- *Event 1* Kept waiting a long time for food at lunch
  Tension level: Moderate to high
  Emotion: Impatience/anger
  Self-talk: *Damn it! I'm not coming here again and I don't see why I should pay for such shoddy service*
- *Event 2* Tutor asks me questions I can't answer
  Tension level: High.
  Emotion: Discomfort/embarrassment.
  Self-talk: *She must think I'm an idiot*

- *Incompatibility*. Substituting behaviours that are incompatible with tension can diminish the experience of stress. For example, speaking very slowly is normally incompatible with speaking loudly, therefore when people find themselves shouting they should try to speak more slowly and this should reduce the noise levels and the stress too.
- *Control*. Expressing needs and complaints verbally, in a non-hostile manner produces more control over the situation.

The third stage in the programme features the cognitive correlates of stress called 'self-talk'. The daily diary is made up of the usual components such as events and tension levels, only the responses are now the links between emotions and self-talk (see Table 8.5).

The aim of this is to make people more aware of what they say to themselves when they experience tension. As we have seen earlier on in this chapter, how we interpret events is very important. The student who receives poor marks for an essay can think 'Well, win some, lose some, let's see what went wrong here' or 'I can never write anything that seems to get reasonable marks.' The type of self-talk used will affect the student's feelings about themselves, their tutor and the desirability of trying hard next time. It is important to substitute new self-talk for unproductive self-talk, as shown in the examples in Table 8.6.

In some cases, stressful situations such as having to queue at the bank on Friday afternoons or waiting in a traffic jam going home every night can be predicted. When stress can be predicted it is useful to adopt a problem-focused coping strategy to either avoid the stressful situation entirely (go to the bank at a less crowded time) or plan an appropriate response to it (use the time being held up by the traffic to plan the next day's activities). Sometimes stress occurs at unpredictable moments where 'emergency braking' procedures are required. For example:

Table 8.6. *Productive versus unproductive self-talk*

Modifying emotions
- *Event 1* Unsuccessful meeting
Tension level:	Medium
Emotion:	Despair
Unproductive self-talk:	*This meeting is a real disaster*
Productive self-talk:	This meeting is not as good as I would like
New emotion:	Disappointment.
- *Event 2* Argument with colleague
Tension level:	High
Emotion:	Anger
Unproductive self-talk:	*Nasty, vindictive, little beast*
Productive self-talk:	I wonder what's eating her?
New emotion:	Curiosity

Modifying behaviour
- *Event 1* Dropped patient's food all down me
Tension level:	High
Stressed behaviour:	Clench teeth/swear
Unproductive self-talk:	*What an idiot I am. I can't do anything right*
Productive self-talk:	Well nobody is perfect. How can I fix myself up?
New behaviour:	Change clothes
- *Event 2* Huge queue at the checkout in the supermarket
Tension level:	Medium/high
Stressed behaviour:	Mutter, look daggers at supermarket staff
Unproductive self-talk:	*Incompetent shower. They take the money but can't put extra staff on to cope with a rush*
New self-talk:	I don't like it, but there's not much I can do about it
New behaviour:	I think I'll amuse myself by looking at the other people in the queue

---

- *Event.* Getting carried away in an argument and starting to raise one's voice.
- *Signs of stress.* Tightness at shoulder and neck, thinking 'he's totally missed the point of what I've been saying', raising voice.
- *Braking signal.* Visualise a red light and say 'Stop' to myself. Strategies to regain control: Deep diaphragmatic breathing, try to relax muscles. Stop speaking for five seconds then restart slowly.

In summary, the focus of multimodal stress management programmes is to 'fine tune' the detection of the physiological, behavioural and cognitive constituents of stress and then to substitute adaptive procedures tailored to each individual's specific circumstances. This can be achieved only with a great deal of practice and therefore takes quite a time to accomplish – there are no quick, easy stress management techniques (Niven and Johnson, 1989).

The use of effective stress management programmes in nursing has taken on increasing significance with evidence that health care professionals in the United Kingdom have higher absence and sickness rates than staff in other sectors (Edwards and Burnard, 2003). Also stress may be a significant factor contributing to nurses leaving the profession. Edwards and Burnard (2003) conducted a systematic review of research between 1966 and 2000 on stress management interventions in the context of mental health nursing. Overall they found that 'relaxation techniques, training in behavioural techniques, stress management workshops and training therapeutic skills were effective stress management techniques' but they added an important proviso – that whilst a great deal is known about stress in the work context what seems to be lacking is the translation of the findings into practice.

Organisational stress

Just as we refer to some individuals as being in good health, so too can we refer to organisations being in good health. Bennis (1962) proposes that we view organisational health in the same as we view individual health and borrows Jahoda's (1958) attempt to characterise the constituents of positive mental health in its analysis. He proposes the following criteria of a healthy organisation:

- *Adaptability*. The ability to solve problems and to react with flexibility to changing environmental demands.
- *A sense of identity*. Knowledge and insight on the part of the organisation of what it is, what its goals are, and what it is to do.
- *Capacity to test reality*. The ability to search out, accurately perceive, and correctly interpret the real properties of the environment, particularly those which have relevance for the functioning of the organisation.
- *Integration*. A state of integration among the subparts of the total organisation, such that the parts are not working at cross-purposes.

Whilst these criteria apply to all organisations, some systems are prone to particular types of problem. One which has received considerable attention over the past few years is the problem of staff burnout.

Burnout

Burnout may be defined as 'the process where professional attitudes and behaviour change in negative ways in response to some form of job stress'. There have been many articles on burnout in a wide range of health care journals, from the stress symptoms, burnout and suicidal thoughts of Finnish physicians (Olkinuora *et al.,* 1992) to the coping strategies used by Canadian ward nurses to deal with job stress (Ogus, 1992). This illustrates the concern of health professionals about the problem and also provides us with a number of different interpretations of the phenomena.

Some of the characteristics that have been put forward to describe the burnout syndrome are:

- labelling patients;
- feeling unappreciated and guilty;
- a sense of failure;
- intolerance of colleagues and patients;
- hating going to work every day;
- cynicism and dislike of patients;
- illness and absenteeism;
- clock-watching;
- exhaustion;
- isolation and withdrawal;
- 'going by the book' all the time;
- lack of concentration boredom;
- sleep difficulties;
- depersonalisation.

One of the first studies to examine burnout in nurses was conducted by Dewe (1989). A sample of 1,801 general nurses were examined for evidence and frequency of tension and tiredness at work. There were five main sources of stress:

- *Work overload.* Problems of staff shortage and dealing with too many patients were the most stressful experiences, allied to trying to maintain high standards at the same time.
- *Difficulties in relating to other staff.* Arguments and conflict with colleagues were found to be the next stressful events.
- *Problems with nursing critically ill patients.* Some of the reported difficulties were having to respond to demands for instant action, operating unfamiliar equipment and working with new procedures or treatments.
- *Anxiety and concern over patient treatment.* Not knowing when and how much to tell patients about their condition comes fourth in the list of stress factors. Also in this category was working with doctors who did not appear to understand the needs of the patients.
- *Patients' condition.* Finally, the least stressful events were related to nursing patients who failed to improve, such as patients with chronic pain and the terminally ill.

A positive feature of this piece of research is that, whilst it is probably impossible to eradicate chronic pain and terminal illness, it is not impossible to develop ways to improve relations between staff, reduce role ambiguity and address work overloads. Indeed, Llewelyn (1989) says that this is exactly what should occur but organisational and political changes need to take place before the imbalance between perceived demands and perceived resources can be achieved. 'Hence, nurses need to be taught about how organisations function, and why change is difficult and threatening to those who work in organisations. Only then will nurses be able to reduce their feelings of powerlessness and hence their experience of stress.'

Problems of definition

Many people would agree that burnout involves some form of change in attitude towards one's job, but many would also disagree on the nature how this change occurs. For Edelwich and Brodsky (1980) burnout consists of four stages of disillusionment:

- Enthusiasm, over-identification with patients and inefficient expenditure of one's energy.
- Stagnation, where one merely conducts the work.
- Frustration with the work.
- Apathy used as a defence against the frustration.

Maslach and Pines (1979) propose phases of fatigue:

Phase 1
- emotional exhaustion (feeling tired when thinking about going to work);
- physical exhaustion (sleeping poorly, prone to colds, headaches, aches and pains).
Phase 2
- develop negative cynical, dehumanised. Attitudes about co-workers feel negative about patients/clients dislike themselves for these negative feelings;
- withdraw into a shell and do a minimum of work.
Phase 3
- total disgust with self, everything and everyone.

It is important to point out that burnout is not just a response to work overload, for individuals can also become disillusioned as a result having too little to do. Burnout is essentially a response to any factor that changes a person's attitude to his or her job in a negative way.

Transactional model

Cherniss (1980, 1992) wants us to view burnout as a transactional process. By this he means that burnout is a process consisting of three stages. The first stage is characterised by resources not meeting demand. The second stage is the emotional response to this deficit – anxiety, tension, tiredness and finally exhaustion. The third stage is a change in attitude and behaviour such as becoming detached and increasingly cynical.

Thus a person who is experiencing high levels of job stress will utilise appropriate coping mechanisms and change her attitude or behaviour to provide a psychological escape. This often manifests itself in detachment from the situation and can lead to an impersonal attitude to patients and their problems. Probably the most harmful feature of the syndrome is the degree to which it reinforces itself. Once the process of negative attitude change is initiated it not only destroys that individual's commitment, it is also extremely infectious and can lead to other members of the organisation developing similar attitudes. It is therefore very important to set up mechanisms whereby the early detection of any disaffection is a priority rather than an option to be incorporated if one has the time.

Therefore not only are patients treated in a detached and mechanical fashion but colleagues will also suffer the consequences of the 'burnt out' individual in the form of lack of co-operation, criticism of attitudes to care and inability to construct a positive approach to problem solving.

Unfortunately, owing to the differences in the way burnout has been defined, and as a result of its popularity, it has become a catch-all phrase to describe a variety of conditions. Jones and Klarr (1985) compared a number of community mental health departments and, not surprisingly, found incidences of burnout. But in one department they noted that:

> The staff worked with an even more difficult and demanding population. The staff in this department worked with equal intensity and for longer hours. Management in this department had less interest and concern for the problems of burnout. Few precautionary or intervention measures were implemented. Despite this, there was little or no evidence of staff burnout. A staff member who had been with the department for twelve years commented, 'We don't have time for burnout.' In the face of bureaucratic pressure and patient demands, this department manifested a minimal amount of burnout.

Herein lies the problem with the concept of burnout; how do we explain its absence in circumstances ideal for its growth? The plethora of definitions give little help in explaining away these findings. Maslach (1982) recognises some of the difficulties and proposes that the fascination with burnout has increased the number of phenomena to which it refers. This can impair understanding of the concept and be a major reason why some people have become so cynical and reject it altogether.

The answer lies not in rejecting the concept altogether, but in seeking to delve deeper into specific features of the relationship between individuals and their workplace. Negative changes in attitude can result from a number of factors and occur at a number of different levels. So in order get a better idea of burnout we must examine its growth at four different levels: individual, group, organisation and institution. In other words, people can become 'burnt out' because of themselves, because of the people they work with, because of the work setting itself and finally because of the way the institution is organised. Unfortunately in some cases individuals may be suffering not just at one level, but at a combination of all four at the same time. Let us start by examining how individual factors contribute to the ways in which people view their work.

Individual factors

Realistic expectations

Many of the underlying causes of job stress and burnout can be examined in terms of inadequate staff development programmes. A great deal of stress is caused by the excessive demands that workers impose on themselves. For instance, new workers can bring unrealistically high goals to a job, such as thinking that they can cure, or at least help in some way, all the people that they come into contact with. Norris (1982) feels that it is a delusion or myth that nurses can significantly influence patients' lives. She considers it irrational to think that change is possible for a patient during a three- to five-day hospital spell. When staff fail to achieve their goals they often abandon them, adopting the most minimal of custodial roles. However, through constructing carefully designed staff development programmes, workers can be helped to become more aware of what their personal goals are in order to alleviate the problems of unrealistically high or low expectations.

Rewards

It is also important to help people to adopt new goals, as well as providing alternative sources of gratification. They may be helped to see the potential dangers of becoming too dependent on work for need fulfilment and encouraged to develop other sources of gratification outside the job. This process is best accomplished during the training phase. Weitz, as long ago as 1956, reported how one company successfully reduced 'reality shock' and turnover in its sales personnel by providing new trainees with a booklet that described typical examples of the kinds of frustrations and disappointments that they might encounter in the job. The company had previously used a booklet that emphasised the positive features of the job in the hope that prospective employees world not be scared away by mentioning difficulties and problems right at the beginning. They found that those who had received the realistic booklet were much more likely to remain in their job than those who had received the positive booklet.

It is heartening to note that this careful attention to initial orientation is in fact present in many of the training programmes in operation at the moment. For instance, a number of community nursing and health visiting courses try to give their trainees a realistic idea of what their job is going to be like at the beginning of the course. In addition to attending various lectures and seminars, students are encouraged to accompany experienced staff on their rounds 'in the field'. Gradually the students begin to assume responsibility, working with the patients themselves whilst being observed by their supervisors. Inevitably at some stage there is bound to be some form of assessment of the trainees' practical skills. It is useful if the practical work teachers and supervisors do not have to provide these assessments until late on in the training programme. In this way one can avoid certain amounts of ambiguity, concern about performance and feelings of being ill at ease in the training environment.

Sometimes the problems have not so much to do with individuals having excessively ambitious goals, but relate to difficulty in realising that they have had any positive effect. How many times does a patient provide her GP with positive reinforcement by going back after the treatment and saying thanks? It would seem very odd. It seems those who keep returning are the unsuccessful cases. Thus in behavioural terms there is little positive reinforcement. When levels of reinforcement become critically low, people will become increasingly disenchanted by lack of apparent progress. So it is very important to construct a system which is able to monitor small gains in treatment and feed these back at frequent intervals to the health professionals involved.

Pines and Aronson (1988) have highlighted the importance of positive conditions in the work place: 'Stress research has concentrated on the presence of negative conditions in the environment as a source of stress and has virtually ignored stress reactions that result from the lack of positive conditions.' They conclude that the absence of positive conditions constitutes a unique source of stress that is independent of the presence of negative conditions.

Problem solving

Durlack (1983) provides a model of professional frustration which has, as a central theme, the inability to pinpoint problems and identify necessary information and organise it in a problem-solving manner. An obvious way to increase psychological success is to help staff develop their skill and ability in their work by providing opportunities to learn new techniques for working with patient problems, to refine old techniques or to develop greater theoretical sophistication in diagnosis and treatment.

One particularly useful focus for training is conflict resolution and organisational problem solving. Much of the frustration and stress that occur is a response to conflict between the needs and goals of staff on the one hand and the demands of the profession on the other. When these conflicts occur, people often feel helpless because they know little about how the system works and have not acquired the skills for negotiating it. Conflicts with supervisors, colleagues and people from other professions are a common source of job stress and it is the knowledge and skill involved in handling these conflicts that could help staff feel more confident and competent.

Kramer (1974) developed a successful training programme in organisational problem solving and conflict resolution for nurses. She designed the programme by collecting examples of typical organisational conflicts and frustrations from experienced nurses.

She also asked the most organisationally adept and successful nurses how they would handle those incidents. These problems and solutions then formed the basis of a training programme for novices. Kramer (1974) found that new nurses who were exposed to this programme experienced less role strain and maintained initial enthusiasm and commitment to a greater extent than did a control group. Planned in-service training programmes that are designed to give staff the ability to confront their problems can significantly decrease dissatisfaction.

Developmental counselling

Another way to influence job satisfaction is to have periodic counselling sessions with individuals who have been trained in staff development and who have no supervisory role. In such a way, current sources of frustration, stress and dissatisfaction may be discussed in a confidential manner without fear of the contents of any discussion being used by other people. Staff are helped to assess how job pressures night be affecting attitudes and performance and some form of action plan can then be discussed.

Holding a series of counselling interviews may help to prevent burnout amongst staff, especially those working in particularly stressful environments. During the interviews the staff member should be encouraged to ventilate their feelings and to self-investigate their negative reactions to patients and colleagues. There may be some initial resistance but often a process of opening up, and ultimately a dramatic change in attitude, follows. This form of developmental counselling does not only help the individual, it can also benefit other members of staff who respond positively to the changes in their colleague.

The power of groups can also be utilised to great effect. Many staff believe that their problems, feelings and reactions are unique. They rarely have the opportunity to discuss these work-related difficulties with others in a setting that encourages both emotional support and positive problem solving. Through carefully planned and skilfully run support groups, staff in these settings can be helped to cope adaptively with the stress associated with their jobs. Leakey et al. (1994) describe a staff counselling service set up in north Derbyshire. Following a survey which found high levels of distress among the staff, counsellors were employed from departments of clinical psychology, psychiatric nursing, occupational health and the chaplaincy to provide a counselling service to all members of staff on free and self-referral basis. A wide range of problems were presented, but does counselling work? Cooper and Sadri (1991) say 'yes'. They found that in comparison with a group who did not receive counselling, those that did reported higher levels of self-esteem, job satisfaction and organisational commitment; lower levels of anxiety and depression; changes in lifestyle; and finally lower absence from work.

Exchanging resources

An important feature of community psychology in recent years has been the establishment of resource exchange networks. Sarason (1977) indicated that the exchange of ideas and experiences in such contexts as conferences, interdisciplinary seminars and task-oriented action programmes can help all concerned in furthering their interests and ability to cope with problems in their work. Staff can receive concrete help that reduces the burden of their jobs, and horizons are broadened as they come to know people involved in different settings working with different types of problems. Just the process of sharing information and exchanging resources reduces the sense of isolation that so often characterises work in the health services. Sarason (1977) says that individuals who participate in such networks experience a sense of community and participation that increases their sense of efficacy, renews hope and optimism, and counteracts the sense of helplessness that all too often contributes to a negative attitude change. Thus the formation of resource exchange networks within and across organisations represents another useful way of promoting a healthy working environment.

Social factors

The approach of Maslach, Pines and Jackson has been to emphasise the social nature of difficulties work. In a series of studies over the 1970s, 1980s and 1990s they found that the most useful analysis of job stress was provided by a social psychological perspective. Maslach and Jackson (1982) say that:

> It is an approach that identifies the crux of the problem not as psychological stress *per se*, but as a particular type of stress arising from the social relationship between providers and recipients. It directs attention to certain classes of variables, such as perceptual biases, attributional inferences, and group processes, which provide many insights into possible solutions for burnout.

They point to a number of variables that affect development of burnout.

Degree of contact

Maslach and Jackson (1982) found a direct relationship between the amount of time spent in direct care of patients and emotional exhaustion. They administered the Maslach Burnout Inventory (MBI) to a number of staff physicians at a health maintenance organisation and then got them to give estimates of the amount of time they spent in various professional activities. They found that the greater the amount of time spent in direct contact with patients the higher the physicians' scores on the MBI subscale of emotional exhaustion. Scores were lower for those who spent some time in teaching and administration. Patient care is emotionally demanding in a number of ways: sometimes it can be due to the feelings and behaviours of the patients themselves; sometimes it is the nature of the patients' health problem; and sometimes it is due to communication problems, on the part of health professional and patient alike. Also, dealing with members of the patients' families can prove stressful in its own right.

Control

In health care settings, many aspects of the professional's environment are beyond his or her control and, as we have seen in previously in this chapter, the ability to be able to predict and control events in one's environment is extremely important in reducing the effects of stress. Frustration is produced by the inability of modern medicine to control the diseases of all the patients and by reluctance of some patients to co-operate with prescribed treatments. However, it is coping with lack of control over decisions made by doctors and administrators that formed the basis of nurses' feelings of exhaustion in the Maslach and Jackson (1982) study. Emotional exhaustion was higher for nurses who felt that they were unable to influence decisions of doctors and the policies of administrators. There were frequent complaints about (1) having no opportunity to be creative, and (2) doctors who failed to turn up for appointments, or disappeared without leaving word where they could be contacted. Similar relationships between perceptions of control and burnout have been found in a study of hospital nurses in the United States (Glass, 1997). Nurses were found to have one advantage over the doctors, and that was their freedom to have more time off and their ability to reschedule patients. Nurses were much more likely to report taking time off as a way of coping (61 per cent of nurses, 12 per cent of doctors). When asked whether they rescheduled their work in order to spend more time with those patients with whom they felt they were being more successful, 83 per cent of nurses said 'yes' as compared with 48 per cent of doctors. The authors suggest that time off and rescheduling are effective methods of coping with the stresses and strains of patient care.

Role ambiguity

This is a major cause of poor performance and job stress (Abraham and Shanley 1992). Therefore to what extent does role ambiguity exist among health professionals? Stein (1967) says there is a 'doctor–nurse game'. The rules are not out in the open and the game must be learnt through trial and error. The nurse's objective is to 'be bold, have initiative, and be responsible for making significant recommendations, while at the same time she must appear passive. This must be done in a manner so as to make her recommendations appear to be initiated by the physician.' There are no 'points' awarded for playing the game well, but penalty 'points' are gained for playing the game badly. The nurse is thus placed in the invidious position of uncertainty and ambiguity about the quality of her performance. This lack of positive feedback in an ambiguous situation, not surprisingly, produces emotional exhaustion. Although nursing has changed considerably since 1967, the extent to which the game is still played will be left for the reader to judge.

Attribution errors, or, 'It's the patient's fault'

This item needs little introduction since attribution errors were discussed in detail in Chapter 2. Maslach and Jackson (1982) suggest that the fundamental attribution error is made worse by utilisation of the medical model. That is, there is a tendency to see individuals in isolation about their problems and thus concentrate on what it is about that person that is causing the difficulty rather than investigating situational factors. The way patient records are kept also contributes to an emphasis on person-centred evaluations of problems, and there is little room for noting the circumstances in which the illness developed.

The process of blaming the patient continues when the health professional gradually develops a depersonalised, detached and often cynical view of patients. The general impression develops that, no matter what one does or how hard one works, patients will continue to disregard medical advice and abuse themselves. This attitude inevitably affects helping behaviour and the quality of patient care. It represents an important shift in the practitioner's view of health care: from a positive, humanised orientation to negative and depersonalised one.

Social support

Different people adopt different ways of coping with the stresses and strains of work, but two methods that have been found to be effective are isolation and social support. It might seem at first that those who use isolation as a means of coping are a different group from those who use social support, but this need not be the case. In fact, both techniques can be used to advantage by the same person.

Firth and Britton (1989) conducted a long-term analysis of the relationship between role ambiguity, perceived support and factors related to burnout such as absence and 'turnover' among British nurses. They concluded that emotional exhaustion and lack of perceived support both influenced motivation. Further, ambiguity about the limits of authority led nurses to avoid some situations. If emotional exhaustion has resulted from the continuous close contact with people, then it is not surprising that one way of coping is to get away from them completely. This can be achieved by physically distancing oneself from the 'interpersonal melee' such as by taking more time off or, if that proves impracticable, to at least have a period of time after work to unwind. Some of the distancing techniques include going for a run, listening to music, meditation or relaxing in a hot bath. Equally important as physical isolation is psychological isolation, for it is no good separating yourself physically from the job if you are going to think about it all the time.

Many psychologists would argue that isolating oneself is only an appropriate coping strategy as long as it is used in conjunction with social support (Duck 1998). Putting a certain amount of distance between us and the job is similar to what Lazarus and Launier (1978) term a *palliative* coping style. Coping in this fashion helps because it changes our internal response to the stress though it does little actively to reduce the stress stimulus itself. Social support, in the form of organised peer-group discussion meetings, can go a long way to actually changing the individual's perception of the stressful stimuli.

Sharing one's feelings with other people who are in the same position serves a number of functions:

- It can make one realise that certain problems are not necessarily unique to one individual.
- The meetings can serve as a reference point, that is, they can give information about what may be a normal reaction to a particular situation.
- Peers can provide the positive feedback that is so often absent from work with patients.
- They serve to save individuals from thinking everything is their fault and highlight the situational nature of problems.
- They can act as an outlet for simply talking about similar difficulties.

Dewe (1987) found that expressing feelings and frustrations was one of six strategies that nurses in New Zealand used to cope with job stress.

Maslach and Jackson (1982) report that those doctors and nurses who scored low on their scale of emotional exhaustion and depersonalisation were actively involved in peer support groups. They were also more likely to seek advice from other staff, discuss with patients the limitations of their professional relationship and try to view circumstances from the patients' point of view. Thus the social approach emphasises the interpersonal side of job stress and suggests that we look towards an analysis of our relationships with others if we want to come to a clearer understanding of the dynamics of job stress.

Work setting

Although reducing role conflict and reducing role ambiguity are important strategies for preventing dissatisfaction, there are a number of other features of the work setting that may be manipulated to facilitate a positive working environment. Just as important as reducing overload is the concept of increasing involvement and interest in the job. Merely eliminating the nasty and distasteful elements of the job is not good enough, for under these circumstances employees may lack a sense of purpose and direction, which can be equally destructive in organisational terms. However, the way in which a person's job is organised can have a significant impact on their attitude towards it (Hawkins, 1987). Role structure is as important as role ambiguity and role conflict.

Overload and shift work

Maslach and Pines (1977) found that they could significantly reduce the effects of overload by manipulating responsibility. Suppose four staff share the responsibility for twenty patients. They can share the responsibility for all of them or they can each be responsible for five patients. Maslach and Pines (1977) found that when the load was divided so that each member of staff was responsible for a small group of patients, there was less stress and fewer reported feelings of being overloaded. Even though the actual ratio of patients to staff was exactly the same in both circumstances, when the responsibility was divided into small groups it resulted in less stress. Some of the reasons put forward for this result were that the role structure probably contributed to a closer and more meaningful relationship with the patients, and the staff probably felt a greater sense of personal responsibility, autonomy and control when they were responsible for a small group of patients. Limiting the number of people for whom staff are responsible appears to be an effective method of reducing overload.

Not all patients require the same amount of care. There are some who may be labelled 'difficult' to work with and exercise more mental and physical energy than others. Therefore it makes sense to share the load among all members of staff even though there may be some people who openly express a desire to work with 'problem patients', for it is often these individuals who experience high levels of burnout. Similarly, it is important to try to balance the rewarding and unrewarding activities throughout the day, for concentrating all the 'dirty jobs' either at the beginning or the end of the day can increase stress. There are always going to be aspects of jobs that are distasteful and those that are rewarding but spreading and balancing the load throughout the day reduces the amount of strain that they may cause any one individual.

Most human functions have a rhythm and these circadian rhythms are geared to activity during the day and rest at night. Shift work leads to a destruction of these rhythms, leading to internal desynchronisation, which can lead to headaches, loss of appetite, fatigue and difficulty in sleeping (Waterhouse 1993). Barton (1994) Surveyed 587 nurses and midwives and found fewer health, sleep, social and domestic complaints among permanent night shift nurses than among rotating shift staff. Problems were further reduced by people who had chosen to do night work. These findings illustrate that it may not be shiftwork *per se* that causes problems but rotating shifts allied with a lack of opportunity to choose shifts.

Taking a break

No matter what the job, whether it be health professional or bringing up children, if one does not get a rest every now and then, pressure and strain will mount up till the burden reaches a critical level. Opportunities for taking some time off, no matter how brief, should be built in to any job programme. Apart from giving staff a rest from their work, time off can also provide an opportunity to reflect on one's position. However, in times of limited resources there is a problem in finding the time to give personnel a rest.

It may seem strange to say that sometimes it is necessary to encourage people to take a break, but such is in fact the case. Allowing holiday or vacation time to accumulate is regarded by some individuals as a status symbol that they can parade around work. Also there are some workers who take great pride in announcing that they have worked twelve or fourteen hours that day. It may illustrate dedication, but the long-term consequences of such action are detrimental to both staff and patient alike and it should be discouraged.

Staff development

Much lip service is paid to this concept in many organisations, but often the opportunities open to staff for development are limited. The words 'personal and professional growth' are sometimes used to refer to staff development and it is important to realise that development is important in both the professional and the personal spheres. The main issue is how to gauge individuals' needs in this particular domain. One method often used is the 'developmental interview', sometimes known as developmental counselling. Here staff are invited from time to time to discuss, usually with their superiors, issues relating to their development. The success of these sessions depends almost entirely on the attitude of the person conducting the interview, for if members of staff feel inhibited in discussing important matters relating to their job the usefulness of the session is limited. Therefore it is incumbent on supervisory staff to create an atmosphere of mutual trust and confidentiality in order to reduce the amount of suspicion that is often created by the very nature of the unequal status of the participants (De la Cour, 1992; Driver, 1994).

An important factor to consider in creating a feeling of active involvement is establishing the opportunity for individuals to become involved in developing ideas, projects and programmes of their own. This serves the dual purpose of providing a creative outlet for members of staff and some form of improvement in the functioning of the organisation itself.

In similar vein, the provision of some form of career ladder that is directed to both professional and academic development provides a necessary form of reinforcement. As Schein (1980) points out, financial and verbal rewards are not good enough in themselves for generating appropriate levels of motivation. There needs to be a clear programme by which people see how they may progress from one stage to the next. Individuals should be encouraged to take time off to attend academic courses relevant to their particular discipline in order that they to may progress up the career ladder and bring new knowledge to their professional practice. It is equally important for those institutions that provide the courses to construct a programme that is available to all, no matter what the initial qualification, so that individuals may progress to degree and master's level.

Management development

One consequence of progressing up the career ladder is that eventually one is more likely than not to find oneself in some form of managerial role, often with little experience of management itself. Good health practitioners may not make the best managers. In-service training programmes can help develop the skills and attitudes necessary for managing people. In this way managers can be helped to develop their awareness of their own operational philosophy and alternative philosophies and the consequences of adopting such alternatives. They may not even know about ways of preventing staff burnout.

Feedback is just as important for managers and administrators as it is for their subordinates. Hegarty (1974) found that when anonymous feedback was provided to managers their managerial style improved. Staff were provided with questionnaires which asked them to evaluate their superiors on a number of criteria. They were also asked to provide information about the qualities they most valued in a superior. The information was anonymous and only the managers saw the results. Some months later the survey was repeated with the same group; the evaluation scores on this occasion had risen. Managers are not immune to the effects of job stress; there is often ambiguity and role conflict in their position.

Conflict resolution

Problems with interpersonal and organisational conflict at their core will always occur, no matter what the management structure. However, mechanisms may be built in to organisations to alleviate conflicts. Filley (1975) recommends three courses of action:

- the creation of a formal mechanism for group problem solving and conflict resolution;
- staff training in the skills of interpersonal problem solving and conflict resolution;
- the determination of an optimal level of staff participation in decision making.

Building formal group problem-solving mechanisms into programmes means that there should be times during the week when all staff meet to discuss any problems. The meetings should be organised so as to encourage staff and supervisors alike to take part and promote an atmosphere of mutual support.

Developing training programmes for staff in the area of interpersonal problem solving and conflict resolution serves to benefit individuals themselves in the handling of their everyday problems and conflicts as well as to facilitate the process of group problem-solving sessions.

The third recommendation concerns the extent to which staff should be allowed to take part in the decision-making activities of the organisation. Whilst there is evidence to suggest that more staff participation leads to less conflict and higher morale (Cherniss and Egnatios 1978), it is often difficult to put it into practice. Therefore each situation must be organised so as to accommodate an optimum level of staff participation. This need not necessarily mean more committees, more meetings, for if it is organised properly it can actually lead to less work. It is also wise to take note of the findings of the experiments on group decision making that were discussed earlier on in Chapter 3.

A sense of direction

Clear, consistent and, most of all, realistic goals provide the focus that staff need to overcome the negative effects of vague, inconsistent or even conflicting institutional philosophies. Where an organisation refuses to give its members a clear sense of purpose, then staff are bound to ask questions about what they are meant to be doing, or even what they are doing there. Reppucci (1973) states that the development of a guiding philosophy of treatment or service is a particularly effective method for creating a sense of purpose. It should not be left up to individuals themselves to try to develop their own philosophy or approach in the absence of direction from the institution. In such cases people can become very quickly disillusioned.

Exercise 8.3 *Twenty Statements Test*

In Chapter 1 the topic of self-disclosure was discussed. Kuhn and McPartland (1954) developed a Twenty Statements Test (TST) to acquire data on self-identification. The test consisted of a page headed by 'Who am I?' and people were required to make twenty different statements in response to the simple question. The authors noted that individuals disclosed personal information which they hesitated to disclose to family members, friends and acquaintances. Locatelli and West (1995) adapted the test, suggesting it could be applied to the organisation. So. rather than giving statements about themselves, they were asked to produce statements beginning 'This department . . .' and 'This organisation . . .'. They found that the TST generated the most information and the largest number of themes as compared with other measures such as the repertory grid technique and group discussions.

With respect to the individual, group, work setting organisation, try to do the same. Try to think of ten statements beginning 'I am . . .' in relation to your work, followed by ten on the people you work with 'They are . . .' then, perhaps, the work setting 'The department is . . .', and finally 'The organisation is . . .'. Of course you can use other headings such as 'The NHS is . . .' depending on your circumstances. You can do this exercise on your own, or in groups. However, if the latter, anonymity must be ensured. Computers are good for this. People tend to concentrate on the negative aspects of others and the less negative aspects of themselves. Compare this with the attribution errors discussed in Chapter 2. This is an example of developing a symbolic interactionist perspective of organisational culture.

Finally, it may be necessary under certain circumstances to redefine the aims and goals of organisations. For instance, Seymour Sarason, a leading figure in community psychology, has said repeatedly that we set our goals too high and that organisations must redefine their goals specifically when scarce resources are in demand. Rather than assume responsibility for a whole population's health, it is more practical to offset some of this load on to the individuals themselves. By sharing the responsibility for health one redefines a number of roles, hopefully to the benefit of all concerned.

In practice this means that people should be encouraged to be less dependent on health professionals, to think and do more for themselves and ultimately to be able to engage in a mutual decision-making process about their own health care. Many 'self-health centres' see this as one of their fundamental aims. According to Sarason (1977) one of the key features of community psychology is to produce 'the competent community'. It seems reasonable that this competence should encompass health as well as other areas of psychological well-being.

Summary

Although some hospital procedures and nursing practices may be unpleasant for patients, there are a number of things nurses can do to alleviate pain and reduce stress for patients in their care. This chapter has explored the theoretical basis for current pain management and stress reduction strategies.

Methods of assessing pain include self-report measures, psychophysiological measures and behavioural assessment scales. A number of pain management strategies have been described, including acupuncture, hypnosis and cognitive restructuring.

Stress has been described from both physiological and psychological perspectives. Coping mechanisms tend to depend on individual styles of coping and may be either problem-focused or emotion-focused. A range of techniques can be taught to manage stress more effectively and these include relaxation techniques, the use of biofeedback and a range of cognitive behavioural techniques.

For both stress and pain management nurses need to be able to draw on a range of strategies in order to take account of individual needs and coping styles.

? Questions for further consideration

1 Discuss the psychological factors that influence pain.
2 Examine the effectiveness of psychological techniques in the management of pain.
3 What is the placebo effect?
4 How can stress be measured?
5 Describe a cognitive behavioural approach to stress management.
6 What is meant by 'cognitive appraisal'?

References

Aaronson, L. S. (1989). Perceived and received support: effects on health behaviour during pregnancy. *Nursing Research, 38,* 4–9.

Abraham, C. and Shanley, E. (1992) *Social psychology for nurses.* London: Edward Arnold.

Ader, R. and Cohen, N. (1993). Psychoneuroimmunology: Conditioning and stress. *Annual Review of Psychology.*

Argyle, M. (1987). *The Psychology of Happiness.* London: Methuen.

Bakal, D. A. (1992). *Psychology and Medicine.* 2nd edn. London: Tavistock.

Barber, J. (1982). Hypnosuggestive procedures in the treatment of clinical pain. In: Millan, T., Green, C. and Meagler, R. (eds) *Handbook of Clinical Health Psychology,* New York: Plenum.

Barber, J. (1986). Hypnotic analgesia. In: Holzman, A. D. and Turk, D. C. (eds) *Pain Management: A handbook of psychological treatment approaches.* Oxford: Pergamon Press.

Barefoot, J. C., Dahlstrom, W. G. and Williams, R. B. (1983). Hostility, CHD incidence and total mortality: A twenty-five-year follow-up study of 255 physicians. *Psychosomatic Medicine, 45,* 559–563.

Barton, J. (1994). Choosing to work at night. *Journal of Applied Psychology, 79,* 449–454.

Beales, J. G. (1979). The effects of attention and distraction on pain among children attending a hospital Casualty. In: Oborne, D. J., Gruneberg, M. M. and Eiser, J. R. (eds) *Research in Psychology and Medicine.* London: Academic Press.

Beecher, H. K. (1959). *Measurement of Subjective Responses: Quantitative effects of drugs.* London: Oxford University Press.

Bennis, W. G. (1962). Toward a truly significant management: the concept of organizational health. *General Systems Yearbook, 7,* 269–283.

Blanchard, E. B., McCoy, G. C., Wittrock, D., Musso, A., Geradi, R. J. and Pangburn, L. (1988). A controlled comparison of thermal biofeedback and relaxation training in the treatment of essential hypertension: effects on cardiovascular reactivity. *Health Psychology, 7,* 19–33.

Borkovec, T. D. and Sides, J. (1979). Critical procedural variables related to the physiological effects of progressive muscular relaxation. *Behavior Research and Therapy, 17,* 119–125.

Brown, S. M. (1990). Quantitative measurement of anxiety in patients undergoing surgery for renal calculus disease. *Journal of Advanced Nursing, 15,* 962–970.

Budzynski, T. (1973). Biofeedback procedures in the clinic. In: Birk, L. (ed.) *Biofeedback: Behavioural medicine.* New York: Grune and Stratton.

Callaghan, P. and Morrissey, J. (1993). Social support and health: a review. *Journal of Advanced Nursing, 18,* 203–210.

Camp, L. D. and O'Sullivan, P. S. (1987). Comparison of medical, surgical, and oncology patients' descriptions of pain and nurses' documentation of pain assessments. *Journal of Advanced Nursing, 12,* 593–598.

Chapman, C. R., Casy, K. L., Dubner, R., Foley, K. M., Gracely, R. H. and Reading, A. E. (1985). Pain measurement: an overview. *Pain, 22,* 1–31.

Cherniss, C. (1980). *Staff burnout.* Beverly Hills: Sage.

Cherniss, C. (1992). Long term consequences of burnout. *Journal of Organisational Behavior, 13,* 1–11.

Cherniss, C. and Egnatios, E. (1978). Clinical supervise in community mental health. *Social Work, 23,* 219–223.

Cohen, S., and McKay, G. (1984). Social support, stress and the buffering hypothesis: A theoretical analysis. In: Baum, A., Taylor, S. E. and Singer, J. E. (eds) *Handbook of Psychology and Health.* Hillsdale NJ: Erlbaum.

Connolly, A. M., Pancheri, P. and Luchetti, L. (1978). Clinical psychoneuroendocrinology in reproduction. In: Carenza, L., Pancheri, P. and Zichella, L. (eds) *Clinical Psychoneuroendrocinology in Reproduction.* London: Academic Press.

Cooper, P. J., Bawden, H. N., Camfield, P. R. and Camfield, C. S. (1987). Anxiety and life events in childhood migraine. *Pediatrics, 79,* 999–1004.

Cooper, C. L. and Sadri, G. (1991) The impact of stress counseling at work. *Journal of Social Behavior and Personality, 6,* 411–423.

Craig, K. D. and Prkachin, K. M. (1978). Social modelling influences on sensory decision theory and psychophysiological indices of pain. *Journal of Personality and Social Psychology, 36,* 805–815.

Curry, S. L. and Russ, S. W. (1985). Identifying coping strategies in children. *Journal of Consulting and Clinical Psychology, 14,* 61–69.

Daruna, J. H. (2004). *Introduction to Psychoneuroimmunology.* London: Academic Press.

Davitz, L. L. and Davitz, J. R. (1985). Culture and nurses' inferences of suffering. In: Copp, L. A. (ed.) *Perspectives on Pain.* Edinburgh: Churchill Livingstone.

De la Cour, J. (1992). Assessment of the staff appraisal systems. *British Journal of Nursing, 1,* 99–102.

Dewe, P. J. (1989). Sressor frequency, tension, tiredness and coping. *Journal of Advanced Nursing, 14,* 308–320.

Driver, M. J. (1994). Careers: a review of personal and organizational research. In: Cooper, C. L., Robertson, I. T. (eds) *Key reviews in managerial psychology.* Chichester: Wiley.

Durlack, J. A. (1983). Social problem-solving. In: Felner R. D. *et al.* (eds) *Preventive psychology.* New York: Pergamon.

Duck, S. (1998). *Human Relationships.* 3rd edn. London: Sage.

Eccleston, C., Morley, S., Williams, A., Yorke, L and Mastroyannopoulou, K. (2002) Systematic review of randomised controlled trials of psychological therapy for chronic pain in children and adolescents with a subset meta-analysis of pain relief. *Pain, 99,* 157–165.

Edelwich, J. and Brodsky, A. (1980). *Burnout: Stages of Disillusionment in the Helping Professions.* New York: Human Sciences Press.

Edwards D. and Burnard P. (2003) A systematic review of stress and stress management interventions for mental health nurses. *Journal of Advanced Nursing, 42 (2),* 169–200.

Fernandez, E. (1986). A classification system of cognitive coping strategies for pain. *Pain, 26,* 141–151.

Ferrell, B. R., McCaffery, M. and Rhiner, M. (1992). Pain and addiction: an urgent need for change in nursing education. *Journal of Pain and Symptom Management, 7,* 117–124.

Filley, A. C. (1975). *Interpersonal Conflict Resolution*. Glencoe, IL: Scott Foresman.

Firth, H. and Britton, P. (1989). Burnout, absence and turnover among British nursing staff. *Journal of Occupational Psychology, 62,* 55–59.

Fields, H. L. and Levine, J. D. (1984). Placebo analgesia: a role for endorphins? *Trends in Neuroscience, 7,* 271–273.

Francis, I. W. (1987). The physiology of pain. In: Boore, J. R. P., Champion, R. and Ferguson, M. C. (eds) *Nursing the Physically Ill Adult.* Edinburgh: Churchill Livingstone.

Glass, D C. (1997) Perceived control, depressive symptomatology, and professional burnout: a review of the evidence, *Psychology and Health, 12,* 435–436.

Gottlieb, B. H. (1985). Social support and the study of personal relationships. *Journal of Social and Personal Relationships, 2,* 351–375.

Hamilton, J. and Edgar, L. (1992). A survey examining nurses' knowledge of pain control. *Journal of Pain and Symptom Management, 7 (1),* 18–26.

Harrison, A. (1991). Assessing patients' pain: identifying reasons for error. *Journal of Advanced Nursing, 16,* 1018–1025.

Hawkings, L. (1987). Anergonomic approach to stress. *International Journal of Nursing Studies, 24,* 307–318.

Hegarty, W. H. (1974). Using subordinate ratings to elicit changes in supervisors. *Journal of Applied Psychology, 59,* 764–766.

Hilgard, E. R. and Hilgard, J. R. (1975). *Hypnosis in the Relief of Pain.* Los Altos CA: Kaufman.

Jacobson, E. (1929). *Progressive Relaxation.* Chicago: University of Chicago Press.

Jahoda, M. (1958). *Current Concepts of Positive Mental Health.* New York: Basic Books.

Johnson, J. E. (1975). Stress reduction through sensation information. In: Sarason, G. and Spielberger, C. D. (eds) *Stress and Anxiety* III. Chichester: Wiley.

Johnson, M. and Wallace, L. (1990). *Stress and Medical Procedures.* 3rd edn. Oxford: Oxford University Press.

Jones, P. and Klarr, A. C. (1985). *A Comparison of Burnout in Eight Mental Health Departments.* Paper presented to 'Burnout in health care conference' University of Newcastle.

Karoly, P. and Jensen, M. P. (1993). *Multimethod Assessment of Chronic Pain.* London: Allyn Bacon.

Karoly, P. (1985). The assessment of pain: concepts and procedures. In: Karoly, P. (ed.) *Measurement Strategies in Health Psychology.* Chichester: Wiley.

Kiecolt-Glaser, K. and Glaser, R. (1992). Psychoneuroimmunology: Can psychological interventions modulate immunity. *Journal of Consulting and Clinical Psychology, 60,* 569–575.

Kleinknecht, R. A. and Bernstein, D. A. (1978). The assessment of dental fear. *Behavior Therapy, 9,* 626–634.

Kramer, M. (1974). *Reality shock: why nurses leave nursing.* St Louis: Mosby.

Kuhn, M. and McPartland, T. (1954). An empirical investigation of self attitudes. *American Sociological Review, 19,* 58–76.

La Montagne, L. L., Johnson, B. D. and Hepworth, J. T. (1991). Children's ratings of postoperative pain compared to ratings by nurses and physicians. *Issues in Comprehensive Pediatric Nursing, 14,* 241–247.

Lander, J., Hodgins, M. and Fowler-Kerry, S. (1991). Children's pain predictions and memories. *Behavior Research Therapy, 30,* 117–124.

Lazarus, R. L. (1966). *Psychological Stress and the Coping Process.* New York: McGraw Hill.

Lazarus, R. L., Opton, E. M., Nomikos, M. S. and Rankin, N. O. (1965). The principle of short-circuiting of threat: further evidence. *Journal of Personality, 33,* 622–635.

Lazarus, R. S. and Launier, R. (1978). Stress-related transactions between person and environment. In: Pervin, L. A. and Lewis, M. (eds) *Perspectives in Interactional Psychology.* New York: Plenum.

Leakey, P., Littlewood, M., Reynolds, S. and Bunea, D. (1994). Caring for the carers. In: Cooper, C. L. and Williams, S. (eds) *Creating Health Work Organizations.* Chichester: Wiley.

Leventhal, H. (1990). Emotional and behavioural processes. In: Johnson, M. and Wallace, L. (eds) *Stress and Medical Procedures,* 3rd edn. Oxford: Oxford University Press.

Llewelyn, S. (1989). Caring: the costs to nurses and their relatives. In: Broome, A. (ed) *Health Pscyhology.* London: Chapman & Hall.

Locatelli, V. and West, M. (1995). A comparison of methods for assessing culture in organizations. Unpublished paper. Memo 1482, Institute of Work Psychology, University of Sheffield.

Loeser, J. D. and Fordyce, W. E. (1983). Chronic pain. In: Carr, J. E. and Dengerink, H. A. (eds) *Behavioural Science in the Practice of Medicine.* New York: Elsevier Biomedical.

Lohaus, A., Klein-Hessling, J., Vogele, C., Kuhn-Hennighausen, C. (2001). Psychophysiological effects of relaxation training in children. *Br J Health Psychol,* May 6 (Pt 2), 197–206.

Lyn, B. (1984). The detection of injury and tissue damage. In: Wall, P. D. and Melzack, R. (eds) *A Textbook of Pain.* Edinburgh: Churchill Livingstone.

Mandy, A. and Tinley, P. (2004). Burnout and occaptional stress. *Journal of the American Podiatric Medical Association, 94 (3),* 282–291.

Maslach, C. (1982). Job burnout: how people cope. In: McConnell, E. A. (ed) *Burnout in the Nursing Profession.* St Louis: Mosby.

Martelli, M. F., Auerbach, S. M., Alexander, J. and Mercuri, L. G. (1987). Stress management in the health care setting: matching interventions with patient coping styles. *Journal of Consulting and Clinical Psychology, 55,* 201–207.

Maslach, C. and Pines, A. (1979). Burnout: the loss of human caring. In: Pines, A. and Maslach, C. (eds) *Experiencing Social Psychology.* New York: Knopf.

Maslach, C. and Jackson, S. E. (1982). Burnout in health professions. In: Saunders, G. S. and Suis, J. (eds) *The social psychology of health and illness.* NJ: Erlbaum Hillsdale.

McCaffery, M. (1983). *Nursing the Patient in Pain.* London: Harper and Row.

McCaffery, M. (1990). Nursing approaches to nonpharmacological pain control. *Journal of Advanced Nursing, 27,* 1–5.

McCaul, K. D. and Malott, J. M. (1984). Distraction and coping with pain. *Psychological Bulletin, 95,* 516–533.

Meichenbaum, D. (1976). Toward a cognitive theory of self-control. In: Schwartz, G. E. and Shapiro, D. (eds) *Consciousness and Self-regulation: Advances in research* I. New York: Plenum.

Meichenbaum, D. (1977). *Cognitive-behaviour Modification: An integrative approach.* New York: Plenum.

Meichenbaum, D. and Cameron, R. (1983). Stress-inoculation training: toward a general paradigm for training coping skills. In: Meichenbaum, D. and Jaremko, M. E. (eds) *Stress Reduction and Prevention.* New York: Plenum.

Melzack, R. (1973). *The Puzzle of Pain.* Harmondsworth: Penguin.

Melzack, R. and Wall, P. D. (1965). Pain mechanisms: a new theory. *Science, 150,* 971–979.

Melzack, R. and Wall, P. D. (1982). *The Challenge of Pain.* Harmondsworth: Penguin.

Miles, M. S. and Mathes, M. (1991). Preparation of patients for the ICU experience: what are we missing? *Children's Health Care, 20,* 132–137.

Miller, N. E. (1978). Biofeedback and visceral learning. In: Rosenzweig, M. R. and Porter, L. W. (eds) *Annual Review of Psychology* XXIX. Palo Alto CA: Annual Reviews.

Miller, S. M. (1987). Monitoring and blunting: validation of a questionnaire to assess styles of information seeking under threat. *Journal of Personality and Social Psychology, 52,* 345–353.

Murray, J. J. and Niven, N. (1992). The child as a dental patient. *Current Opinion in Dentistry, 2,* 59–65

Niven, C. A. and Murphy-Black, T. (2000) Memory for labor pain: a review of the literature. *Issues in Perinatal Care, 27,* 244–253.

Niven, N. and Johnson, D. (1989). Taking the lid off stress management. *European Journal of Management, 17,* 14–17.

Norris, C. M. (1982). Delusions that trap nurses. In: McConnell as above.

Novaco, R. W. (1975). *Anger Control: The development and evaluation of an experimental treatment.* Lexington MA: Heath.

Ogus, E. D. (1992). Burnout and coping strategies: a comparative study of ward nurses. *Journal of social behavior and personality, 7,* 111–124.

Okinura, M. et al. (1992). Stress and burnout in Finnish physicians. *Scandanavian Journal of Work Environment and Health, 18,* 110–112.

Pearlin, L. I. and Schooler, C. (1978). The structure of coping. *Journal of Health and Social Behaviour, 19,* 2–21.

Pennebaker, J. W. (1982). *The Psychology of Physical Symptoms.* New York: Springer.

Pennebaker, J. W. (1984). Accuracy of symptom perception. In: Baum, A., Taylor, S. E. and Singer, J. E. (eds) *Handbook of Psychology and Health.* Hillsdale NJ: Erlbaum.

Peveler, R. C. and Johnston, D. W. (1986). Subjective and cognitive effects of relaxation. *Behavior Research and Therapy, 24,* 413–419.

Pines, A. and Aronson, E. (1988). *Career burnout: causes and cures*. London: Collier Macmillan.

Rappaport, N. B., McAnulty, D. P., Waggoner, C. D. and Brantley, P. J. (1987). Cluster analysis of Minnesota Multiphasic Personality Inventory (MMPI) profiles in a chronic headache population. *Journal of Behavioural Medicine, 10,* 49–60.

Reppucci, N. D. (1973). Social psychology of institutional change. *Journal of Community Psychology, 1,* 330–341.

Richards, J. S., Nepomuceno, C., Riles, M. and Suer, Z. (1982). Assessing pain behaviour: the UAB pain behaviour scale. *Pain, 14,* 393–398.

Rodin, J., Solomon, S. K. and Metcalf, J. (1979). Role of control in mediating perceptions of density. *Journal of Personality and Social Psychology, 36,* 988–999.

Roskies, E. (1987). *Stress Management for the Healthy Type A: Theory and practice*. New York: Guilford Press.

Sanders, S. H. (1985). Chronic pain: conceptualisation and epidemiology. *Annals of Behavioral Medicine, 7,* 3–5.

Sarason, S. (1977). Community psychology, netwoks and Mr Everyman. *American Psychologist, 31,* 317–328.

Seyle, H. (1956). *The Stress of Life.* New York: McGraw Hill.

Stein, L. (1967). The nurse–doctor game. *Archives of General Psychiatry, 16,* 699–703.

Steptoe, A. and Vogele, C. (1986). Are stress responses influenced by cognitive appraisals? An experimental comparison of coping strategies. *British Journal of Psychology, 77,* 243–255.

Suinn, R. M. (1980). Pattern A behaviours and heart disease: intervention approaches. In: Ferguson, J. M. and Taylor, C. B. (eds) *The Comprehensive Handbook of Behavioural Medicine* I. Jamaica, NY: Spectrum.

Taylor, B. and Barling, J. (2004). Feature article identifying sources and effects of carer fatigue and burnout for mental health. *International Journal of Mental Health Nursing, 13 (2),* 117.

Turk, D. C., Meichenbaum, D. and Genest, M. (1983). *Pain and Behavioural Medicine: A cognitive behavioural perspective*. New York: Guilford Press.

Van Tulder, M. W., Ostelo, R., Vleeyan, J. W. *et al.* (2000) Behavioural treatment for chronic low back pain. *Spine, 25,* 2688–2669.

Varni, J. W. and Thompson, K. L. (1986). Biobehavioural assessment and management of pediatric pain. In: Krasnegor, N. A., Arasteh, J. D. and Cataldo, M. F. (eds) *Child Health Behaviour: A behavioural pediatrics perspective*. Chichester: Wiley.

Volicer, B. J., Isenberg, M. A. and Burns, M. W. (1977). Medical-surgical differences in hospital stress factors. *Journal of Human Stress, 3,* 3–13.

Walding, M. F. (1991). Pain, anxiety and powerlessness. *Journal of Advanced Nursing, 16,* 388–397.

Walmsley, P. N., Brockopp, D. Y. and Brockoppo, G. W. (1992). The role of prior pain experience and expectations on postoperative pain. *Journal of Pain and Symptom Management, 7,* 34–37.

Waterhouse, J. (1993). Cicadian rhythms. *British Medical Journal, 306,* 448–451.

Weiss, J. M. (1972). Influence of psychological variables on stress-induced pathology. In: Porter, R. and Knight, J. (eds) *Physiology, Emotion and Psychosomatic Illness*. New York: American Elsevier.

Weitz, J. (1956). Job expectancy and survival. *Journal of Applied Psychology, 40,* 245–247.

Wortman, C. B. and Dunkel-Schetter, C. D. (1979). Interpersonal relations and career: a theoretical analysis. *Journal of Social Issues, 34,* 120–155.

Wynd, C. A. (1992). Relaxation imagery used for stress reduction in the prevention of smoking relapse. *Journal of Advanced Nursing, 17,* 294–302.

Zborowski, M. (1969). *People in Pain.* San Francisco: Jossey Bass.

Further reading

Horn, Sandra and Munafo, Marcus (1997) *Pain: Theory, Research and Intervention*. Milton Keynes: Open University Press. A concise account of the main theories and research on pain. Also contains practical aspects of intervention that are particularly directed to nursing care.

Roskies, Ethel (1987) *Stress Management for the Healthy Type A*. New York: Guilford Press. I still think that this is one of the best books on stress management. Directed at 'Type As', but I think the basic principles can be applied to us all.

Decision Making and Communication

A practice conundrum

Few student nurses would deny that practice placements and learning within practice is potentially stressful – but just why is that? Practice is surely the place where we learn the most authentic skills that we will use in the future. Practice is where we have the opportunity to meet patients and to provide the care that we hope will seem excellent.

If you are reading this textbook as a pre-registration learner think about practice placements and make notes regarding what it is about them that can seem so stressful. If you are reading the book as a qualified nurse, think of practice placements for students from the mentor's perspective. What do you anticipate students will find most stressful and why?

As you read through this chapter, consider the ways in which what you have learnt about the processes of decision making and problem solving help you to understand why learning in practice might seem more difficult.

Elsewhere (Niven, 2000) I have described a 'process of communication'. This process starts with deciding to do something and determining what action to take. Hence the key psychological components are decision making and problem solving. This may result in you, the protagonist, actually doing something or it may involve you having to communicate some course of action to someone else. But merely presenting people with information will not ensure 'a result', as they may not understand what you are talking about. Here it is important to know about how people learn and remember information. Finally, how you present information can also influence the ways people will respond to you. For years salesmen have been able to get us to do all sorts of things that we would probably not have done in the first place by cunning manipulation. We usually see this as fair enough even though we may have been duped, but should nurses use these techniques to get patients to do what they want? Also, how do we learn? Is it better to learn by reading how to do something or actually doing it? Hopefully at the end of this chapter some of these issues may be answered.

John and his wife Jean have gone to their doctor to get the results of some tests John has had. The doctor informs them that John has cancer but says that there are a number of things that can be done. He goes on to describe them in some detail. When John and Jean get home all they can remember of the interview is that John has cancer. They know they were told about various treatments but cannot recall what they were.

- Imagine that you and a friend are on your way to the theatre. You have spent £20 on two tickets for the performance. However, in the foyer of the theatre you discover that you have lost the tickets. Would you spend another £20 on two more tickets?
- Imagine that you are on your way to the same theatre but haven't yet bought the tickets, when you discover that you have just lost £20 in cash. Would you still buy tickets for the play?

You may consider both situations equivalent and indeed in objective terms they are – you have lost £20 in either situation. However, when people are presented with both scenarios they tend to say that they would be more likely to buy new tickets if they had lost the money than if they had lost the tickets.

Decision making

We make decisions every day of our lives. Some are more important than others, but all decisions resolve some sort of problem and many take up considerable amounts of time and effort. But how good are the decisions that we make each day? Unfortunately, according to many statisticians and mathematicians, most of them are not very good at all, indeed mathematicians would describe us as irrational decision makers. For example, if I say that for every time I toss a coin and it turns up heads I will give you £5 but for every time the coin turns up tails *you* have to give *me* £2, you will probably accept the offer. However, if I then say that in order to play the game with me you have to give me £1 for every toss of the coin, you might think twice about it. A rational decision-maker would jump at the chance to make some money, because if the coin were fair, over the course of two tosses you would be likely to win £5 and lose £2, leaving £3. You would have made £1.50 for each toss of the coin. Subtract your entrance fee of £1, and you have made a profit of £0.50 per game. If the entrance fee was increased to £2 *you* would be ill advised to play the game, because you would be likely to average a loss of £0.50 per game.

Consider the same situation but with the stakes increased a hundredfold – heads I give you £500 and tails you give me £200, with a £100 entrance fee. A rational decision maker would still play the game because the odds have not changed. However, we may be reluctant to play since the 'psychological risk' involved is too great; when the stakes are very high, psychological factors play an increasing role in decision making.

This chapter examines why we are not rational in making decisions and looks at the psychological factors involved in the decision-making process. It examines decision making from the nurse's perspective, and from the point of view of the public who have to make frequent decisions about their own health care.

Mistakes

There is a distinction between the 'clinical decision' and the 'statistical decision'.

- *The clinical decision* involves the nurse making a prediction about the effectiveness of a particular care programme based on his or her knowledge and experience of the patient and their condition. The decision-making process sometimes involves intuition, and often the nurse is unaware how he or she came to make the decision. (Luker and Kenrick, 1992, found that although community nurses consider a large proportion of their work to require a scientific basis, their practice is largely founded on experiential knowledge.) Hoffman *et al.* (2004) looked at some of the factors that might influence nurses' clinical decision making and found that, contrary to common expectation, educational level and experience did not seem to play as significant a role as factors such as holding a professional orientation. Although, the authors point out that this was a study of Australian nurses, who may have experienced a different educational process from nurses in other countries.
- *The statistical decision* is based on established mathematical rules. Thus, a prediction about the effectiveness of a care programme depends on statistical probabilities based on previous research studies, rather than on intuition.

People who favour the clinical decision-making approach emphasise the unique properties of the human brain, whereas those who advocate the statistical decision-making method point to the vague, often unscientific nature of these same unique properties. Of course, both approaches are perfectly compatible and need to be used in conjunction with each other. The human brain is far more complex than any computer and thus able to produce exceptional solutions to many problems. However, the use of statistics can supplement the decision-making process to good effect.

If the nurse is aware of the typical mistakes that can be made in the process of making decisions, she can combine the benefits of her intuition with the sophistication of statistical analysis in order to produce logical *and* human results.

Representativeness

Sometimes irrelevant information can obscure judgements otherwise based on reliable details. Consider the following description provided by Tversky and Kahneman (1974):

Intelligent but lacks creativity. Is a neat and tidy, but rather a dull, mechanical person. Does not mix well with others but has a high need to achieve. He has a deep moral sense of purpose.

This is a description of a person chosen at random from a group comprising thirty engineers and seventy social scientists. What is the probability that the person described is an engineer? If you think the probability is quite high, you have been misled by the description; there is a seven in ten chance that the person described is a social scientist. Pairing the subjective personality sketch with the actual statistics distracts us from a true representation of the odds; a rational decision maker would ignore the relatively worthless personality profile and concentrate on the 30 : 70 ratio of engineers to social scientists.

Lalljee *et al.* (1993) conducted a similar sort of study in a health and illness context. They gave students descriptions a various people such as:

Mr C is 53 years old and has quite a 'high-powered' job which he says gives him little time for relaxation or exercise. Mr C tends to like his food and is known to be a bit of a gourmet. Accordingly he has been overweight for some time. Mr C feels he doesn't have the same stamina that he used to have. At the moment he becomes breathless and sometime has chest pains after a small amount of physical exertion.

The students were asked to select an illness from the following list that they thought Mr C. might be suffering from. If the illness was not there, then to denote another: AIDS, arthritis, heart disease, influenza, leukaemia, mumps, pneumonia. The majority (95.8 per cent) selected heart disease because the symptoms, such as lack of stamina, breathlessness and chest pains, matched the prototype of the man as a bon viveur with a high-powered job, etc. But what would happen if the same symptoms were prescribed to someone else such as a child or someone from a 'Third World' culture? A different prototype. Diagnoses of heart disease fell to 35 per cent when the person was described as young and 5 per cent when the symptoms were ascribed to someone from the 'Third World'. In this case Lalljee *et al.* (1993) illustrated that the nature of the person was a more important factor in determining illness than the symptoms.

Unrelated events

People have a tendency to view unrelated events as related. Suppose a coin is tossed five times and it turns up tails every time. If you had to predict the outcome of the sixth toss, would you choose heads or tails? It might feel right to say that it is about time heads turned up, but in fact the odds are still 50 : 50; there is just as much chance that the result will be heads as it will be tails. The coin cannot 'remember' the five previous tails, so each toss of the coin is unrelated to the next one. However, if one uses a model such as a *theoretical sampling distribution*, which shows the theoretical expectation of obtaining runs of a certain length given a fair coin, then Holloway (1974) provides the following probabilities.

Runs of heads:

Toss	P
First	0.05
Second	0.25
Third	0.125
Fourth	0.063
Fifth	0.031
Sixth	0.016
Seventh	0.008
Eighth	0.004
Ninth	0.002
Tenth	0.001

A probability of 1 denotes certainty. This is because the model is based on taking a coin and spinning it thousands of times Essentially, when one is dealing with short sequences, people expect random events. Confused? Then think carefully how you might respond to a patient's request for the odds on some condition recurring.

 Exercise 9.1 *Transitivity: influencing the job selection interview*

The principle of *transitivity* can be used to secure a person's preferred candidate in job selection interviews. The principle of transitivity states that a person who prefers outcome A to outcome B, and who prefers outcome B to outcome C, should prefer outcome A to outcome C. Bearing this in mind consider the following scenario.

You are chair of a committee whose task is to select a new lecturer for the department. The committee is comprised of five members: Jacky, David, Hilary, Peter and Francis. There are three candidates (A, B and C) and you know the committee's preferences based on interviews and CVs. They are as follows in order of preference:

Jacky	A	B	C
David	A	C	B
Hilary	B	C	A
Peter	C	A	B
Francis	C	A	B

Secretly you would like candidate C to get the job but there is not much difference between the candidates. In fairness you put it to the vote.

The committee members are unaware that the manner of comparison (the Principle of Transitivity) is crucial in determining who should get the job. So you must avoid any direct comparison between B and C because three of the five committee members prefer B to C. Instead you ask them to compare A or B, then when A wins you should ask for a second vote between A and C. Or should you prefer B, first ask for a vote between A and C, and after C has won, a vote between C and B. As long as the comparisons are based on pairs and thus intransitive, you have control.

Availability of information

In each of the following pairs, which cause of death is more likely?

- Lung cancer or stomach cancer?
- Murder or suicide?
- Diabetes or a motor vehicle accident?

Lichtenstein *et al.* (1978) established that people overestimate the frequency of medical conditions which receive a large amount of publicity, and underestimate the frequency of those conditions which don't receive so much publicity. Lung cancer is thought to be more common than stomach cancer, murder more common than suicide and diabetes more common than motor vehicle accidents. In fact in each case the opposite is true. Events are judged to be more likely to occur if examples of them come easily to mind. Nurses should be careful when considering probable outcomes and be aware of the possible effects of a heavily publicised or widely available background of information.

Gains and losses

Imagine that we are threatened by a rare disease which is expected to kill 600 people. Preparations have begun to cope with its outbreak and two alternative programmes (A and B) have been proposed to combat the disease.

The exact scientific consequences of the disease are these. If programme A is adopted, 200 people will be saved; if programme B is adopted, there is a one in three probability that 600 people will be saved and a two in three probability that no one will be saved. Which of the two programmes would you choose?

Most people will choose programme A because of the risks involved in programme B. However, consider the same problem reformulated as follows. If programme C is adopted, 400 people will die; if programme D is adopted, there is a one in three chance that nobody will die and a two in three probability that 600 people will die. Which of the two programmes would you choose now?

Under these circumstances most people choose the risk-seeking alternative; the certain death of 400 people is less acceptable than the chance that 600 people will die. However, the two versions of the problem describe identical outcomes, the only difference being that in the first situation the death of 600 people is the reference point and the outcome is evaluated in terms of lives saved or gained. In the second situation, the reference point is no deaths, and so the programmes are evaluated in terms of lives lost. How decisions are framed to patients can determine outcome.

Base-rate neglect

This feature of decision making is related to framing and concerns the disproportional influence of base rates when assessing risk. For example, when people are presented with two different statements about cancer:

- it is likely to kill 1,286 out of 10,000 people;
- it is likely to kill 24.14 out of 100 people;

they judge the first statement as being much more risky despite the level of risk in the second statement being twice as high. Niven (2002) illustrated that health professionals were susceptible to this bias. He presented them with a series of statements about causes of death, supposedly representing data from a Far Eastern study. Again the results indicated a preference to report more risk when the data were presented with a high baseline despite the actual odds being less risky. This study, and others, illustrates the care that must be taken when handling statistical data.

In the previous example the reference point is fixed – deaths or lives. Sometimes the reference point may be determined by events that are only imagined, as in the following example. Two nurses were about to go away for the weekend from the same train station but to different destinations. Since their departure times were the same, they decided to share a taxi. Unfortunately their taxi was held up in traffic and they arrived thirty minutes after the scheduled departure of their trains. Dorothy was told that her train left on time. Mary was told that her train had been delayed and had left five minutes ago. Who was the more upset?

Most people would say Mary, yet both nurses' objective conditions and expectations of missing their trains were the same. If Mary is more upset, it is because, in the act of imagination, she came closer to catching her train. The frustration increases when a more desirable alternative is imagined. Kahneman and Tversky (1974) state:

An individual's experience of pleasure or frustration may therefore depend on an act of imagination that determines the reference level to which reality is compared.

How good are nurses at making decisions? Dowding and Thompson (2003) say that first of all one has to distinguish between judgements and decision making and that, whilst they are closely linked, it is useful to deal with them separately. They say that until now the measures of nursing judgements have been based on 'rather simplistic measures of patient outcome as a criterion'. Also, decision making has been characterised by problems with measurement such as comparisons with expert panels and their inherent bias. They acknowledge that measuring the quality of decision making in nursing is a complex one so perhaps it is best to concentrate on becoming more aware of the pitfalls rather than becoming an expert decision maker.

Implications for nursing

The research on decision making has considerable implications for the nurse as a rational decision maker. To summarise the main findings, it seems that:

- Background details can give useful information concerning a decision, but it is crucial that the nurse is aware of the influence of subjective, irrelevant personality profiles.
- The research on decision making indicates the desirability of avoiding casino games and machines because of adverse odds, but more importantly it should be noted that where there is a high degree of risk, people are less likely to follow rational decision-making rules. Decisions relating to patients which involve a high degree of risk require careful consideration.
- Real and imagined reference points can have a significant effect on decision-making strategies and on the nurse's objective experience of outcomes.

Health decision making

Every day people make important decisions about their health. These decisions can range from whether to make an appointment to see a doctor to deciding whether to continue with a therapeutic programme. A number of models have been proposed to try to account for the individual's decision-making behaviour in a variety of circumstances. I will look at *conflict theory* here and other, more general models of health behaviour, in the next chapter.

Conflict theory

Janis and Mann (1977) present five different plans for coping with stress and crisis and five stages of decision making. The plans for coping stemmed from observing people, examining research data and monitoring public health messages. The decision maker can adopt one of the following five patterns of coping.

- *Unconflicted persistence.* Details about risks are ignored, and the individual continues to behave complacently.
- *Unconflicted change.* A course of action is adopted without any challenge or discussion.
- *Defensive avoidance.* The situation is avoided either by shifting responsibility to someone else or by procrastinating over the decision. Another avoidance technique is selective attention, that is, hearing only what one wants to hear.
- *Hypervigilance.* Under conditions of pressure or panic, the individual selects the first solution that appears to work, without considering alternative courses of action.
- *Vigilance.* A carefully considered action pattern is considered and compared to alternative plans before making a decision.

Let us consider the patterns of coping in relation to the following example.

You have taken your three-month-old son to the baby clinic for his injections. The health visitor asks if you are going to have him immunised against whooping cough. She tells you that your baby will be safer if you have him immunised against whooping cough, as the disease is dangerous. You know that the whooping cough vaccine has caused brain damage in some babies. The health visitor is waiting for your decision.

- *Unconflicted persistence.* You do nothing and complacently decide to ignore the advice of the health visitor about vaccination.
- *Unconflicted change.* You uncritically adopt the advice of the health visitor and do not think any more about it.
- *Defensive avoidance.* You believe that there are risks to your baby's health either way. You don't see how you can make a decision under these circumstances and ask the health visitor to decide for you.
- *Hypervigilance.* You are aware of the risks but believe that there must be a way to safeguard your baby's health. However, you don't feel that you have had enough time or information upon which to base your decision but you make a decision as you feel under pressure to do so.
- *Vigilance.* You accept that there are risks involved in either course of action but feel that there is a way to safeguard your baby's health and that you must have enough time and information upon which to base your decision under these circumstances.

Janis and Rodin (1980) state that:

While the first two patterns are occasionally adaptive in saving time, effort and emotional wear and tear, especially for routine or minor decisions, they often lead to defective decision-making if the person must make a vital choice.

Janis (1984) says that occasionally a vigilant action pattern may not work, specifically if a split-second response is required, but in the majority of situations it leads to decisions of the best quality. Janis provides three conditions for the vigilance pattern to take place.

- Awareness: specifically of the risks of each alternative.
- Hope: of finding a better alternative.
- Belief: in having adequate time to arrive at a desirable decision.

Thus, if awareness does not occur, unconflicted persistence or change will take place; if hope is not met, defensive avoidance is to be expected; if belief that there is adequate time does not come about, then hypervigilance will be the foremost coping pattern.

If the vigilant action pattern is adopted, the individual can proceed to make a stable decision. If any of the other patterns are dominant, then:

the decision maker will fail to engage in adequate information search and appraisal of consequences, overlooking or ignoring crucial information about relevant costs and benefits.

(Janis, 1984)

Problem solving

Keighley (1993), in discussing the management of care in nursing, cites the work of Allinson (1971), who proposed that one way to describe decision making is to use the rational decision-making process. After agreeing the definition of a problem, the second stage of this process is to discover all the solutions. However, little advice is given on how to achieve this goal. How *does* one go about discovering solutions to problems?

Brainstorming

This is a technique which can be used to generate solutions to problems. Initially it involves sitting down and producing as many solutions to the problem as possible (Osborn, 1963). The rules are as follows.

- *No criticism.* Write down any idea or possible solution without judging it good or bad. Evaluation comes later.
- *Encourage quantity.* Try and produce as many solutions as possible. If you run out of ideas, put your list down and come back to it.
- *Be bizarre.* Do not be afraid to write down what may seem to be wild or crazy ideas.
- *Combine suggestions.* Some ideas may be combined or improved.

- *General strategies.* Do not worry about the 'nuts and bolts' of the solution; keep to general strategies for the achievement of goals.

The following is an example of brainstorming.

John is 52 years old and has just had a heart attack. There is a history of heart disease in his family, he is overweight, works hard and smokes thirty to forty cigarettes a day. He has been told that it is imperative to stop smoking, and he understands the need to quit but has absolutely no idea how to do so. John comes to you and says, 'How on earth am I going to give up smoking?' You sit down with him and start to brainstorm some strategies. He could:

- cut down by one cigarette a day;
- have his hands put in casts so he can't hold the cigarette;
- try hypnotism;
- suck non-sugar sweets;
- just stop;
- look at films of people dying of lung cancer;
- buy some cigarettes, smoke one and throw the rest away;
- tell everybody he knows that he's giving up;
- try to avoid people who smoke;
- try and avoid places where smoking takes place;
- send £1 for every cigarette smoked to a cause he hates;
- smoke and smoke till he vomits;
- join a 'stop smoking' group;
- chew nicotine gum;
- pair smoking with electric shocks;
- give points for not smoking and a present for every 50 not smoked;
- visit a ward where people are dying through smoking;
- give himself a big reward if he stops for three weeks;
- switch to a low-tar brand;
- place 'You will die if you smoke' notices everywhere.

If John gets stuck, he should think of people who can help, places and times where the problem occurs, and his own ability to cope with situations.

The next stage is to go over the strategies and apply commonsense criteria for selection. The suggestions John decides to keep are:

- just stop;
- join a 'stop smoking' group;
- give points for not smoking and a present for every fifty cigarettes not smoked;
- a big reward if he stops for three weeks;
- chew nicotine gum.

Discuss with John his reasons for choosing these strategies. Then apply practical criteria to each strategy to see whether it will work.

- Determine whether the strategy is clear enough to follow.
- Compare the positive and negative consequences of applying the strategy.
- Decide whether the strategy will actually achieve the goal.
- Establish the extent to which the person can follow it. Is it realistic?
- Does the strategy conflict with the individual's values? Do they like it?
- Award points out of ten for the usefulness of the strategy.

John decides to investigate the strategy of giving points for not smoking and a present for every fifty not smoked.

- 'The strategy is clear enough and I can see myself gradually cutting down'. (70 per cent probability of success.)
- 'I can see myself getting the rewards but will they be good for me?'. (40 per cent probability of success.)
- 'It will stop me smoking but only if I manage to keep it up.' (30 per cent probability of success.)
- 'I like the idea of stopping slowly but I am convinced of the harm of cigarettes and think that I have the willpower to stop immediately'. (10 per cent probability of success.)

John concludes that the point-awarding strategy really is not for him and decides to investigate the 'just stop' proposal with the added incentive of rewards after a specified period of time. Of course John's chosen plan may not work, and he may have to try again, but at least he has alternatives and is not in the powerless position of not knowing what to do.

Mental ruts

 ### Exercise 9.2 *Mental ruts*

The problem given is to measure out quantities of water by pouring water from one jug to another. You have one jar that holds twenty-nine pints and another that holds three pints. If your task is to measure out twenty pints, the solution is to fill up the large jar and pour water from it into the small jar until it is full. This would leave twenty-six pints in the large jar. If you repeat this procedure twice you will have twenty pints in the small jar. Easy. Try to work out solutions to the following problems. This time there are three jars, and their capacity differs with each problem.

Problem	Jar A	Jar B	Jar C	Desired amount
Example	29	3	–	20
1	21	127	3	100
2	14	163	25	99
3	18	43	10	5
4	9	42	6	21
5	20	59	4	31
6	23	49	3	20
7	15	39	3	18

In each case the problem can be solved by filling up jar B, pouring water into jar A, then pouring water into jar C twice The solution may be represented mathematically thus: B – A – 2C. However, if you used this to solve problems 6 and 7, you have become 'stuck in a mental rut', a much easier strategy would have been A – C (for problem 6) and A + C for problem 7), eliminating the need for B altogether.

Intuition

Getting stuck in a mental rut can also occur when dealing with objects and people as well as with mathematical processes. Maier (1930) posed the following problem.

Two pieces of string are dangling from the ceiling. The goal is to tie them together. However, they are too far apart and too short for a person to keep hold of one while reaching for the other. Scattered about the room are numerous objects, including a pair of pliers. Could the pliers be of any help in solving the problem?

Most people, when faced with this problem, need hints from the experimenter in order to find the solution. The answer is to tie the pliers to one of the pieces of string and swing it to form a pendulum. On the backswing, catch it and tie it to the other piece of string. The normal function of pliers is to act as a tool and not as a pendulum, so most people fail to solve the problem immediately.

This inclination to view objects as having fixed uses is called *functional fixedness*. We can also view people in a functionally fixed way. Think back to the story about the surgeon described in Chapter 2. We tend to think of surgeons as being male and therefore overlook the fact that the surgeon could be the boy's mother.

One factor related to an individual's ability to solve these sorts of problems is prior experience. If a person were building a wall and mislaid the plumb line, they might tie some pliers on to the end of a piece of string and use it in place of the plumb line. This type of prior experience of using objects in different ways can help in problem solving.

Exercise 9.3 *Problem solving*

Take two groups of people. Give one group the following problem.

A lorry driver is travelling the wrong way down a one-way street. A policeman sees him and does nothing. Why?

Ask the other group to write down as many different ways of travelling from A to B as they can think of, and then give them the same problem to solve.

Were there any differences between the ability of the two groups to solve the problem? If the second group were better at solving the problem, then the 'travelling' task served to break the functional fixedness of seeing the lorry driver in his lorry and driving up the one-way street.

Problem solving in social settings

An area in which problem-solving skills are particularly useful is the social domain. Many problems occur through our interactions with other people in specific situations. The purpose of the next section is to help you identify the issues, problems and concerns of your own life in order that you might help patients do the same.

Positive and negative

Often a very simple structure can help with the identification of the major constituents of a problem.

Write down the things in your life that you feel positive about and the things that you feel negative about. Make sure you write down at least two positive features of your life for every negative feature and don't worry about the importance of each issue. For example:

Positive
- I'm not too badly off as far as money is concerned.
- I get along OK with my parents.
- I think I have a reasonable amount of intelligence and ability to be a nurse.
- I have some very good friends.

Negative

- I think I'm a bit too shy.
- I hate it when others tell me I'm doing something wrong.

Now do the same for the following specific headings. The questions will give you some guidelines to start you thinking.

- *Ability*. How good am I? Am I going to be able to get things done? Do I have what it takes to be a good nurse? Have I the ability to deal with everything life throws at me?
- *Identity*. What do I believe in? In what ways does my life have meaning? Do I have a clear sense of purpose and direction in life? What am I confused about?
- *Relationships*. How do I relate to others. What social settings influence the way I act sexually? What are my views on long-term relationships?
- *Nursing*. How do I feel about the way things are going in my career? What do I get out of nursing? What am I like, and how do others see me, as a nurse?
- *Community*. What do I do at home or with friends? Do I contribute anything to the community? Do I have enough free time? What do I do with it? What is my neighbourhood like?

Finally, it is important to review problems in specific social settings. The first stage is to write down all the social settings you can think of, as in the following example.

- *Social settings*. Friends; parents, nursing college; badminton club; student union; tutors; family; church group; friends outside college.
- *Analysis*. Take each of these settings and determine what people think about how you should act; the demands they place upon you; your thoughts; how satisfied you are.
- Action. Finally, action has to be taken. Therefore choose one problem and try to think through some possible strategies. Use techniques similar to the brainstorming action plans described earlier and discuss them with friends if possible.

Practice problems

The term 'practice' problems could mean 'Here are some problems for you to practice' or it could refer to problems encountered by nurses during the course of their practice – it depends on your frame of reference. Price (2003) refers to the importance of frames of reference in solving nursing practice problems. He uses the example of a patient who has diabetes mellitus and is unable to control his diet and weight. How does the nurse go about solving the problem of helping him manage his condition? Price (2003) presents three frames of reference that nurses might consider:

- *Instruction/learning*. Here the emphasis should be on facilitating the learning of the patient with respect to the information and skills required to manage the condition.

It should be 'andragogical', where initially the nurse works with the patient's own particular views and develops them rather than imposing his or her own explanations. This is more difficult than instruction where important information is presented and understanding tested.

- *Risk management*. As nurses are accountable for patients' safety, information concerning acute and life-threatening conditions is important.
- *Moral action*. As it is the patient who must live with decisions, the nurse may consider his or her role in the phrasing consequences. 'This isn't just your health, Mr Jones, it's time and worry for your wife and cost to the country if you need surgery later on' versus 'I think that you need to know the consequences of not adjusting, but only you can make such choices'.

We are presented with problems practically every day of our lives and often are reasonably successful in coming to some sort of solution or resolution, but the process by which we arrive at an end point is not always clear, either to ourselves or, more important, to others. Therefore some time should be given to trying to analyse the basic constituents of the problem, to break it down and recognise the parts, even verbalise the process in order to improve our understanding of how we came by a course of action rather than just why.

Social influence

There are a number of strategies which are used to influence people's decisions about health care. The manner in which information is presented to a person often determines the degree of adherence. Similarly, the presence of others can have a significant effect on health behaviour. Thus the term *social influence* refers to the ways in which people's behaviour is influenced by the presence and actions of others (Cialdini, 2001). The 'others' include the nurse and people of influence, such as partners or friends, in the individual's life. Social influence takes a number of forms:

- *Conformity*. Individuals alter their behaviour to adhere to social norms or socially accepted behaviour.
- *Adherence*. Asking people to alter their behaviour in some particular way.
- *Obedience*. Ordering a person to change his or her behaviour.
- *Modelling*. Behaviour is changed through observing the actions of someone else.

Conformity

Conformity has been discussed more fully in Chapter 3 (pp. 74–7) but is worth looking at again briefly, in the context of social influence. Societies have a number of rules, some formal, some unwritten, which indicate how people should behave in particular circumstances (*social norms*). In some circumstances these norms serve a useful function – forming a queue prevents social chaos, while other norms appear to have no obvious purpose. However, it is clear that there are forceful pressures to conform in many contexts.

Imagine that you are revising for your exams. Whilst engaged in this worthwhile pursuit you become aware that one of your friends is using a totally different revision technique and disagrees with you about which technique is best. This causes a slight degree of apprehension in you, but you are then joined by another friend who also disagrees with you. Do you stick to your original technique or change to the one your friends have adopted? You might chance your luck, but if two more friends arrived and agreed with the other two, you would be under enormous pressure to change and conform.

Nurses are sometimes faced with a situation where they disagree with decisions affecting the care of their clients. They may feel that these decisions are not in the client's best interest and their professional code of conduct requires them to speak out on behalf of their client. This is particularly difficult when other members of the team are perceived as more powerful or of a higher status. The pressure to conform can be infectious; as each group member agrees with the next, personal doubts are suppressed and a false impression of unanimity arises, inevitably leading to irrational and sometimes dangerous decisions being made.

Adherence

Nurses often find themselves asking people to alter aspects of their behaviour. This may seem straightforward, but in many instances people do not do what you wish them to do. However, there are ways of phrasing requests which can significantly affect patient adherence. It is important that nurses are aware of these techniques, as they may be using them unknowingly. If patients become aware that they have been manipulated, all trust in the relationship evaporates.

The 'foot in the door' technique

This technique operates on the principle that a small or petty request followed by a larger, more important request will increase adherence. Freedman and Fraser (1966) conducted a famous study into the 'foot in the door' technique. People were phoned at home and asked a few simple questions about the kind of soap they used. Several days later the same person phoned again, this time asking if they could send five or six people along to make an inventory of all the household products the person contacted had on hand. They explained that it would take about two hours and that access would be needed to all parts of the house. Despite the enormity of the request, 52.8 per cent agreed to the visit, while only 22.2 per cent agreed to a visit when asked without the 'foot in the door' request. One explanation of these results is that once people comply with a small request they experience a small shift in their self-perception, coming to see themselves as 'helpful people'. When a large request follows, they do not want to destroy this self-image.

'Throwing the low ball' technique

If one of your tutors were to say to you 'Could you help me with some work I'm doing on social influence? It starts at 7.30 a.m. and will only take up ten minutes of your time, I promise.' You might think that you would like to. help, but that 7.30 a.m. is much too early. If your tutor phrased the same request as: 'Could you help me with some work I am doing on social influence? It will only take up ten minutes of your time, I promise,' waited for you to say yes or no and then told you it was due to start at 7.30 a.m. he or she might get more volunteers. This approach has been called 'low balling', from the baseball term to 'throw a low ball' (Cialdini, 2001).

Cialdini *et al.* (1978) asked students if they would put a poster up in their rooms. In the low ball condition, they agreed to display the poster and were then told that they had to collect it from the foyer, a considerable distance downstairs. In the control condition, the students were told that they would have to pick the poster up from the foyer when asked to display it in their rooms. Cialdini and colleagues found that 60 per cent of the students in the 'low ball' condition displayed the poster compared with 20 per cent in the control condition. This experiment suggests that it is a good idea to avoid hasty decisions, especially when the alternatives seem simple or easy. If patients are given a limited yet positive piece of information when asked to 'sign up' to some medical regimen, then at a later date are presented with a more detailed specification of the problems associated with taking on the same regimen, they are more likely to go ahead with the procedure as they have been 'low balled' and have made an initial commitment which may be difficult to go back on.

'That's not all' (TNA) technique

This effect is demonstrated at street markets throughout the world and it seems to work: 'Tell you what I'm going to do for you, madam . . .'. Burger (1986) investigated the TNA effect by selling cakes at different prices. The participants in the TNA condition were told that the cakes cost £1, but before they could reply they were told that he would lower the price to 50p as it was near closing time. In the second (control) condition, the cakes were priced at 50p. The third condition was called a 'bargain'. Here the seller told the people that the cakes had originally been priced at £1 but were now reduced to 50p. It was found that 55 per cent of the participants bought the cakes in the TNA condition, compared with 25 per cent and 20 per cent in the bargain and control conditions respectively. It seems that the TNA effect involves something more than merely reducing the price. Burger says that the effect comprises an element of social reciprocity – that there is an obligation to reciprocate when another person makes a concession.

Ingratiation

Simply put, if people like us, they are more likely to yield to our requests. Godfrey *et al.* (1986) asked pairs of unacquainted people to engage each other in conversation. After the first conversation, one subject in each pair was told to try to make the other like him (experimental group), whereas in the control condition no such instructions were given. Individual ratings and video-tapes of the conversations indicated that the participants told to ingratiate themselves succeeded. However, Wortmann and Linsenmeier (1977) caution about the use of too much ingratiation. They found that subtle forms of flattery are more effective. Less direct techniques, such as paying attention and showing concern about what the other person says, enhance attractiveness. Also, sharing people's beliefs and opinions increases affinity.

Implications

The use of these techniques should be avoided if possible as they not only put trust at risk but are also contradictory to the emphasis on promoting self-care and decision making. Phrasing requests in such a manner takes away the patient's ability to make a 'real' decision. The use of covert strategies further reduces the emphasis on providing open, honest, client-centred care.

Obedience

Obedience is concerned with *telling* people to act rather than *asking* them to do so. People often obey commands because they fear punishment if they fail to comply; however, under certain circumstances people will obey others even when there is no obvious need to do so. Milgram (1963, 1965, 1974) devised a series of dramatic and controversial experiments looking into the extent of people's obedience to authority.

He advertised in the local press for volunteers to take part in an experiment on learning at Harvard University. On arrival they were introduced to another person who was to take part in the experiment but who was, in fact, Milgram's accomplice. A coin was tossed to decide who would be the 'experimenter' and who would be the 'subject' in the experiment. It always transpired that the accomplice was the 'subject' and the true volunteer the experimenter. The true 'participants' of the experiment were told that they were taking part in a study of the effects of punishment on learning. Their role was to deliver electric shocks to the other person by means of thirty switches on a control panel in front of them. The strength of the shock was graded in intervals of fifteen, from 15 V (slight shock) to 450 V (marked XXX).

The 'participants' were told to move to the next higher level of shock every time the learner made an error. In reality, the learner never received a shock, but to convince the 'subject' that the apparatus was real, a mild pulse of 45 V was administered to him. It was prearranged that the learner would get gradually worse, and the strength of the shocks increased, until the 'subject' faced a dilemma about whether he should proceed. Milgram then gave one of three graded remarks:

- Please go on.
- It is absolutely essential that you continue.
- You have no other choice; you must go on.

All the 'participants' were volunteers and had been paid in advance. They could have terminated the experiment at any time, yet 65 per cent showed total obedience and proceeded through the entire range to the 450 V level.

In this, and other experiments, Milgram (1974) found that 62.5 per cent of participants would administer lethal doses of shock even when they knew that the learner was suffering from a 'heart condition'. Some (30 per cent) went so far as to force the learner's hand on to the shock plate when he refused to comply. However, many participants protested, verbally attacking the experimenter and displaying signs of anguish, and a fair proportion refused to obey Milgram's commands. Indeed, several participants suffered uncontrollable seizures.

Two main factors were found to be important in resisting obedience to authority:

- *Responsibility*. In some of the experiments carried out by Milgram participants were told that they would have to accept responsibility for their actions. Under these circumstances there was significantly less obedience to authority. Hamilton (1978) found that when people are made responsible for their actions, they are less susceptible to commands to obey.
- *Disobedience*. Exposure to disobedient models also reduces obedience. In Milgram's (1965) initial experiments, the presence of people who visibly disobeyed his requests to increase the shock reduced the adherence figures to 10 per cent.

Even though the participants in Milgram's experiments were given a full debriefing after the experiment, there are serious ethical concerns relating to this sort of study. Bushman (1988) has shown that obedience can be investigated in a less harmful way. A female accomplice of the experimenter ordered passers-by to give money to a young man who needed it for a parking meter. In one condition the accomplice was dressed in a uniform; in another as a business executive and in a third as a vagrant. In the first condition 72 per cent complied with the order, compared with 48 per cent and 52 per cent respectively in the other two. It seems that some outward sign of authority such as a uniform is an important factor in obeying commands.

Slater (2004) found two of Milgram's first 'subjects' and asked them how they felt now about the experiments some forty years later. One had been obedient to the end, the other had disobeyed Milgram's instructions. The latter, it seems, not so much for the pain supposedly inflicted on the stooge as because the stress was causing him to fear for his own health by way of a heart attack. Also, when asked to keep the true nature of the experiment quiet, he thought about going to the police but in the end complied with Milgram's request for secrecy. The 'obedient' participant was asked by Slater if the experiment had caused any long-term emotional harm. He replied that, on the contrary, the experiment caused him to re-evaluate his life and confront his compliance, it had led him to the 'ethical gym'.

After being vilified by the academic community for his experiments, Milgram died at the age of 51 after a series of heart attacks.

Implications

It is important for nurses to recognise the meanings people attach to the wearing of uniforms. A uniform is rarely just an overall to protect personal clothing, and the meanings patients place on a nurse's uniform may well affect the kind of relationship that develops between nurse and patient. Patients for whom a uniform means authority may expect to be told what to do and the nurse needs to be aware of this in order to encourage self care and independence.

Being aware of those factors which are more likely to counteract unquestioning obedience is important. In the light of the studies described previously, consider the likely outcome of increasing a patient's sense of personal responsibility for maintaining their own health. Consider also the effect of your perceived position of authority in relation to the gaining of informed consent from patients. It is not always easy to ensure that patients have a real choice in a climate where nurses and doctors are perceived as having (legitimate) authority.

Modelling

In many instances social influence can be exerted unintentionally. This influence can lead to either inhibition or disinhibition.

- *Inhibition.* Suppose you are waiting in a traffic jam and are late for an important appointment. You are about to pull out and overtake the other cars when you spot someone ahead of you doing just that and then falling back into line. You have second thoughts about overtaking and remain where you are. In this situation, your behaviour has been unintentionally inhibited by somebody else's act.
- *Disinhibition.* Imagine that you are standing in a queue waiting for a bus. Unfortunately the bus cannot stop at the head of the queue and instead stops some yards further on. You are waiting for the person at the front of the line to start walking when someone bursts from the middle of the line and rushes for the bus. You decide that if they can do it so can you, and you rush off as well. Here the person has unintentionally disinhibited your behaviour.

Both these examples illustrate the power of modelling. In each case the models were unaware of the effect they were having on others' behaviour, and thus it is often counterproductive to say one thing and do another, as people may be influenced by your actions even when you are unaware you are being observed.

Modelling is also an extremely useful technique for reducing pain and stress, details of which were given earlier on in Chapter 8 (see p. 270).

Planning and executing effective communication

Once referred to as compliance, then as adherence, then concordance – the extent to which patients do, and should, carry out the advice of the nurse – of has been an important factor in health behaviour. No matter how good the diagnosis or construction of medical regimen, if details are not communicated effectively to patients then all the effort producing them is wasted. The problem with adherence to medical advice has been an issue since the 1960's. Ley and Spelman (1967) found that 48.7 per cent of patients failed to take their antibiotic tablets, 37.5 per cent fail to take their anti-tuberculosis drugs, and, even among those patients who attempted to comply with the instructions given to them, anything from one-quarter to two-thirds may have been taking the wrong dose, with up to 30 per cent making errors that could have been fatal. Of course there are a number of factors involved in non-adherence, such as:

- complexity of treatment procedure;
- degree of change required in one's lifestyle;
- length of time during which the patient has to follow the advice;
- whether the illness is extremely painful;
- whether the illness is seen as potentially life-saving;
- severity of illness as perceived by the patient.

There are some general guidelines in relation to facilitating communication provided by Neuhauser and Kreps (2003). They recommend the following:

- It is important to address patients with regard to their emotions as well as providing 'rational' information.
- A person's social context provides a useful template for communicating information.
- 'Tailored' communication is more effective than a standard message.
- The degree of patient involvement should be ascertained at the beginning of the interaction.

Nurses should be aware that they are not the only source of information. With access to the internet becoming more widespread it is not unusual for patients to get information concerning their situation from various web sites. This can of course be counterproductive if the wrong sites are consulted. Being knowledgeable about sources and the kinds of information available to patients will reduce the chance of compromised advice.

Summary

Making decisions and solving problems are important features of a nurse's work. Chapter 9 has looked at the psychological factors associated with irrational decision making, a range of models which attempt to explain how individuals make decisions about their health behaviour and has looked at strategies for improving the quality of our decision making. Examples of the range of mistakes which people typically make have been provided and the difference between clinical decisions and statistical decisions highlighted. Problem solving in social settings and the use of brainstorming are used as examples of ways of improving the effectiveness of decisions.

Conundrum revisited

We first touched upon the issue of practice decision making in the conundrum presented in Chapter 2. Now we can develop this further by exploring why learning in practice may seem daunting for learners. Anxieties about making mistakes may have loomed large in your account of why practice based learning seems stressful to students. Students are keenly aware of the risks to patients that may attend nursing care measures and are anxious to practice safely. This is well expressed in terms of clinical and statistical decisions. Nurses rarely have enough information available to make a completely statistical decision. Giving an intramuscular injection in the buttock for instance involves estimating the course of the sciatic nerve and inserting the needle at a point where it is least likely to damage the nerve. Nurses are taught how to estimate the safe area for injection, but they do not have the benefit a diagnostic test that proves where the nerve runs. They make a clinical, rather than a statistical, decision and students consequently have to trust that that which was taught in theory will prove robust in practice.

Care decisions are also stressful because the student has to learn how to make decisions based upon information that is considered likely to be representative in other cases and involving other patients. Experienced nurses have learned to do this intuitively and rarely pause to consider what skills they are using. Consider for a moment the ways in which a patient might react when receiving news that he will need to undergo additional and uncomfortable treatment. The experienced nurse remembers how others have reacted to such news in the past and prepares a number of strategies to support the patient, depending upon which reactions occur. Past experiences are considered representative of what is likely to happen in the future. For the student, though, not only has there been minimal prior experience, but she may not have understood that such care cannot reasonably be learnt through reading or lectures. The student may believe that she should have 'picked this information up somehow' and wonders whether the patient or the mentor will evaluate her badly for not intervening sensitively enough.

In practice students learn that decision making is often an art rather than a science. The nurse weighs the merits of different options and works with the patient to achieve the most favourable outcome. The nurse reads situations, learning to be vigilant, rather than hypervigilant, to attend to the important cues and to reason for herself, rather than naively accepting the direction of others. Perhaps it is not surprising that this form of learning is daunting for the student. To enable her to make sense of how to manage health care decisions, she needs a mentor who is willing and able to 'think aloud' his reasoning of care. The art of nursing makes sense the more she can access just how the more experienced practitioner avoids the mistakes described in conflict theory.

You may have noted that the student nurse is unlikely to feel in control of learning in clinical practice. This is frequently true. The variety and complexity of information that she is invited to process means that she senses the locus of control is with others. Practice colleagues determine what she must attend to, how much she should learn and what sequence of learning she should follow. The pace of required learning can seem extremely fast unless the mentor selects practice experiences and lessons that the student can adequately assimilate. Under these circumstances it is extremely tempting to avoid learning through active engagement in care. The student announces that she is here to 'observe' rather than to 'work'. The clinical staff may then misinterpret her anxieties as unwillingness to develop skills through practice or as an arrogant attitude to learning associated with university study. Misconceptions then spiral and learning opportunities are lost.

Whilst it would be inaccurate to suggest that clinical decision making is often conducted using brainstorming, it is fair to argue that some of the most innovative health care arises out of case conferences or team work where this technique is used. Successful team leaders use case conferences, shift handovers, 'teaching rounds' or reviews of care plans to welcome interpretations and suggestions from all members of the nursing team. Exposed to this sort of environment, practice placements can seem considerably less stressful. Not only does the student learn that senior colleagues respect different contributions, but they appreciate that a portion of decisions are made collectively. Contrary to the student's first fears, not all decisions have to be made 'on the spot, without consultation and measured against absolute perfection'.

Mentors should acknowledge learners' anxieties about the pace and variety of learning and 'rehearse aloud' a selection of care measures and associated decisions during the shift that they work with the student. Other care can simply be observed, acknowledging the learners need to see, hear, discuss as well as practise care as a means of learning. Practice placement leaders will assist students if they expose the learner to collective decision making. In turn, students should appreciate that decisions are 'clinical' and that it is legitimate to ask questions that help them to identify the information that their mentor would use to make his or her judgement.

❓ Questions for further consideration

1 Discuss the psychological factors that influence decision making.
2 What is brainstorming? How can it be applied in the nursing context?
3 Outline methods of social problem solving.
4 The way in which a problem is framed determines the response. Discuss.

References

Ajzen, I. (1991). The theory of planned behavior. *Organizational Behavior and Human Decision Processes, 50,* 179–211.

Ajzen, I. and Fishbein, M. (1977). Attitude–behavior relations: a theoretical analysis and review of empirical research. *Psychological Bulletin, 84,* 888–918.

Allinson, G. (1971). *Essence of Decision: Explaining the Cuban missile crisis.* Boston: Little Brown.

Becker, M. H., Haefner, D. P., Kasl, S. V., Kirscht, J. P., Maiman, L. A. and Rosenstock, I. M. (1977). Selected psychosocial models and correlates of individual health-related behaviors. *Medical Care, 15,* 27–46.

Biley, F. C. (1992). Some determinants that affect patient participation in decision making about nursing care. *Journal of Advanced Nursing, 17,* 414–421.

Burger, J. M. (1986). Increasing compliance by improving the deal. *Journal of Personality and Social Psychology, 51,* 277–283.

Bushman, B. (1988). The effects of apparel on compliance: a field experiment with a female authority figure. *Personality and Social Psychology Bulletin, 14,* 459–467.

Cialdini, R. B. (2001) *Influence: Science and Practice.* Boston MA: Allyn and Bacon.

Dowding, D. and Thompson, C. (2003). Measuring the quality of judgement and decision making in nursing. *Journal of Advanced Nursing, 44 (1),* 49–57.

English, I. (1993). Intuition as a function of the expert nurse: a critique of Benner's novice to expert model. *Journal of Advanced Nursing, 18,* 387–393.

Fishbein, M. (1982). Social psychological analysis of smoking behaviour. In Eiser, J. R. (ed.) *Social Psychology and Behavioural Medicine.* Chichester: Wiley.

Freedman, J. L. and Fraser, S. C. (1966). Compliance without pressure: the foot-in-the-door technique. *Journal of Personality and Social Psychology, 4,* 195–202.

Godfrey, D. K., Jones, E. E. and Lord, C. G. (1986). Self promotion is not ingratiating. *Journal of Personality and Social Pscyhology, 50,* 106–115.

Hamilton, V. L. (1978). Obedience and responsibility: a jury similation. *Journal of Personality and Social Psychology, 36,* 126–146.

Heermann, J. A. and Wills, L. M. (1992). Effect of problem-solving instruction and health locus of control on the management of childhood asthma. *Children's Health Care, 21,* 76–83.

Holloway, C. (1974) Experiments and Statistics. In Approaches and Methods DS261. Maidenhead: Open University Press.

Janis, I. L. (1984). The patient as decision maker. In Gentry, W. D. (ed.) *Handbook of Behavioural Medicine.* New York: Guilford Press.

Janis, I. L. and Mann, L. (1977). *Decision Making: A psychological analysis of conflict, choice, and commitment.* New York: Free Press.

Janis, I. L. and Rodin, J. (1980). Attribution, control, and decision making. In Stone, G. C., Cohen, F. and Adler, N. E. (eds) *Health Psychology.* New York: Jossey Bass.

Kahneman, D. and Tversky, A. (1974). The psychology of preferences. *Science, 185,* 136–142.

Keighley, T. (1993). The management of care. In Hinchliff, S. M., Norman, S. E. and Schober, J. E. (eds) *Nursing Practice and Health Care.* 2nd edn. London: Arnold.

Lalljee, M., Lalljee, R., Lamb, G., Carnibella (1993). Lay prototypes of illness: Their content and use. *Psychology and Health, 3,* 172–178.

Lau, R. R., Hartman, K. A. and Ware, J. E. (1986). Health as a value: methodological and theoretical decisions. *Health Psychology, 5,* 25–43.

Lichtenstein, S., Slovic, P., Fischoff, B., Layman, M. and Coombs, B. (1978). Judged frequency of lethal events. *Journal of Experimental Psychology: Human Learning and Memory, 4,* 551–578.

Ley, P. and Spelman, M. S. (1967). *Communicating with the patient.* London: Staples Press.

Luker, K. A. and Kenrick, M. (1992). An exploratory study of the sources of influence on the clinical decisions of community nurses. *Journal of Advanced Nursing, 17,* 457–466.

Maier, N. F. R. (1930). Reasoning in humans I: On direction. *Journal of Comparative Psychology, 10,* 115–143.

Milgram, S. (1963). Behavior study of obedience. *Journal of Personality and Social Psychology, 67,* 317–378.

Milgram, S. (1965). Some conditions of obedience and disobedience to authority. *Human Relations, 18,* 57–76.

Milgram, S. (1974). *Obedience to Authority.* Harper, New York.

Miller, P., Wikoff, R. and Hiatt, A. (1992). Fishbein's model of reasoned action and adherence behaviour of hypertensive patients. *Nursing Research, 41,* 104–109.

Milner, S. (1994). Evaluation of a Drop-in Health Centre. Unpublished PhD thesis, University of Northumbria.

Nemcek, M. A. (1990). Health beliefs and breast self-examination among black women. *Health Values, Health Behaviour, Education and Promotion, 14,* 41–52.

Neuhauser, L. and Kreps, G. L. (2003) Rethinking communication in the e-health era. *Journal of Health Psychology, 8,* 7–23.

Niven, N. (2000). *Health Psychology.* Edinburgh: Churchill Livingstone.

Oberle, K. (1991). A decade of research in locus of control: what have we learned? *Journal of Advanced Nursing, 16,* 800–806.

Osborn, A. F. (1963). *Applied Imagination: Principles and procedures of creative problem solving.* 3rd edn. New York: Scribner's.

Price, B. (2003) Understanding the origin of practice problems. *Nursing Standard, 17, (50),* 47–53.

Rutter, D. (1989). Models of belief: behaviour relationships in health. *Health Psychology Update, 4,* 3–10.

Schmieding, M (1999) Reflective enquiry framework for nurse administrators. *Journal of Advanced Nursing, 30, (3),* 631–639.

Slater, L. (2004) *Opening Skinner's Box.* London: Bloomsbury.

Tiedje, L. B., Kingry, M. J. and Stommel, M. (1992). Patient attitudes concerning health behaviours during pregnancy: initial development of a questionnaire. *Health Education Quarterly, 19,* 481–493.

Tversky, A. and Kahneman, D. (1974). Judgement under uncertainty: heuristics and biases. *Science, 185,* 1124–1131.

Wallston, B. S. and Wallston, K. A. (1984). Social psychological models of health behavior: an examination and integration. In Baum, A., Singer, S. E. and Singer, J. E. (eds) *Handbook of Psychology and Health.* New York: Erlbaum.

Wallston, K. A. (1992). Hocus-pocus, the focus isn't strictly on locus: Rutter's social learning theory modified for health. *Cognitive Therapy and Research, 16,* 183–199.

Wallston, K. A. and Wallston, B. S. (1982). Who is responsible for your health? The construct of health locus of control. In Sanders, G. S. and Suls, J. (eds) *Social Psychology of Health and Illness.* Hillsdale NJ: Erlbaum.

Wortman, C. B. and Linsenmeier, J. A. (1977). Interpersonal attraction and techniques of ingratiation in organizational settings. In: Shaw, B. M. and Salanak, G. R. (eds) *New directions in organizational behavior.* Chicago: St. Clair Press.

Further reading

Berry, Dianne (2004) *Risk, Communication and Health Psychology.* Milton Keynes: Open University Press. We may be given more choice these days but how do we make a decision? Little advice is given on how to make choices. This book examines how the communication of risk factors is important in making choices and decisions.

Cialdini, Robert (2001) *Influence: Science and Practice.* Boston MA: Allyn and Bacon. Really does contain all you would want to know about social influence. Into its fourth edition and written in an extremely interesting and engaging style.

Plous, Scott (1993) *The Psychology of Judgement and Decision Making.* New York: McGraw Hill. Again gives an enormous amount of information on the psychology of decision making with loads of exercises. A great book.

Slater, Lauren (2004) *Opening Skinner's Box: Great Psychological Experiments of the twentieth Century.* London: Bloomsbury. By this time the reader has hopefully looked at some of the classic experiments of Milgram, Asch, Festinger, Rosenhan, Loftus, etc. This book gives an absorbing insight into what went on at the time and why the studies became famous.

10

Changing Attitudes and Behaviour

A practice conundrum

There is now substantial evidence that smoking cigarettes damages human health, that associated with respiratory and cardiac function in particular. Yet health educators face a major dilemma: given that nicotine is addictive and the habit of smoking widely established, how do you persuade patients to give up cigarette smoking? A television health education campaign in Britain portrayed a series of individuals who were manifestly ill talking about their regrets and the costs associated with smoking. One is gravely ill with lung cancer and another has an irreparably damaged heart.

Do campaigns such as these change individual's attitudes towards smoking? If you were in charge of this campaign what might you change to get your message across? Discuss your ideas with colleagues and then read Chapter 9 to identify concepts and theories that might either support or challenge your strategy.

Attempts to define an attitude are often too general to be useful. To describe an attitude as a 'general evaluation', as one of my students did, does not do justice to the complexity of the construct. It is more useful to examine the main components of attitudes.

- The *affective* component of an attitude is concerned with feelings. We have feelings and emotions about people, objects and issues, and thus we may like or dislike anything from pizzas to the Minister for Health.
- The *cognitive* component of an attitude is concerned with thoughts and beliefs. Again, these thoughts can be directed towards objects, people or issues. Pizzas are bad for our health because they are fattening, and the Minister of Health may not always tell the whole story.
- The *behavioural* component of an attitude is concerned with our actions toward others. Despite pizzas being fattening, we may continue to eat them, and we may keep voting for the Minister of Health's political party.

We do not necessarily have an attitude towards everything, and some people and topics command complete ambivalence. However, the strength of the attitudes we do possess is largely determined by the variables which led to their construction or formation.

Attitude formation

Many, but not all, attitudes are formed during childhood. However, the processes involved in attitude formation are the same throughout our lifespan. There are three main ways to form an attitude: *instrumental conditioning* (reward), *modelling* (imitation) and *direct experience.*

Instrumental conditioning

In the last chapter, the role of instrumental conditioning in the learning process was discussed. Attitudes, like other features of behaviour, are learned in the same way. Children are rewarded for having certain attitudes, and not rewarded or even punished, for having 'inappropriate views'. Parents and 'significant others' use rewards to promote what they consider to be good attitudes, and over a period of years the child may gradually be influenced by the views of parents, older children, teachers and other influential people.

Modelling

Individuals acquire new attitudes through observing the actions of others. Children are continually looking at adults and older children for information on how to behave, and thus adults can exert a considerable influence on children by their actions as well as by their words. Examples might be the father who talks about the perils of smoking to his daughter but then proceeds to smoke a cigarette, or the mother who shouts at her son to tidy his room but leaves her own in a mess. There is a clear dilemma between doing as the parents say or doing as the parents do. Unfortunately for the parents in these examples, there is evidence that children tend to be more influenced by actions than by words.

The use of modelling to influence attitudes is apparent in media campaigns aimed at stopping children from smoking. Superheroes, or sometimes sporting heroes, are often seen to despise smoking and favour children who do not smoke. Hopefully the children. will identify with their 'idols' and copy their attitude. Watching television programmes has been found to influence not just attitudes but also behavioural intentions as well (Schofield and Pavelchak, 1989).

However, it is not just parents and the media who are influential in attitude formation; nurses can have an important role to play in the development of appropriate attitudes towards health by giving rewards where appropriate and by setting a good example themselves.

Recent debate about whether or not it is right to prioritise non-smokers over smokers for certain investigations and treatment suggests that there is a general and understandable uneasiness about the ethical implications of directly rewarding individuals for appropriate attitudes and behaviour towards health. The nurse may, however, help the patient identify the intrinsic rewards which can be associated with healthy behaviour. For example, a patient who wishes to give up smoking could be reminded that they will feel fitter and enjoy the taste of their food more.

The nurse's behaviour in relation to his or her own health may affect the way in which the patient receives advice about health maintenance. For example, the nurse who smells of nicotine when working with or talking to a patient will be identified as a smoker and will convey a message to the patient which suggests that it is alright to smoke. Nurses need to be aware of the messages they are conveying to patients by their own behaviour as well as through verbal communication.

In the case of the patient who wishes to give up smoking, direct experience of the health benefits will help to strengthen the patient's feelings and attitudes about the relationship between smoking and ill health. The nurse can play a significant role in drawing to the patient's attention the links between their healthy behaviour and their increasing feelings of well-being.

Direct experience

The third main process of attitude formation is direct experience of the target object or person – one way to form an attitude about pizzas is to eat one. Many people wish to 'see for themselves' when it comes to forming an attitude or an opinion of something new, and there is evidence that attitudes formed by direct experience are stronger and more resistant to change than those formed through indirect experience (Wu and Shaffer, 1987).

Overall, it is much simpler to influence attitude formation than attitude change. Therefore nurses can play a significant role in health education by influencing the three main acquisitional strategies mentioned in a positive way.

Attitude measurement

Attitudes can be determined by observing people's behaviour. If a crowd of people were demonstrating outside a building bearing placards saying GAY RIGHTS, it would not be too big a step to conclude that the demonstrators had a particular attitude towards sexuality. However, in the majority of circumstances people do not outwardly display their attitudes; indeed in some circumstances it requires specific prompting to elicit any reaction at all. One method which is used to measure attitudes and views on general and particular topics is the attitude questionnaire. These questionnaires are sometimes called scales and usually consist of a series of statements about a particular participant. Table 10.1 gives an example of a Likert attitude scale.

Table 10.1 *A Likert attitude scale*

'There is no relationship between the practice of safe sex and AIDS.' Do you:

agree strongly?	agree somewhat?	neither agree nor disagree?	disagree somewhat?	disagree strongly?
1	2	3	4	5

Please encircle your choice.

Exercise 10.1 *Developing an attitude questionnaire*

The first stage in developing an attitude questionnaire is to *select a topic* (as above). In doing so, some sort of hypothesis needs to be constructed regarding the differences that are likely to exist between the groups of people whose attitudes are being measured. The next stage is to create an *item pool.* This is a series of statements about your topic which you think would make good items in your questionnaire. Do not make these statements too long and keep them to one point. Avoid double negatives and technical language. Try and investigate as many issues as you can. You should aim to produce at least twenty-four items, divided between favourable and unfavourable. Assign a '+' for positive or favourable items, and a '–' for unfavourable items.

The next stage is to *see how good the items are.* This is called *validity* and refers to whether your questions actually measure what they are intended to measure. You need to find at least twenty people to answer your twenty-four-item list. Get them to respond to each question in the Likert format described above. If the item has been assigned positively (+), they would score 1 for agree strongly' and 5 for 'disagree strongly'. If the item has been negatively assigned –, they would score 5 for 'agree strongly' and 1 for 'disagree strongly. You can, of course reverse these allocations if you wish.

Add up the scores of your participants and place them in order of highest to lowest in a table of results. Select the top third and call them high scorers, and the bottom third and call them low scorers.

Select item one from your list of twenty-five. Go through your high scorers one by one and see if they scored 4 or 5 on that item. If they did, then a point is awarded. Repeat the procedure for your low scorers; give them a point if they scored 4 or 5, nothing if they didn't. Total the scores for the high and low scorer groups and compare them. If the difference between the scores of the two groups is high then it is a 'good' item, it discriminates between the two groups. If, on the other, there is little or no difference between the scores, it is not very good at discriminating between the two groups and should be discarded. Work through all the items and you will get an indication of how good or bad they are. It is up to you to select how many you want to keep and how many you want to throw away, but you should keep at least twelve.

Your attitude scale now has internal validity but it is not necessarily reliable it is no use developing a scale if it is inconsistent in its measurement of attitudes. You have to show that your scale gives the same results when it is given to the same group of people on two different occasions. After a significant amount of time, usually a few days, give your questionnaire to your participants once more and note their responses. You should now have two sets of results, which should, if your test was 100 per cent, reliable, be the same. Of course in real life this rarely happens, but to see how good a correspondence exists between the two scores, a test of correlation such as Spearman's rho is normally used. A correlation coefficient of 0.9 is good, less than 0.7 means your test is definitely unreliable. If you cannot perform this test you must use your judgement to assess the comparability of the two sets of scores.

You now have a valid and reliable test which you can use to see if different groups of people have different attitudes to your chosen topic. Psychologists would normally use many more items and many more participants. They would also use statistical tests to determine validity and reliability, but this exercise represents the basic processes involved in attitude measurement.

Attitude change

Each day we seem to be bombarded by attempts to change our attitudes to something or other. Advertisers want us to buy their product, politicians want us to share their views, and health professionals want us to adopt a healthy lifestyle. These efforts at persuasion are carried out via newspapers, television, radio, magazines and billboards and some succeed remarkably well in their aims. In many instances, this 'persuasive communication' is being used to encourage people to change their attitudes with little cost to the advertiser. Changing the washing-up liquid to an 'ecological brand', or agreeing with a particular politician, does not take much effort, but changing attitudes to health is much more difficult, as it often involves a person stopping something he or she likes and doing something he or she dislikes.

Faced with a seemingly uphill battle, nurses need to know how to produce the most effective and persuasive communication possible. Over the past three decades, psychologists have conducted a number of experiments into persuasive communication and many of the findings relating to the factors that influence attitude change have stood the test of time.

There are three factors involved in a persuasive communication: *the communicator, the message, the target group.*

Communicator characteristics

There are certain features of a communicator which determine the effectiveness of their attempts to change attitudes. These include *credibility, likability, trustworthiness,* and *speed of presentation of information.*

- A nurse's ability as an effective communicator will depend very much on the extent to which he or she is perceived as credible. As long ago as 1951 Hovland and Weiss demonstrated that experts are seen as more credible than non-experts. They gave a talk based on an article about antihistamine drugs to an American audience. It was found that the audience was more convinced when the source used was given as *The New England Journal of Medicine* as opposed to a popular magazine.
- Another factor which has been found to influence effectiveness is the likability of the communicator. Possessing positive personality traits and physical attractiveness also increase credibility (Kiesler and Kiesler, 1969). Credibility is also enhanced if the 'audience' perceives a nurse to be similar to them, thus increasing their propensity to like him or her.
- The question 'What is this person going to gain from me changing my opinion?' crosses most people's minds when they are faced with someone trying to convince them to change their attitude. Trust and the intentions of the communicator play an important role in the effectiveness of persuasive communication. If a person thinks that the communicator is liable to gain by the message being conveyed, he or she will be less likely to do as the communicator says (Hennigan *et al.*, 1982).
- Finally, people who speak rapidly are usually more convincing than those who speak slowly (Miller *et al.*, 1976). Despite the general impression that 'fast talkers' are untrustworthy, it seems that speaking fast is equated with knowledge of a participant and hence expertise. However, speaking fast can often confuse a patient, so care must be taken.

Therefore, if nurses are to be successful in persuading patients to change their attitudes, they should appear credible; that is, they should try to show expertise whilst eliciting trust and amiability.

Message characteristics

One technique which has been used extensively over the years to change people's attitudes is the use of fear. The question is, 'Does it work?' Evidence suggests that the careful use of fear in a message can induce attitude change, but only under certain conditions.

- McGuire (1969) says that the level of emotional arousal induced by a fearful message must be moderate. Too low, or minimal fear, and the participant will not be aroused by the message. Too high a fear content, and the person may resort to denial mechanisms to deal with the threat (for example, 'that just could not happen to me').
- People must realise that they are at risk if they ignore the message. If they think the consequences of inaction are minor, emotional messages will not work.
- There has to be a belief that if the instructions of the message are carried out, the risks to health will be minimal or significantly reduced. Leventhal (1970) said that if people are given instructions on how to avoid undesirable consequences and believe that their actions will work, then fearful messages will prove effective.

Another feature of the message is the type of argument to employ. Is it best to present both sides of an argument or to stick to just one point of view? The answer is that it depends on the audience. If people are generally well disposed to your point of view then telling them the other side of the argument will be counterproductive. It is best to concentrate on emphasising the main points of your side of the argument, and not highlight any other. If the audience is undecided and also aware of the counter-arguments, it is better to present a two-sided argument. The usual form is to put forward the opposing view and attack it successfully before presenting one's own position.

Finally, continual exposure to a message produces familiarity and often results in favourable evaluations. In a study of politicians, Grush (1980) found that frequency of exposure was related to popularity. In one instance where all the candidates were unknown before the election, those that were given frequent public exposure during their campaigns were the ones likely to be elected.

Target group characteristics

People with a high need for approval and a strong desire to be liked are more susceptible to attitude change (Skolnik and Heslin, 1971). The mood of the target group is also important. Mackie and Worth (1989) found that students who learned that they had just been randomly allocated a cash prize (and not surprisingly were in a good mood) were more susceptible to persuasion than those students who did not receive any money. The experimenters argued that being in a good mood reduces people's ability to engage in systematic analysis of the message. The reduced capacity for active thought can sometimes lead to an increase in susceptibility to persuasion.

The age of the target group is an important factor in attitude change. Krosnick and Alwin (1989) suggested that we pass through a period in our development which can be labelled 'the impressionable years'. They found that during our late teens and early 20s we are more open to change and shifts in our attitudes than at later times in our lives. However, they found no evidence to support the hypothesis that once formed, attitudes remain stable through to old age.

Forrester and Murphy (1992) investigated nurses' attitudes towards patients with AIDS and AIDS-related risk factors. They found that an AIDS medical diagnosis and a history of intravenous drug use were found to increase nurses' negative attitude toward patients and significantly reduced their willingness to interact with patients.

Reactance: bending over backwards to do the opposite

Having taken into consideration all the previously mentioned characteristics, people may still resist attempts to change their attitudes. Most people like to think of themselves as perfectly able to make up their own minds about important issues of the day. If a person is engaged in trying to change attitudes and the audience feel that their autonomy or ability to think for themselves is being restricted, they will do the opposite of what is being requested of them. This is called *reactance* and results in a negative attitude change. This is one reason why attempts at a 'hard sell' may fail.

On many occasions it is known very well that someone is trying to change our attitudes, and this forewarning of an attempt to change attitudes gives time for individuals to prepare counter-arguments and to recall relevant facts from memory (Petty and Cacioppo, 1981).

It should not be assumed that the target group has no preconceived ideas about issues. In many situations people hold particular points of view and previous attempts to change attitudes will affect a person's resistance to change.

Inoculation

Inoculation is one process that can have a significant effect on the success of any persuasive communication. Consider an audience that is about to be addressed by two speakers, Mrs R and Mrs H. Mrs R.is in favour of breast feeding; Mrs H is not. How could Mrs R get her message across to the audience at the expense of Mrs H? She does it by inoculating the audience against Mrs H. Mrs R speaks first and either presents the best argument possible for breast feeding, using all the techniques of attitude change, or produces an argument against the use of breast milk in an incompetent fashion. By presenting the argument using poor ideas and an unsatisfactory presentation style the audience is stimulated into producing counter-arguments which will still be in their minds when it is the turn of the next speaker to talk. In this way Mrs R has inoculated the audience against Mrs H.

In some situations nurses may face patients who have been inoculated against them.

Many attitudes and beliefs concerning health care are transmitted to patients via a *lay referral network*. This is a network or group of people who are usually consulted by the patient when in doubt about a particular issue, and is usually made up of family and friends. If this network has already advised the patient, say in this instance, to forego breastfeeding, it makes the job of the nurse that much harder if she is to convince the patient that it is worth trying.

Counterbalancing inoculation

One way of counterbalancing inoculation of this kind is to help the patient re-examine the sources and rationality of her attitude towards breastfeeding. Of course, attitude change is not always possible, but if the nurse has spent time developing a positive relationship with the patient her credibility and likability may influence the extent to which the patient is able to change her views.

Cognitive dissonance: attitudes and behaviour

Changing people's attitudes does not necessarily change their behaviour. Fishbein and Ajzen (1975) examined the relationship between attitudes and behaviour. Their theory is discussed later; however, another approach which has been used to try to determine the relationship between attitudes and behaviour is *cognitive dissonance* (Festinger, 1957). An example of cognitive dissonance would be a person who smokes a lot and believes that this behaviour will lead to ill health. The smoking behaviour is incompatible with the attitude towards the relationship between smoking and health, and this situation produces a feeling of discomfort or dissonance which individuals will seek to resolve. There are two ways to reduce the dissonance: (1) stop smoking; (2) change the attitude.

In the majority of circumstances, people chose the easier option, which in this instance is usually to change the attitude to smoking and health (Lipkus *et al.*, 2001). This may be achieved by the use of self-statements such as 'Wait a minute, what about Uncle George? He smoked like a chimney and lived till he was 86' or 'Didn't I see a report the other day in the newspaper suggesting that smoking was not as harmful as people made it out to be?'

Cognitive dissonance can also occur when there is a decision to be made between adopting two equally attractive options. Consider the nurse who does not know whether to do the 'Nursing the child', option or to do the 'Nursing people with learning disability option'. Both seem equally desirable, yet a choice has to be made. A decision is made to opt for nursing children and immediately a state of dissonance occurs because the nurse will now miss all the advantages of doing the disability option. In this situation, the dissonance is reduced by rehearsing all the positive features of the 'child' option and all the negative features of the 'disability' option. The result may be an initial overestimation of the chosen course and a devaluation of the rejected one. Thus the forced decision has produced changed attitudes towards nursing children and nursing people with a mental disability.

Another feature of cognitive dissonance is the 'less leads to more' effect. Festinger and Carlsmith (1959) gave people either a small reward ($1) or a large reward ($20) for telling others that the dull, boring task they were doing was in fact very interesting. Afterwards the participants were asked how they felt about the task. Participants reported a greater liking for the boring tasks when they received the small reward than when they received a large one. The small reward had increased the dissonance. The participants in the small reward group could not justify their behaviour by saying, 'Well, I'm getting paid good money for doing this,' and thus rationalised their behaviour by changing their attitude toward the task. Further research on the 'less leads to more effect' has found that there are certain conditions that have to be satisfied for attitude change to take place.

- People must believe that they have not been coerced into the attitude-discrepant behaviour.
- They must feel that they are personally responsible for their actions.
- There must be no hint of bribery.

Dissonance is not always counterproductive; it can be used to help people. Axson and Cooper (1985) used the 'effort justification' effect to help overweight women lose weight. This effect is based on the premise that the harder people work to achieve a goal, the more worthwhile they perceive it to be, even if the end product turns out to be rather disappointing. Axsom and Cooper reasoned that convincing individuals that a specific form of therapy designed to help people lose weight involved a lot of effort would increase its effectiveness. They gave overweight women a 'bogus' therapy which consisted of various tasks. Half the tasks were very difficult and half of the tasks were very easy, but by no stretch of the imagination could these tasks be construed as aiding weight loss. Over a period of three weeks the participants in the high effort condition lost significantly more weight than those in the low effort condition and the difference increased over the next six months. Clearly, exerting considerable effort on their 'therapy' led to a commitment to restructure their diet and lose weight.

In summary, when people find that their attitudes and their actions do not correspond, they may experience pressure for change and it is usually their attitudes that change first.

Behaviour

The last link in the process of communication is action. If a person does not act on the communication then it is useless. It may be that a correct decision has been made and communicated effectively but a change in behaviour does not take place because the person, or people, in question just cannot change the behaviour. Deep-seated habits and routines are very hard to change even when people wish to do so. 'I known I have to lose weight, but I've tried and tried and just can't,' 'You say I have to change, but how?' are statements and questions that typically accompany requests to change behaviour.

Many people lack the skill, or ability, to carry out instructions. There are, however, a number of behavioural techniques which can be used to help people change their behaviour in a desired direction. The next section describes some of these techniques, gives some general guidelines on behaviour change and finally examines how they can be applied in one specific context; that of losing weight.

Techniques of behaviour change

The techniques of behaviour change or modification have their roots in classical and instrumental conditioning (described in the previous chapter). Thus the principles of behaviour change are based on reinforcement and association.

Positive reinforcement

One of the main features of problem behaviour is the provision of inappropriate rewards. A young man in a psychiatric hospital had a particularly debilitating behaviour problem – he used to vomit over his companions at meal times. It appeared as if he could not keep any food down, so the problem became critical. The first act of the nursing staff was to check that there was no physical cause for his behaviour. It appeared that there was nothing physically wrong, so attention was switched to his behaviour. The staff closely examined the young man's behaviour and found that two rewards featured prominently – every time the man vomited he got attention; he also got a warm bath.

The nursing staff decided to remove these rewards, and did not pay the young man any attention when he vomited nor did they give him a nice warm bath. To replace the socially unacceptable behaviours new ones were substituted. Every time the man did not vomit he was given a reward and he was encouraged to get the attention he needed from his companions rather than from the nursing staff. The use of positive reinforcement over a period of months gradually changed the man's behaviour. He was able to retain his food at meal times and also enjoy socialising with his companions.

Punishment

In the case of this man it should be noted that he was not punished for his abnormal behaviour. If the nursing staff had punished him every time he vomited they might have been successful in stopping him vomiting but they would have had no control over any behaviour he chose to replace it. For this reason, punishment on its own should not be used in the context of nursing care.

However, it is recognised that in some circumstances outside the nursing context the use of punishment may have to be considered, but it is hoped that all alternatives will have been exhausted before it is administered. If punishment has to be used, then it should be dispensed as quickly as possible. If punishment occurs too long a time after the event, no connection will be made between the event and the punishment, and in some circumstances an opposite effect to the desired outcome will occur. For instance, if parents spank their children for being naughty a considerable time after the act took place, the children may fail to make the connection between the naughty act and the spanking. Worse, the children may think that it is perfectly acceptable to hit people for no apparent reason since they have seen this behaviour in their parents. Bee and Boyd (2003) say that physical punishment should be avoided wherever possible and gives three good reasons why.

- Children observe adults using force to solve problems and therefore will model their behaviour on what they see. It is no use saying to the child that it is alright for 'grown-ups' to hit but wrong for children to do so, as research on modelling (see *Chapter 7*) indicates that children are influenced more by actions than by words.
- The repeated pairing of a parent with the unpleasant event of being spanked will result in negative feelings towards the parent, not just because of the frustration and pain engendered by the spanking, but because of the parent being frequently associated with disagreeable acts.
- Children may pick up in a parent's face the anger that usually accompanies physical punishment. This produces an atmosphere of rejection and frigidity rather than warmth and caring.

Patterson (1975) has suggested that there are other forms of effective control which do not rely on punishment, and other forms of punishment that do not rely on spanking or hitting.

Systematic desensitisation

An 18-year-old first-year student nurse was very nervous about seeing blood. For several years she had reacted to the sight of blood with discomfort and feelings of nausea. Up to the time she had decided to become a nurse the anxiety had not presented her with any particular problem, but now she was faced with a real quandary. In the course of her training she was shown films depicting a variety of medical conditions and often had to leave the room because she thought she would either faint or vomit if she stayed to watch. She reasoned to herself that if this was the state that she got into watching films, what would it be like when she was faced with the real thing? Her future as a nurse seemed under threat.

This was a case history reported by Rardin (1969) who used systematic desensitisation to help this nurse deal with her phobia. The technique was developed by Wolpe (1958) and involves the following four stages.

- Learning how to relax.
- Listing all your fears.
- Constructing a hierarchy of threatening scenes.
- Working through the scenes.

The student nurse constructed a fear hierarchy, including items such as blood from surgery, blood from injury and blood from childbirth. Then the nurse was asked to visualise the least anxiety-provoking situation and rate her anxiety on a scale from 1 to 10. During this period she was given help with relaxation and provided with positive reinforcement. Slowly she worked through her fear hierarchy, visualising progressively more anxiety-provoking events until she was able to cope with visualising the most threatening situations. After one year of practising the technique the nurse was successfully able to manage her fear of blood.

Some researchers have suggested that graded hierarchies are not necessary and a close relationship between therapist and patient is not important (Miller and Morley, 1986). Nevertheless, the full technique has proved successful in a number of cases of fear and anxiety.

Exercise 10.2 *Desensitisation*

Although the nurse in the example had someone to help her through the technique, it can be practised on one's own. Try the following exercise but do not expect to master the technique straight away; most skills require time and effort to perfect.

Fear inventory

- Construct a fear inventory by listing objects or experiences that bother you. What makes you embarrassed? What would make you leave a room or cross the street to avoid? What makes you feel uneasy? Here are some examples to start you off

Human blood	Going to the dentist
Crawling insects	People who seem insane
Open wounds	Sight of fighting
Enclosed spaces	Witnessing surgery
Sight of hypodermic needles	Looking foolish
Snakes	People with deformities
Being touched	Aggressive people
Heights	Speaking in public
Being alone at night	Crowds
Dead people	Medical smells

Taking exams	Flying
Cemeteries	Mice in the hair
Nude men or women	Being ignored
Lack of control	Being teased

Having listed as many 'fears' as possible, assign each one a value between 1 and 5 according to the extent to which they disturb you:

Not at all	*A bit*	*A fair amount*	*A lot*	*A great deal*
1	2	3	4	5

- If the items are related to each other, group them according to themes.
- Construct a threatening scene hierarchy. Pick one area of considerable importance and assemble some scenarios. List the scenes in ascending order of discomfort.

Example: fear of hypodermic needles:

1 Watching a film with someone getting an injection.
2 A friend talks to you about the jabs he needed to go abroad.
3 You prick your finger with a needle or pin.
4 You have to give a blood sample at the health centre.
5 Driving to the health centre and parking your car.
6 Thinking about injections in the waiting room.
7 A nurse with a tray of syringes walks past.
8 Entering examination room.
9 Doctor says he wants a small sample of blood.
10 Doctor picks up syringe.
11 Smell of alcohol on cotton ball.
12 Hypodermic poised in doctor's hand
13 Needle goes in.
14 Pain starts.

Visualising the scenes
Get into a comfortable position and close your eyes. Put on some relaxing music if you wish and start to relax all the muscles in your body. You could use the progressive muscular relaxation described in Chapter 8). Try to imagine lying in a soft meadow on a sunny summer day, watching the clouds slowly floating by. Each cloud takes some of your tension with it.

When you are completely relaxed, select your first scene and start to visualise it. Try to make it as real as possible. Ask yourself what colours are there in the scene. Is the light bright? What details are there – chairs, carpets, a table, pictures? Listen for sounds such as traffic noises, the wind or even your own voice. Reach out and feel some of the objects. Are they rough or smooth Touch your clothes and feel your skin. What smells are present? Flowers? Chemicals? Perfume? Are you eating or drinking anything? If so, what does it taste like?

Note any tension and assign it a value from ie Take a deep breath, hold it, and release it slowly, saying over to yourself, 'Relax, calm, let go.' Note any tension relief, switch off the scene and return to your 'meadow'.

Repeat this procedure until your tension has decreased. It may take a few goes to do this and then you can go on to the next scene in your hierarchy. Stop when you are tired or bored.

The technique is a skill and therefore practice is needed. Do not be disappointed if you are unsuccessful at first; keep trying. If you happen to experience the threatening scene in real life, note any tension and use it as a signal to relax. Take deep breaths and repeat your calming statement to yourself.

Programmes of behavioural change

Most programmes of behavioural change specify distinct stages. Usually there is a progression from one to the next, however, this is not always the case and people can either become 'stuck' or even oscillate between them. What follows are two examples of behaviour change strategies or programmes, one concerning weight loss the other relationships. It can be seen that both contain a number of similarities but the main feature of each of the programmes is the concentration on the specific manipulation of particular behaviours.

Weight loss

The first behavioural change programme comprises three stages: assessment; treatment; maintenance.

Assessment

The most important feature of any behavioural change programme is to define exactly where the problem lies. Mistakes at this stage are critical. The problem may be that the patient has insufficient information about what to do, in which case providing relevant details may suffice. If lack of information is not the problem, then one needs to decide whether there is a skill deficiency or a management deficiency. Again, skill deficiencies can be remedied by tuition. Management deficiencies require further investigation.

Pinpointing. Before any change in behaviour can take place it is necessary to identify the precise behaviours that need to be changed. People tend to speak about their problems in general terms. Sentences such as 'He just doesn't care for me any more' or 'I just can't stop snacking' are of little use, since they do not identify precise behaviours. Much better comments would be 'He doesn't hug me enough' or 'Every time I see a biscuit I have to eat it.' Here the problems are clearly stated in behavioural terms and can be addressed. Pinpointing may be achieved by interviewing and keeping diaries. A typical behavioural management programme would have three stages.

- *Stage 1*. An initial interview concerned with establishing the nature of the problem, previous attempts to change, habits, reasons for wanting to change and the effects of any social networks. A daily diary, or record, is kept to assemble a 'baseline' of behaviour.
- *Stage 2*. The second interview evaluates the self-monitored behaviour patterns. The diary is discussed and any shortcomings illustrated.
- *Stage 3*. The third interview establishes some form of commitment, or contract, by the patient to the programme. At this stage the patient is free to opt out and leave. If a decision is made to continue, usually an agreement is signed by those taking part in the programme.

Treatment

The first stage in the treatment phase is to set realistic goals. Too often people wish to 'run before they can walk'. Thus small, manageable changes in behaviour should be encouraged at first. If the goals set become too difficult, the patient will soon lose heart and give up. The events that precede an act are called *antecedents* and must be considered as well; entering a newsagent to buy a magazine can be a trigger for buying sweets.

A behavioural change regimen is constructed listing appropriate rewards for targeted behaviours and family and friends are encouraged to take part. After a while, the patient is seen again to discuss problems with the treatment programme in an attempt to stabilise the change programme.

Maintenance

Despite motivation and good intentions, there are bound to be drawbacks and failures. Therefore it is important to maintain contact with the client for at least a year to help resolve problems as they occur so that the individual does not slide back into undesirable habits. Let's look at the following example.

Jane knows that she has to lose weight and feels that she has tried everything. She has spoken to you about getting her stomach stapled but does not know if she could go through such a procedure. She is willing to give losing weight one last try.

Assessment. Jane is asked to list:

- when she started to put on weight;
- previous attempts to lose weight;

- eating habits in the form of a diary;
- exercise patterns (diary);
- weight (diary);
- prospective social and family support.

You emphasise to Jane the importance of keeping an exact record of her behaviour.

At the next meeting you analyse her diary and find that she has been making some mistakes and point these out to her. You evaluate Jane's self-monitored weight, eating and exercise habits. Items such as snacking, 'binges' and particular situations that trigger eating are given prominent attention. You discuss with her the advantages and difficulties of dealing with her weight problem. A contract is prepared which specifies the exact guidelines and the consequences of failure to follow them. An amount of money is deposited, which will only be returned on completion of various stages of the programme. Jane is asked to go away and think about it.

At the third meeting, you review the programme and the contract. At this stage Jane may decide that she no longer wishes to continue with the programme; however if she decides to go ahead, the contract is finalised and the treatment starts.

Treatment. Initially, you give Jane advice on the sorts of food that she should eat and construct a system to exchange the new for the old foods. A weekly weight loss of 1–4 lb is targeted and Jane can eat her favourite food as long as this objective is achieved.

Jane's food buying habits are investigated; you tell her to prepare a list before going shopping and to buy only those foods that have been agreed in the food exchange plan. You also suggest that she never shops when she's hungry and that she should avoid buying extra quantities of foods. Having brought the food home, she should store it away from sight in cupboards or in opaque containers. (Out of sight is out of mind.) Together you construct menus which include some favourite foods and Jane is encouraged to serve small portions of food on small plates.

You advise Jane to change the way that she eats by taking more time to chew her food and savour each bite; after all eating is meant to be a pleasurable experience. Placing small amounts of food on a fork and pausing between mouthfuls helps reduce the speed of consumption. As soon as a meal is over, Jane is urged to leave the table and not to 'finish off' any leftovers.

Snacking between meals is a major factor in becoming overweight. The effects can be reduced by substituting low-calorie foods for the usual snacks but a better method is encouraging Jane to eat at regular intervals.

Family and friends can play an important role in altering the antecedents of Jane's eating behaviour. By avoiding continual talk about food and engaging in non-food activities, the temptation to eat is reduced. Family and friends should be asked to reward Jane for her progress and never to criticise her obesity.

Exercise is not only useful for reducing weight but it is also a good way to manage stress. Therefore an exercise plan should be constructed with the help of one of Jane's friends. If Jane tackles stress and anxiety by eating more food, alternatives have to be found and substituted.

As the treatment progresses, encourage Jane to discuss problems with the programme and to determine and provide her own rewards when she achieves her desired weight loss goals. As the desired goals are achieved, a proportion of the money deposited at the beginning of the treatment programme should be returned to Jane.

Maintenance. The meetings with Jane should become shorter and shorter as the programme proceeds. However, if there are problems, it should be ensured that Jane experiences no difficulty in making contact with you. If the eating and exercise habits to preserve weight loss are maintained for the period specified in the contract, Jane should be given the rest of the money. It should be stressed that the programme will only succeed if there is genuine motivation on Jane's part to lose weight; coercion will not work and little can be done for those who refuse to co-operate.

Living together

The behavioural approach to relationships is based on mutual reward. Relationships are maintained as long as both members continue to supply each other with positive reinforcement. If both partners cease to provide appropriate rewards, the relationship breaks down and the couple drift apart. Unfortunately, married people have signed a contract to stay together for life and there are legal, social and religious sanctions to prohibit them from divorcing. Many couples stay together in the most disharmonious circumstances rather than go through a divorce. Although approximately one marriage in three ends in divorce, it is quite surprising that the numbers are not greater. A couple may have to face illnesses, financial difficulties, changes in home and jobs, the needs of children, the attractiveness of others, etc. If one considers the lack of practice in learning how to live together in difficult circumstances, the divorce rate might not seem so surprising.

An example of an unsatisfactory relationship in behavioural terms is provided by Hops (1976) who cites the case of the husband who comes home from work and, as the marriage is in its infancy, is eager to discuss his day at work with his wife. However, as the marriage progresses the frequency of this behaviour decreases. The husband, who is talking and interacting with people all day, is satiated but his wife is anxious to talk and starts to ask lots of questions. Unfortunately, the husband is exhausted and just wants to put his feet up in front of the television and maybe read a newspaper. A likely result of this behaviour is the continual nagging of the wife to try to get some response from her husband. Hops (1976) says this is one of the most frequently noted scenarios reported by marital therapists. A sequel to this behaviour pattern is the establishment of mutual punishment rather than reinforcement. In order to get some reaction from her husband, the wife may punish him in some way. He in turn may respond with some verbal jibe and mutual punishment is established. The result is often long silences at mealtimes and boring, lifeless evenings.

A behavioural programme designed to help couples is described by Hops (1976).

There are four stages: pinpointing; communication skills training; problem-solving and negotiation; contingency contracting.

Pinpointing

Before any change in behaviour can take place, it is necessary to pinpoint the behaviours that need changing. Many couples are unable to discriminate between positive and negative behaviour and use broad undefined statements to describe each other. 'He always treats me like dirt' and 'She doesn't love me any more' are statements that fail to define precisely the problem. Statements like 'He never kisses me or hugs me' are much more precise and pinpoint the problem in behavioural terms. Couples are taught to specify behaviours precisely and are give the task of recording behaviours that produce pleasure or displeasure in their partner. In this way, a list is produced of the exact behaviours that need to be changed by the couple.

Communication skills training

One result of pinpointing may be an increase in communication between the partners, but in the majority of circumstances, some training in communication skills is required. Sometime people are so intent on getting over their own point of view that they fail to listen to what their partners are saying. The first communication skill to learn is the ability to listen. In certain situations it is necessary to teach a person to paraphrase his or her partner's last few sentences in order to ensure active listening.

Sharing the time spent speaking to each other is another important communication skill. Many interactions are dominated by one person so that the partner cannot 'get a word in edgeways'. Training can take the form of both partners speaking for a set period of time, say two minutes, with active listening to the content of the conversation.

Some people have non-verbal responses that are 'put down' behaviour. Often individuals who behave in this way are unaware of the effect they are having on their partners. Therefore, it is necessary to give them feedback about their manner when they are behaving in this way. Couples are taught to reduce their aversive verbal behaviours. They are asked to think of something positive the spouse has done during the week and state it. If a verbal or non-verbal put down occurs as a response, it is pointed out to him or her.

Problem solving and negotiation training

The goal of this stage is to provide couples with the skills necessary to solve problems together. A woman complained to her partner that he never hung up his clothes in the bedroom. He replied that he would hang them up if the wardrobe was not full up with all her clothes that she never used. The argument continued until the woman compromised by saying that she would make space in the wardrobe if he would agree to hang his clothes up more often. He agreed. The solution was facilitated by the woman's ability to compromise and seek a mutual solution to the problem.

Contingency contracting

If the previous three procedures have failed to help the couple reconcile their problems, contingency contracting can be used. This represents the final stage in the behavioural approach to relationships. Contracts are set up between the two individuals concerning their behaviour toward each other. The couple get together and discuss those features of each other's behaviour that they find rewarding. They then discuss the rewards they would like if they behave accordingly and the punishments that will occur if they fail. (see Figure 10.1 for an example of a contingency contract drawn up between a couple in the 1960s and 1970s in the United States).

Notice that there is no mention of love and affection in this approach. Psychologists who adopt the behavioural perspective are solely concerned with the modification of observed behaviours; they do not study the thoughts and emotions of people and have been criticised for neglecting to do so. However, both procedures contain some sound advice on practical ways to reduce weight and get along with each other.

Models of behaviour change

Kasl and Cobb (1966) make a distinction between three different types of 'health behaviour':

- *Health behaviour*: An activity undertaken by person believing himself to be healthy for the purpose of preventing disease or detecting it in asymptomatic stage.
- *Illness behaviour*: Any activity undertaken by a person who feels ill, to define the state of his health and to discover a suitable remedy.
- *Sick-role behaviour*: Activity undertaken for purpose of getting well, by those who consider themselves ill. It includes receiving treatment from appropriate therapists, generally involves a whole range of dependent behaviours and leads to some degree of neglect of one's usual duties.

The models of behaviour change to be discussed in this chapter are essentially concerned with understanding and predicting behaviour and the first is the health belief model.

Health belief model

This was developed by four psychologists – Hochbaum, Kegeles, Leventhal and Rosenstock (Rosenstock 1974) – to predict individuals' preventive health behaviour. It was subsequently modified by Becker and Maiman (1975) to incorporate sick-role behaviour and compliance with medical regimens. Readiness to take action and to engage in health-related behaviours depends on a number of factors. The first two are

NAME: *Dick*   NAME: *Jane*

CONVERSATION AND SEX

Accelerate: 10 minutes of talk about Dick's Day as it concerns studies and future - every day.

Accelerate: Sleep in nude every night except during periods.

Reward: 1 bottle of beer per 10 minutes.

Reward: 30¢ a day to be spent in any way I see fit.

Penalty: Write two letters, e.g., to friends or relatives.

Penalty: Heavy housework, e.g.,
1) wash windows in 1 room
2) clean oven
3) wax floors
4) shampoo rug

HOME TIME AND CHILD TRAINING

Accelerate: Dick will be home four evenings per week, explicitly Monday, Wednesday, Friday, and Saturday. Of these, Jane will have one night out, one at her option, and two will be shared family nights.

Accelerate: Jane will spend involved, meaningful time with children, reading, art projects, excursions, reading readiness, etc., at the rate of 7 half-hour periods per week.

Reward: One-half hour sense relaxation exercises with Jane.

Reward: Late cooking or dinner together with Dick is earned for 3 points (one point per half-hour with kids). One point may also be exchanged for 15 minutes help from Dick.

Penalty: Complete the whole kitchen shebang alone after dinner.

Penalty: Complete RCAF exercises at my level for failure to spend time with kids on any day.

Figure 10.1 A contingency contract

concerned with the extent to which individuals feel vulnerable to a particular illness. This involves whether they feel susceptible to contracting the illness and their thoughts about how severe it is:

- *Susceptibility*: an individual's beliefs about whether he or she is likely to contract an illness.
- *Severity*: the degree to which an individual perceives the consequences of having an illness to be severe.

Together these two factors constitute what is known as the perceived threat of an illness, sometimes known as vulnerability. Vulnerability comprises the extent to which one believes that his lifestyle is likely to result in heart disease and also the extent to which he believes the consequences of contracting heart disease are particularly severe. If one perceives oneself's vulnerable, then this represents the first stage in doing something about his condition.

The next two factors concerned with the pros and cons of taking some action to combat the illness. 'What is to be gained? What do I have pay?'

- *Benefits*. This refers to the potential to be gained from a particular course of action that will reduce the health threat.
- *Barriers*. Any decision to act will have a certain lumber of consequences. There may be a degree of physical, psychological or financial stress associated with any form of action.

In this next stage, one has to 'weigh up' the benefits that might accrue from a change in lifestyle against the cost to one in terms of the extent to which one may be 'put out' by such actions. After considering these four factors, one may decide to take some form of action, there are two further factors that may stimulate one to do something about the condition.

- *Cues to action*. Cues are stimuli that trigger appropriate health behaviour. They can either be internal (perception of bodily states), or external, (stimuli from the environment such as the mass media)
- *Diverse factors*. These include demographic, ethnic, social and personality factors that may influence health behaviour.

One may be spurred into action by abnormally severe chest pains, by listening to the advice of his colleagues at work, or by the concern of family and close friends about his condition.

Becker *et al.* (1977) include a seventh factor in their revision of the model which is the pre-disposition, or motivation, of people to engage in health-related practices. Becker *et al.* (1977) state that the health belief model is a useful tool in predicting the degree to which individuals are likely to play an active role in their, and others' health care. They provide as an example of the model in action an attempt to predict whether mothers of obese children would keep their clinic appointments. The participants in the experiment were 182 mothers of children newly diagnosed as obese. Over a twelve-month period, the participants were required to visit the clinic four times – this was a measure of their actual behaviour. They also measured the amount of weight change that occurred during this period. A questionnaire was used to gain information about the mothers' health beliefs regarding such items as how easily the child became ill (susceptibility) extent to which being overweight caused serious illness (severity); how attention diet could help alleviate obesity problems benefits); whether there were problems adhering a diet when the children did not want to have anything to do with it; an assessment of the mothers' own concern about health care in general and the extent to which their willingness to engage in health-related practices affected compliance (motivation). The results suggested that there was a relationship between the mothers' health beliefs and a reduction in obesity over the twelve-month period. More than half the correlations between the questionnaire items and the attendance at clinic plus subsequent weight loss were significant. However, the health belief model seemed to be better at predicting actual behavioural outcomes (weight loss) than behaviour per se (keeping appointments at the clinic). Here is no doubt that the health belief model can be a useful guide to health behaviour under certain circumstances (Rosenstock and Kirscht 1979), but there are a number of criticisms. First, the reformulations proposed by Becker and Maiman (1975) make the theory unnecessarily unwieldy with eleven 'readiness' factors and twenty-three 'enabling' factors. This clearly constitutes more variables than can be included in any one study. Second, the model treats people as rational decision makers. Janis (1984) says, 'The important point is that the health belief model, like other models of rational choice, fails to specify under what conditions people will give priority to avoiding participative discomfort at the cost of endangering their lives, and under what conditions they will make a more rational decision.'

Locus of control

Consider the following statements.

> When I become ill, it is a matter of fate.
>
> It seems my health is influenced by accidental happenings.
>
> When I stay healthy, it is just luck.

If you agree with these statements then you believe that we are not masters of our own fate and that we are prone to destiny or to powers outside our control (*external locus of control*).

If I become ill I have the power to become well again.

My physical health depends on how well I take care of myself.

I am directly responsible for my health.

If you agree with these statements, then you believe that you have the ability to determine the factors affecting your life (*internal locus of control*).

Wallston and Wallston (1984) adapted the concept of locus of control to health-related behaviours (the Multidimensional Health Locus of Control Scale). They contend that an individual's locus of control will influence decisions made such that if an external locus of control is adopted then a decision to adopt a *laissez-faire* attitude to health will take place. If an internal locus of control is adopted, it will lead to a decision to do things for oneself and to take a significant role in how decisions about one's health are made.

However, Wallston and Wallston divided the external locus of control into two separate sections, 'chance' and 'powerful others'. 'Chance' refers to fate or God as being the agents of control, but it was recognised that often people depended on significant or powerful others to control their lives. Thus, a reliance on nurses and doctors to determine one's health outcomes would be classed as a 'powerful others' locus of control. Ogden (2004) cites the work of Murray and McMillan (1993) on predicting women's cancer screening behaviour as providing support for both the health locus of control and health belief models, in particular the 'barriers' component of the HBM was found to be most useful in predicting behaviour.

Self-efficacy

Self-efficacy can be defined as the extent to which people believe they are competent to confront the challenges in life. Self-efficacy forms part of Bandura's social cognitive theory (Bandura, 1986) which holds that behaviour is learned through modelling, visualising, self-monitoring and skill training. Behaviour is determined by expectancies and incentives. Expectancies are categorised into:

- expectancies about *environmental* cues – beliefs about how events are connected;
- *outcome* expectancies – beliefs about how behaviour is likely to influence outcomes;
- *efficacy* expectancies – expectancies about one's own competence to perform the behaviour needed to influence the outcome.

Incentive is the value of a particular object or outcome (health status, approval of others, economic gain). Thus people with a weight problem will attempt to change their diet if they believe that their current eating habits pose a threat to any personally valued outcome such as health or appearance (environmental cues); that particular changes in eating habits will reduce the threats (outcome expectations) and they are capable of adopting new eating habits (efficacy expectations). Bandura (1989) says that expectations of personal efficacy determine whether coping behaviour will be sustained in the face adversity. In the case of people with weight problems, a strong sense of self-efficacy will result in adherence to a particular diet regimen even though there is only a small change in weight. Those with a weak sense of self-efficacy, in the same circumstances, would be more likely to become discouraged and give up. Linn (1988) related the ability to tolerate pain to self-efficacy. Those participants with high self-efficacy were able to tolerate more pain than those with low self-efficacy. Bandura *et al.* (1988) say that self-efficacy enables people to cope with stressors because it activates the production of endogenous opioids that block the transmission of pain and allow the person to function more effectively. Schwarzer (1992) has claimed that self-efficacy is the single best predictor of intentions and behaviour change across a wide range of behaviours, from dental flossing to drug addicts' intention to use clean needles. However, the assumption that people are rational processors of information should not be taken for granted.

Protection motivation theory

As with the HBM, Protection Motivation Theory (Rogers, 1985) was developed over a number of years 1975–85. Essentially, PMT is an extension of the HBM with some additions: response effectiveness (Stopping smoking would improve my health), self-efficacy (I really believe I can give up smoking) and fear (I'm scared stiff of getting lung cancer). Behavioural intentions are partly made up of threat appraisals (severity, susceptibility and fear) along with coping appraisals (response effectiveness and self-efficacy).

On the face of it, the constituents of PMT all seem reasonable features of a person's intentions to behave in a particular way. However, as with the HBM, this reasonableness contributes to the theory's inability to deal with non-reasonable behaviour – something that characterises a great deal of health behaviour. On a more specific note, Floyd *et al.* (2000) reviewed sixty-five studies that had used PMT and found that of the five factors, self-efficacy and responsiveness were good predictors of behavioural intentions but the theory was better at describing present behaviour rather than predicting future behaviour.

Theory of reasoned action/planned behaviour

The main contention of this theory is that intention is the best predictor of behaviour. Suppose you are in a restaurant with a friend who has just given up drinking alcohol. The waiter asks your friend would she like a glass of wine with her meal. You wonder whether she will accept. According to the theory of reasoned action (Ajzen and Fishbein,

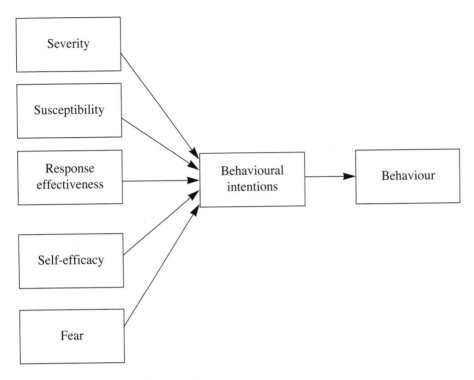

Figure 10.2 Protection motivation theory

1980) it would depend on her intentions. But what determines intentions? The theory says that intention to perform a behaviour is determined by beliefs and attitudes. Let us take an example of a person with a weight problem who wants to shed a few pounds. The behavioural intention is 'I would like to lose some weight.' The two attitudes influencing this intention are:

● The attitude regarding the behaviour of eating: 'Eating certain foods would be a good thing to do.'
● The participative norm of eating: 'Eating certain foods is seen by many people as an appropriate act.'

In turn these attitudes are influenced by beliefs, so that the attitude regarding the behaviour of eating is affected by:

● Beliefs about the outcomes of eating: 'If I eat well I will improve my health and be more attractive.'
● Evaluations regarding the outcomes of eating: 'Being healthy and good looking are enjoyable, satisfying and pleasant.'

The participative norm is influenced by:

- Beliefs about others' opinions: 'My family and friends think I should eat certain foods.'
- Motivation to comply with others' opinions: 'I would like to do what my friends and family want.'

Ajzen (1985) added another concept to the theory and called it the *the theory of planned behaviour* (TPB). He proposed that perceived control was an important factor in behavioural intention. Thus one of the best predictors of weight loss is perceived control over one's weight. It involves beliefs about abilities, opportunities and obstacles to the behaviour. The theory has been applied to smoking (Fishbein 1982), losing weight (Schifter and Ajzen 1985) and breast self-examination (Lierman *et al.* 1990). Norman and Smith (1995) used the TPB to predict exercise behaviour. They found that although the TPB factors of strong desire to exercise and pressure from others to exercise were related to future behaviour, the strongest predictor of future exercise behaviour was previous exercise behaviour indicating a significant habitual component.

Stages of change

Proshaska and Di Clemente (1982) put forward *a transtheoretical model* of behaviour change. They said that people are in a particular stage of change with respect to smoking, drinking, diet, etc. For example, people may be in a stage of:

- *Precontemplation*: not intending to make any changes.
- *Contemplation*: considering making changes.
- *Preparation*: starting to make small changes.
- *Action*: actually engaging in new behaviour.
- *Maintenance*: maintaining the change over time.

Again, there are strengths and weaknesses to this model. First, the changes do not always recur in a linear fashion. People may move back and forward between stages. Second, the stages not be so discreet (Sutton, 2000) and the cross-sectional designs of many studies rules out causal factors. However, broadly speaking if someone is toward the 'front end' of the model, interventions should be based on changing attitude. If a person wants to change but is having difficulty then one needs to concentrate on developing cognitive/behavioural techniques. Thus to summarise:

- If the person lacks knowledge about health behaviour, then health education is the appropriate intervention.

- If the person could not care less about what she is doing, then attitude change is the approach
- If the person is trying to change, but are having difficulty, then cognitive/behavioural techniques might prove successful.

An assessment

First, these are by no means all the models of 'health/illness behaviour'. And many continue to provide the basis of research into health issues such as using the theory of planned behaviour to shed light on exercise and healthy eating (Payne *et al.*, 2005). Also, many of the models' components are implicated in aspects of health behaviour. But when we investigated some of the models' applicability to an intervention programme for healthy eating in the north-east of England (Niven *et al.*, 2003), we found that social rather than psychological factors were more likely to play a part.. For instance, intention to eat healthy food is certainly important, but when you are a one parent family with little money and have three young children to look after, the prospect of a long bus ride to the nearest 'healthy' shop/supermarket is not an option. Further, whilst more sophisticated statistical analyses seek to tease out specific components of models as responsible for behaviour change, they neglect to actually ask the people themselves why they are doing what they are doing. Essentially this is a plea for less quantitative approaches and more qualitative approaches to researching changes in attitudes and behaviour.

Summary

Whilst some may feel that changing attitudes to health and health care is the most important feature of health promotion and illness prevention, it is not. Changing behaviour is the ultimate goal. From the evidence it seems that changing attitudes and developing intentions to act in a particular way are the prerequisites of behavioural change programmes, not the end point of change. People need much more than good intentions to change their behaviour.

There are perhaps two cardinal rules that nurses should keep in mind when constructing behavioural change programmes. These are:

- Make sure you know the exact behaviours and rewards. Many of us had a school-teacher who punished children by sending them outside the classroom to stand in the corridor. Sometimes it did not work because a fair proportion of children actually wanted to stand outside the classroom!
- Do not bite off more than you can chew. Start with something very simple so that initial success is virtually guaranteed.

Models of health behaviour give a limited view of the reasons why people do and do not indulge in healthy behaviour but this does not mean that we should abandon concepts such as self-efficacy, merely we should try to incorporate them in more meaningful research designs.

Conundrum revisited

You may not surprised to discover that television health education messages are but part of the campaign to help people stop smoking cigarettes, but they do represent a useful case study associated with this chapter. The first point is that using 'personal stories' does work with all three components of attitude. In the affective component the viewer is invited to identify with the individuals on screen: 'That could be me.' The individuals talk to the viewer: 'You've got to stop smoking, do it now.' The appeal is emotional, highlighting risk and the onus of decision making. The adverts operate in the cognitive component by emphasising information that may be new to the viewer. Smoking affects your heart as well as your lungs. It can leave you unable to play with your children and your wife a widow in waiting. Here the challenge is subtle but effective: 'Did you really think that it was just your lungs you're risking?' Finally, the message, do it now, stop smoking is reinforced both as a strap line on screen and verbally. The emphasis is upon behavioural change and yes, here are the contact details for people to help you.

In this particular television campaign all the role modelling is negative – don't be like me. Equally though, much could be made of featuring people who are successful and who consistently do not smoke cigarettes. It is though more difficult to present abstract, healthy outcomes quite so visually on screen. Energy, fitness and appearance may be taken for granted by young smokers who for a considerable period of time perceive little or no impact from cigarettes on their fitness and physical attractiveness. Instead, the television campaign with its folk next door approach features individuals who are chosen to have direct appeal and to be 'just like us' in all other regards. They wear casual clothes, talk in accents similar to our own and come from our communities.

You may have suggested that it is important to judge the impact of health messages upon attitudes and decided to prepare a follow up questionnaire. Likert scale questionnaires are described in Chapter 9 but it is notoriously difficult to judge whether such scales measure deep seated attitudes or whether what is recorded upon them will predict how the individual will feel, think or behave in weeks to come. Questionnaires take a 'snap shot picture' of attitudes and it may be more fruitful to plan television adverts and/or associated literature and questionnaires that attend to the profile of individuals who's attitudes you seek to change. For example, women smokers might arguably respond to different messages or images to men and teenagers might respond differently to older smokers. Health educators regularly profile their target groups, whether this is associated with safe sex, giving up cigarettes or the risks associated with injury at work.

This brings us to the question of anticipated and unanticipated results of health education campaigns. Over a number of decades now health promoters have debated the merits of scaring people with stark messages. You may have witnessed television images of badly diseased lungs, the volume of fat squeezed from the diseased arteries of smokers or images of nails and coffins. One argument against outright scare tactics is that they consign the established smoker to a 'no hope' category. The smoker reasons, if my lungs are that badly damaged already, there is no point in giving up now. I might as well take what little pleasure is left to me.

Because of this health educators have sometimes employed cognitive dissonance to try and influence the smoker's behaviour. Instead of saying 'damage already done' they offer 'this is what you *could* have had if you didn't smoke'. The usual mechanism for this is to describe what the money spent on cigarettes could have bought you and that which you can still attain if you kick the habit now. It works well where money and alternative material rewards appeal to individuals. It works less well where the addictive component of smoking is not also addressed or where the smoker is already wealthy and not motivated by additional material benefits.

Perhaps you concluded that extreme behaviour requires extreme ends. At present the costs of smoking are portrayed as a form of Russian roulette. You *might* get lung cancer, you might suffer from peripheral vascular disease. We know that you know, that health care treatments might militate against such risks. The risks might seem 'not so bad'. Some exasperated health care professionals wonder whether smokers should be told that they will not be eligible for treatment that is adjudged smoking related. Peripheral vascular surgery becomes off limits for smokers. In this way the profile of fears associated with smoking are accentuated. Significant risk of illness and little chance of treatment is the message here. Such an approach though poses significant moral dilemmas and assumes that we are able to objectively assess illness associated with smoking as separate from that associated with ageing or genetic factors for instance. In practice it places the health educating nurse in conflict with a portion of the public and removes the opportunity of working on the affective component of behaviour in future. 'Why should I trust you, you don't value me'.

? Questions for further consideration

1 Discuss the problems associated with overcoming resistance to attitude change.
2 Distinguish between positive reinforcement, negative reinforcement and punishment, giving examples where appropriate.

3 Outline the processes involved in systematic desensitisation.
4 Discuss the relationship between attitudes and behaviour.

References

Ajzen, I. (1985). From intention to actions: A theory of planned behavior. In: Kuhl, J. and Beckman, J. (eds) *Action-control: From Cognition to Behavior.* Heidelberg: Springer.

Ajzen, J. and Fishbein, M. (1980). *Understanding Attitudes and Predicting Social Behavior.* Englewod Cliffs, NJ: Prentice-Hall.

Axsom, D. and Cooper, J. (1985). Cognitive dissonance and psychotherapy: the role of effort justification in inducing weight loss. *Journal of Experimental Social Psychology, 21,* 149–160.

Bandura, A. (1986). *Social foundations of thought and action: a social cognitive theory.* NJ: Prentice-Hall.

Bandura, A., Cioff, D., Taylor, C. and Brouillard, M. (1988). Received self-efficacy in coping with cognitive stressors and opiod activation. *Journal of Personality and Social Psychology, 55,* 479.

Bandura, A. (1989). Perceived self-efficacy in the exercise of personal agency. *The Psychologist, 10,* 411–424.

Becker, M. H. (1975). Maiman IA Sociobehavioral compliance with health and medical care recommendations. *Medical Care, 13,* 10–24.

Becker, M. H. et al. (1977). Selected psychosocial models and correlates of individual health-related behaviors. *Medical Care, 15,* 27–46.

Bee, H. and Boyd, D. (2003*) The Developing Child.* 10th edn. New York: Allyn and Bacon.

Festinger, L. (1957). *A Theory of Cognitive Dissonance.* Evanston IL: Row Peterson.

Festinger, L. and Carlsmith, J. M. (1959). Cognitive consequences of forced compliance. *Journal of Abnormal and Social Psychology, 58,* 203–210.

Fishbein, M. (1982). Social psychological analysis of smoking behavior. In: Eiser, J. (ed) *Social psychology and behavioural medicine.* Chichester: Wiley.

Fishbein, M. and Ajzen, I. (1975). *Belief Attitude, Intention and Behaviour: An introduction to theory and research.* Reading MA: Addison Wesley.

Floyd, D. L., Prentice-Dunn, S. and Rogers, R. W. (2000) A meta-analysis of research on protection motivation theory. *Journal of Applied Social Psychology, 4,* 67–79.

Forrester, D. A. and Murphy, P. A. (1992). Nurses' attitudes towards patients with AIDS and AIDS-related risk factors. *Journal of Advanced Nursing, 17,* 1260–1266.

Grush, J. E. (1980). The impact of candidate expenditures, regionality and prior outcomes on the 1976 Democratic presidential primaries. *Journal of Personality and Social Psychology, 38,* 337–347.

Hennigan, K. M., Cook, T. D. and Gruder, C. L. (1982). Cognitive tuning set, source credibility, and the temporal persistence of attitude change. *Journal of Personality and Social Psychology, 42,* 412–425.

Hops, H. (1976). Behavioral treatment of marital problems. In: Craighead, W. E., Kazdin, A. E. and Mahoney, M. S. (eds) *Behavior modification.* Boston: Houghton Mifflin.

Janis, I. L. (1984). The patient as decision maker. In: Gentry, W. (ed) *Handbook of behavioral medicine*. New York: Guilford.

Hovland, C. I. and Weiss, W. (1951). The influence of source credibility on communication effectiveness. *Public Opinion Quarterly, 15,* 635–650.

Kasl, S. V. and Cobb, S. (1966). Health behaviour, illness behaviour and sick role behaviour. *Archives of Environmental Health, 12,* 246–266.

Kiesler, C. A. and Kiesler, S. B. (1969). *Conformity.* Reading MA: Addison Wesley.

Krosnick, J. A. and Alwin, D. F. (1989). Aging and susceptibility to attitude change. *Journal of Personality and Social Psychology, 57,* 416–425.

Leventhal, H. (1970). Findings and theory in the study of fear communications. In: Berkowitz, L. (ed.) *Advances in Experimental Social Psychology* V. New York: Academic Press.

Lierman, L. M., Young, H. M., Kasprzyk, D. and Benoliel, J. (1990). Predicting breast self-examination using the theory of reasoned action. *Nursing Research, 39,* 97–101.

Linn, M. W. (1988). Psychotherapy with cancer patients. In: Goldberg, R. (ed) *Psychiatric aspects of cancer*, vol 18, Basel: Karger.

Lipkus, I. M., Green, J. D., Feaganes, J. R. and Sedikides, C. (2001) The relationships between attitudinal ambivalence and desire to quit smoking among college smokers. *Journal of Applied Social Psychology, 31,* 113–133.

Mackie, D. M. and Worth, L. T. (1989). Processing defects and the mediation of positive affect in persuasion. *Journal of Personality and Social Psychology, 57,* 27–40.

McGuire, W. J. (1969). The nature of attitudes and attitude change. In: Linzey, G. and Aronson, E. (eds) *Handbook of Social Psychology* III. Reading MA: Addison Wesley.

Miller, E. and Morley, S. (1986). *Investigating Abnormal Behaviour.* Chichester: Erlbaum.

Miller, N., Maruyama, G., Beaber, R. J. and Valone, K. (1976). Speed of speech and persuasion. *Journal of Personality and Social Psychology, 34,* 615–624.

Murray, M. and McMillan, C. (1993). Health beliefs, locus of control, emotional control and women's cancer screening behaviour. *Br J Clin Psychol, Feb. 32 (1),* 87–100.

Niven, N., Adamson, A. and Hay, F. (2003) Psychological factors influencing increased intake of starch and decreased intake of fat in a sample of NE England families. *Proceedings of the British Psychological Society, 11,* 37.

Norman, P. and Smith, L. (1995) The theory of planned behaviour and exercise. *European Journal of Social Psychology, 25,* 403–415.

Ogden, J. (2004) *Health Psychology.* 3rd edn. Maidenhead: Open University Press.

Patterson, G. R. (1975). *Families: Applications of Social Learning to Family Life.* Champaign IL: Research Press.

Payne, N., Jones, F. and Harris, P. (2005) The impact of job strain on the predictive validity of the theory of planned behaviour: an investigation of exercise and healthy eating. *British Journal of Health Psychology, 10,* 115–131.

Petty, R. E. and Cacioppo, J. T. (1981). *Attitudes and Persuasion: Classic and contemporary approaches.* Dubuque IA: Brown.

Proshaska, J. and Di Clemente, C. (1982). Transtheoretical therapy: Toward a more integrative model of change. *Psychotherapy: Theory, Research and Practice, 19, 276–288.*

Rardin, M. (1969). Treatment of a phobia by partial self-desensitization. *Journal of Consulting and Clinical Psychology, 33,* 125–126.

Rogers, R. W. (1985). A protection motivation theory of fear appeals and attitude change. *The Journal of Psychology, 6,* 143–151.

Rosenstock, I. M. (1974). The health belief model and preventative health behavior. *Health Education Monographs, 2,* 354–386.

Rosenstock, I. M. and Kirscht, J. P. (1979). Why people seek health care. In: Stone, G., Cohen, F. and Adler, N. (eds) *Health Psychology.* New York: Jossey Bass.

Schifter, D. and Ajzen, I. (1985). Intention, perceived control and weight loss: An application of the theory of planned behaviour. *Journal of Personality and Social Psychology, 49,* 843–851.

Schofield, J. W. and Pavelchak, M. A. (1989). Fallout from *The Day After*: Impact of a TV film on attitudes related to nuclear war. *Journal of Applied Social Psychology, 19,* 433–448.

Schwarzer, R. (1992). *Self-efficacy: Thought Control of Action.* Washington: Hemisphere Pub. Corp.

Skolnick, P. and Heslin, R. (1971). Approval dependence and reactions to bad arguments and low credibility scores. *Journal of Experimental Research in Personality, 5,* 199–207.

Sutton, S. (2000) Interpreting cross-sectional data on stages of change. *Psychology and Health, 15,* 163–171.

Wallston, B. S. and Wallston, K. A. (1984). Social psychological models of health behavior. In: Baum, A., Singer, S. E. and Singer, J. E. (eds) *Handbook of Psychology and Health.* NJ: Erlbaum Hillsdale.

Wolpe, J. (1958). *Psychotherapy by Reciprocal Inhibition.* Stanford CA: Stanford University Press.

Wu, C. and Shaffer, D. R. (1987). Susceptibility to persuasive appeals as a function of source credibility and prior experience with attitude object. *Journal of Personality and Social Psychology, 52,* 677–688.

Further reading

Bohner, Gerd and Waenke, Michaela (2002) *Attitudes and Attitude Change.* London: Psychology Press. Presents a great deal of recent research in this area. Requires some application, as there is a lot of detail.

Kazdin, Alan (2000) *Behaviour Modification in Applied Settings.* Belmont CA: Wadsworth. Looks at the practical application of basic behaviour modification in many applied settings including health and nursing.

Norman, Paul (2000) *Understanding Change in Health Behaviour.* London: Psychology Press. There are so many models of health behaviour these days; it needed someone like Paul Norman to make some sense of them.

Community Health Psychology

A practice conundrum

Patients, persons and places? An investigation of status, circumstances, roles and help in hospital and the community

What does it mean to be a patient and under what circumstances and conditions do we need care from a nurse? Contact with nurses, in their different roles and locations, can represent a status transition and force the individual to reconsider what help they need and from just where they might obtain it. Patients make transitions between home and hospital, hospital and clinic and have different experiences *en route*. Our conundrum on this occasion focuses upon a particular assertion made by a nurse:

Wherever the patient is, nursing remains the same. We're there to help and patients know what they can expect from professional carers.

Do you support this assertion? Is it equally true regarding patients and their experience of hospital or care in the community? Make a note of points in support of your answer and then read Chapter 10 to discover what psychologists offer regarding the experience of different health care environments and their impact upon access to social support from other sources.

Marks (2005) defines community health psychology as 'Advancing theory, research and social action to promote positive well-being, increase empowerment, and prevent the development of problems of communities, groups and individuals.' Whilst some aspects of this definition are all-encompassing (prevent the development of problems of communities, groups and individuals), the focus is clear – on the community rather than just the individual member and on promoting positive well-being and empowerment. To do this a knowledge of different areas is needed, such as environmental psychology, cross-cultural psychology, health promotion and community development.

Environment and behaviour

Lewin (1951) emphasised the importance of the environment by saying that all behaviour was a function of the interaction between person and environment. People do not exist in a vacuum but are part of their surroundings; they shape, and are shaped by, their environment. Therefore, when studying nursing in the community, it is necessary to construct a model of human behaviour that reflects the relationships between people and their habitat. Moos (1979) put forward a 'social ecology' model which represents this *person–environment fit.*

- *Physical setting.* Temperature, rainfall, pollution and architectural design are all important features of health behaviour. Arthritic patients who were exposed to stormlike pressure and humidity experienced increasing pain sensations (Hollander and Yeastros, 1963).
- *Organisational factors.* The size of an organisation and how the work space is structured can affect people's health.
- *Human aggregate.* This factor is concerned with the characteristics of the inhabitants of a particular environment. Gender, age, income, background and culture are some of the main components of the human aggregate. Some people refer to this factor as *social epidemiology.*
- *Social climate.* The extent to which people interact with and support each other are important dimensions of community care. The presence of functional social networks and support groups creates a positive social climate where people feel they have more control over their circumstances.

There are other features of Moos's 'social ecology' model, but these four variables represent the main categorisation of the environmental system and provide a useful template for assessing factors influencing health behaviour in the community. A clearer picture of the social ecology model can be obtained by selecting one area and looking at it within this framework.

Crowding and health

The physical setting

Galle *et al.* (1972) distinguished between four different elements of population density and crowding in Chicago: the number of persons per room, the number of rooms per housing unit, the number of housing units per residential structure and the number of residential structures per acre. They found a relationship between all four components and fertility, delinquency and hospital admission rates. Fuller *et al.* (1993) suggest that two major factors are thought to be involved in the relationship between health and crowding:

- High levels of crowding lead to an increase in stress which has an adverse effect on health.
- People living in close proximity with each other are likely to be more prone to communicable disease.

Organisational factors

Social density, or the number of people in a group, affects the influence of crowding on behaviour. Higher social density has been thought to increase complaints of illness, raise blood pressure and increase the number of psychiatric admissions (Paulus *et al.,* 1978). However, one has to take into consideration the ways in which space is used as well as the level of dwelling unit density. This last point is particularly relevant to the next factor, the human aggregate.

Human aggregate

A wellknown experiment by MacDonald and Oden (1973) illustrated how the use of space could mediate the effects of crowding. They examined three married couples who were trying to simulate the conditions they were about to experience during their work with the Peace Corps. The couples had to live together in one room 30 ft square for three months. This would seem to be a recipe for confrontation and conflict, yet, because the couples developed a high degree of co-operation with each other, they experienced little stress. Indeed, they were found to show enhanced marital relationships, were chosen as social-emotional leaders (see Chapter 6) by other volunteers and regretted leaving their accommodation more than those who had been assigned to living in a hotel. The co-operation between the couples had led to the development of decisional control over their environment which diminished the effects of the crowded space.

Social climate

Groups who show social cohesion are less likely to experience stress in crowded conditions than groups who do not get on well together. In a review of studies on crowding in dormitories, Karlin *et al.* (1979) found that uncohesive groups of individuals experienced more stress, acted more competitively, performed less well in exams and felt more helpless than their counterparts who had formed into socially cohesive groups.

Thus it appears that the effects of physical crowding can be tempered by the amount of perceived control that inhabitants have over their surroundings and in the personal relationships between residents. Living in crowded conditions need not produce stress and ill health if people get on well together and determine, as a group, to do something to improve the situation. Nurses working in the community can play a crucial role in facilitating the development of cohesive groups who can then evolve an agenda for dealing with their specific problems.

Noise, pollution and heat

Another way of investigating the environment is to examine the effects of specific features on health and behaviour. Just as noise, pollution and heat are important in a hospital context, so do they play an equally distinct role in the community. It is important for those nurses who work in the community to be aware of the ways in which certain features of the environment affect health and behaviour.

Noise

Cohen *et al.* (1986) reviewed the effects of environmental noise on health and behaviour. They found that people who, for instance, live near busy airports suffer a wide range of health disorders, such as cardiac insufficiency, pregnancy complications, high blood pressure, nervous and gastrointestinal diseases. Furthermore, unpredictable and uncontrollable sound levels have been described as more stressful than those under one's control (Evans and Cohen, 1987).

In one study which examined children from four primary schools situated beneath the flight path of Los Angeles airport (over 300 flights per day; one every two and a half minutes during school hours) the effects of the noise were found to increase the children's blood pressure and decrease their motivation for school work, compared with a matched sample of children from 'non-noisy' schools (Cohen *et al.,* 1979). Some people who live in noisy environments say that after a while they become unaware of the noise and adapt to it. However, these same children were examined a year later with similar results, indicating that adaptation to noise does not necessarily occur.

Pollution

The presence of high levels of photochemical oxidants (smog) in the atmosphere has been linked to people suffering from depression, hostility, anxiety and the increased use of healthcare facilities. Evans and Jacobs (1984) found that people suffering from stress were more susceptible to the negative effects of high levels of smog than those who reported less stress. Furthermore, the perception of the effects of pollution was tempered by how long the residents had lived in the area. People who had lived in areas with smog for a period of time regarded it as less of a problem, exaggerated their health and had a higher locus of control than those residents who had only recently moved into the area. Despite the physical and emotional dangers of smog, long-term residents seem to come to accept the pollution psychologically and not perceive it as a problem.

Thunder and lightning storms, wind and other atmospheric conditions that split ions into positive and negative do seem to affect individuals' moods. Baron (1987) found that the presence of negative ions increased whatever emotion was being experienced at the time. Thus, when negative ions were present, Type A individuals experienced more aggression, and people with similar attitudes liked each other more than those with dissimilar attitudes. Nurses working in the community should be aware not only of the effects of atmospheric pollution on physical health, but of the consequences for human behaviour as well.

Temperature

There seems to be a positive relationship between temperature and aggression, and people tend to become more irritable and unco-operative as the temperature rises. Simpson and Perry (1990) found in a study conducted in the United States that as the average monthly temperature rose, incidences of rape and aggravated assault also increased. Carlsmith and Anderson (1979) found that the most dangerous outbreaks of violence occurred when temperatures were in the mid-80s. Milder forms of aggression, such as car drivers beeping their horns, also increased with temperature. Kenrick and McFarlane (1986) measured the amount of horn beeping at a driver of a car that remained stationary at a green traffic light, and found the amount of beeping increased with increases in temperature during spring and summer days.

However, care must be exercised if causal connections are to be made between aggression and temperature, as other factors may be involved. For example, as the temperature rises people may increase their consumption of alcohol to quench their thirst, which may be the real cause of heightened interpersonal aggression.

The hospital environment

Hospitals have not always existed. The ancient Roman army was one of the first groups of people to provide 'hospitals', in the form of separate barracks for its ill or wounded soldiers. From about AD 542 Christian monasteries took on the role of caring for the sick, in addition to sheltering the poor and needy. During the eighteenth and nineteenth centuries, hospitals became much more specialised and established wards for different categories of illness. These institutions still catered mainly for poor people, who often died of their afflictions, and so most people, if they could afford it, were treated at home by private physicians. With the advances in medical knowledge and treatment at the end of the nineteenth century and the beginning of the twentieth, the reputation of hospitals improved and they became widely accepted as institutions with a variety of functions such as treating disease and injuries, preventing illness, conducting tests and research, teaching and assisting patients' rehabilitation. However, while the physical experience of hospital has vastly improved, the psychological experience of the hospital is still found to cause problems for both patients and staff.

Stress rating scales

Volicer *et al.* (1977) devised the Hospital Stress Rating Scale to assess the degree of stress patients experience during periods of hospitalisation. Medical and surgical hospital patients were asked to rate events in terms of their perceived stressfulness (see Table 11.1). From these results it can be seen that some of the most stressful events involved lack of communication – not being told the nature of the diagnosis (34.1 per cent); having one's questions ignored (27.6 per cent); not knowing the results of, or reasons for, treatment (31.9 per cent); and staff talking too fast or using difficult words (26.4 per cent).

Maslach (1982) used the Maslach Burnout Inventory (MBI) to measure the stress experienced by nurses in the hospital environment. She found that there was a relation-ship between the amount of time spent taking care of patients and emotional exhaus-tion. Emotional exhaustion was defined as 'feeling tired when thinking about going to work'. Guppy and Gutteridge (1991) looked at the factors that were associated with perceptions of stress reported by nurses in a general hospital. The main factors concerned with the sources of stress were: interpersonal relations, resource problems and dealing with death. There were no differences between the wards in the hospital in relation to stress; however, there were differences according to grade of nurse, and job satisfaction was correlated with nursing experience.

A positive feature of surveys such as those conducted by Volicer *et al.* is that the prob-lems that have been identified as important by patients are not insoluble. However, communication and understanding *can* be improved, as the following experiment by Ley *et al.* (1976) illustrates. Patients on three wards of a general hospital were assigned to three conditions.

- *Ward A.* Patients were given an extra visit by nurses or doctors every ten days. During these visits attempts were made to ensure that the patients had understood what they had been told about their condition and treatment. No new information was provided, as the purpose of the visit was to clarify existing information..
- *Ward B.* Patients were given extra visits to discuss their welfare and food, but received no clarification of the information given.
- *Ward C.* No extra visits were given.

The results of this experiment indicated that the patients from Ward A were approxi-mately twice as satisfied with the way they had been treated as patients from the other two wards. In Ward A 80 per cent of patients were satisfied with communication; in Ward B 41 per cent were satisfied and in Ward C 48 per cent were satisfied. The results of this study indicate that one of the main problems facing patients in hospital is that of uncertainty over procedures and information given, but with a little more effort from both nurses and doctors, this uncertainty can be significantly reduced.

Surgery-related stress

Uncertainty may be particularly apparent in those patients waiting for surgery or inva-sive medical procedures. In Chapter 10, techniques for coping with stress were found to

Table 11.1 *Perceived stressfulness of events experienced during hospitalisation*
(adapted from Volicer et al., 1977)

Stress-scale events	Mean rank score
Unfamiliarity of surroundings	
Having strangers sleep in the same room as you	13.9
Having to sleep in a strange bed	15.9
Having strange machines around	16.8
Being awakened in the night by the nurse	16.9
Being aware of unusual smells around you	19.4
Being in a room that is too cold or too hot	21.7
Having to eat cold or tasteless food	23.2
Being cared for by an unfamiliar doctor	23.4
Loss of independence	
Having to eat at different times than you usually do	15.4
Having to wear a hospital gown	16.0
Having to be assisted with bathing	17.0
Not being able to get newspapers, radio or television when you want them	17.7
Having a room mate who has too many visitors	18.1
Having to stay in bed or the same room all day	19.1
Having to be assisted with a bedpan	21.5
Not having your call light answered	27.3
Being fed through tubes	29.2
Thinking you may lose your sight	40.6
Separation from spouse	
Worrying about your spouse being away from you	22.7
Missing your spouse	28.4
Financial problems	
Thinking about losing income because of your illness	25.9
Not having enough insurance to pay for your hospitalisation	27.4
Isolation from other people	
Having a room mate who is seriously ill or cannot talk to you	21.2
Having a room mate who is unfriendly	21.6
Not having friends visit you	21.7
Not being able to call family or friends on the phone	23.3
Having the staff be in too much of a hurry	24.5
Thinking you might lose your hearing	34.5

Table 11.1 *(continued)*

Lack of information
- Thinking you might have pain because of surgery or test procedures — 22.4
- Not knowing when to expect things will be done to you — 24.2
- Having nurses or doctors talk too fast or use words you can't understand — 26.4
- Not having your questions answered by the staff — 27.6
- Not knowing the results or reasons for your treatments — 31.9
- Not knowing for sure what illnesses you have — 34.0
- Not being told what your diagnosis is — 34.1

Threat of severe illness
- Thinking your appearance might be changed after your hospitalisation — 22.1
- Being put in the hospital because of an accident — 26.9
- Knowing you have to have an operation — 26.9
- Having a sudden hospitalisation you weren't planning to have — 27.2
- Knowing you have a serious illness — 34.6
- Thinking you might lose a kidney or some other organ — 35.6
- Thinking you might have cancer — 39.2

Separation from family
- Being in the hospital during holidays or special family occasions — 22.3
- Not having family visit you — 26.5
- Being hospitalised far away from home — 27.1

Problems with medications
- Having medications cause you discomfort — 26.0
- Feeling you are getting dependent on medications — 26.4
- Not getting relief from pain medications — 31.2
- Not getting pain medication when you need it — 32.4

fall into behavioural, cognitive and emotional control categories. Similarly, styles of coping with surgery and unpleasant invasive techniques also fall into these categories.

Cognitive control is concerned with enabling patients to focus on the positive aspects of the medical procedure, such as the benefits, whilst ignoring the unpleasant features. Langner *et al.* (1975) investigated the use of cognitive control in patients waiting to undergo types of surgery which typically had favourable prognoses, such as hernia and hysterectomy operations. One group of patients received training in the use of cognitive control. This involved discussion about what the positive aspects of the surgery might be, and then patients were encouraged to think about these positive features when feeling distressed about the surgery. The control group of patients spent an equal amount of time engaging in general conversation. Nurses rated the behaviour of both groups of patients before and after surgery and kept a note of patients' requests for pain relief. Those patients who received the cognitive control training were found to have lower levels of both pre- and post-operative stress, and made fewer requests for medication than the patients in the control group.

Behavioural and informational control reduce discomfort by getting the patients to perform actions that are incompatible with the stress of the procedure, such as relaxation, breathing and coughing exercises. These also provide knowledge about the sort of sensations to expect during the procedure. Anderson (1987) found that giving male cardiac patients waiting for coronary bypass surgery both informational and behavioural control reduced the patients' anxiety before and after the operation. The patients were given the standard preparation for surgery, which consisted of the patient and the nurse discussing two pamphlets outlining the procedures relating to the surgery. Patients then watched a video about the procedure, which included interviews with patients who had successfully recovered from the operation. They were also given an audio-tape describing sensations they might experience. Finally the patients were taught how to perform behaviours such as coughing exercises and ways to turn in bed after the operation. Generally speaking, if patients have a limited opportunity to take an active role in coping, informational and cognitive control are particularly effective preparations for surgery and for stressful medical procedures. When patients can take some form of direct action in relation to their condition, behavioural control should be used to reduce discomfort.

Corney *et al.* (1992) interviewed 105 patients who had undergone major surgery for carcinoma of the cervix or vulva in the previous five years. They found a high proportion of their sample depressed and reporting chronic sexual problems. Both the patients and spouses indicated that they would have liked more information on the after-effects of the operation, including the physical, sexual and emotional aspects.

Social domain and surgery

The social domain should also be considered in the context of preparation for surgery. Kulik and Mahler (1989) studied patients who were scheduled for coronary bypass surgery. Two nights before the operation the patients were asked whether they would like to share a room with a person who was scheduled to undergo the same operation; a person who was recovering from the same operation; or if it made no difference who they shared with.

The results indicated that 60 per cent of patients preferred to share a room with someone who had just had the operation compared with 23 per cent who had no preference, and 17 per cent who would prefer to share with a person waiting for the same operation. This would seem to support the patient's need to be provided with accurate information, in this instance about what the operation actually feels like from a patient's perspective.

Stages in patient care

To indicate that hospitalisation involves a period of preparation for admission as well as a period of readjustment after discharge, Kincey (1989) provided a model that considers these stages in the care of patients.

The pre-operative stage

It is important to realise that the cognitive and emotional reactions of patients vary enormously and high levels of anxiety may interfere with their ability to understand and make decisions about information. Certainly the patient needs to be clear about whether the surgery is essential or optional.

A patient's level of understanding should be ascertained and any gaps or misconceptions corrected. It is probably a good idea at this stage to find out the coping style of the patient and tailor the information given on procedural details accordingly.

If probabilities are used in relation to outcomes, then care should be taken to consider the difficulties patients may experience in understanding the implications of certain courses of action, especially if they are feeling nervous or anxious.

The pre-operative admission information should not only give clear, relevant, factual information about hospital policy and self-preparation, but should also make patients feel free to ask about procedures and conduct.

Post-operative hospitalisation stage

After recovery from the anaesthetic, the patients should be given clear verbal feedback about the surgical procedure that has been undertaken.

Nurses should be aware that patterns of pain experience vary considerably between patients undergoing the same surgical procedure. The absence of verbal requests for pain relief may not correlate with non-verbal signals:

> Ward staff should recognise that patients are assessing their own recovery in terms of comparisons with other patients whom they perceive as undergoing a similar process, and in terms of their own expectations of how rapidly they should recover after surgery.
>
> (Kincey, 1989)

Therefore it is important for nurses to be able to correct misinterpretations and point out appropriate progress comparisons.

The self-care information presented to patients before discharge should be framed in specific behavioural terms. That is (when it is possible to be exact), information should be given about when it would be safe to engage in walking, resume sexual activity, lifting, and so on. Patients should be told if it is impossible to predict the exact timing of activities.

Post-discharge stage

Psychological, as well as physical, progress should be assessed post-discharge. Major surgery can engender loss of physical function, changes in self-image and numerous other psychological sequelae. Reactions may include anger, depression and anxiety, all of which should be dealt with in an accepting manner.

At some point the opinion of either specialist or lay support groups should be considered. However, this action should not be forced on patients, and if they are uncertain about whether to seek help a familiar person and setting should be used to set up initial contact.

Wilson-Barnett and Carrigy (1978) monitored patients' daily emotional reactions from the time that they were admitted to a general hospital ward to the time when they were discharged. Emotional reactions were measured using a mood adjective checklist, interviews with the patients and the Eysenck Personality Inventory. The first finding to emerge was that patients' anxiety scores were significantly higher during the first twenty-four hours of their hospital stay than the average of the scores during their entire stay in hospital. This occurred for both anxious and non-anxious patients. Factors that did not seem to be important were age, sex and whether the patients had been admitted from the waiting list or as emergencies. Some of the reasons given by the patients for their anxiety included 'not wanting to leave the family'; 'fear of hospitals'; and 'worries about illness'. Those patients who rated themselves as 'not so ill' felt more negative about their admission to hospital.

A significant finding of the study was the relationship between the patient's personality and the time taken to adjust to the hospital. Those patients who scored highly for emotionality took longer to adjust, and in many cases it took these patients up to five days to become attuned to the hospital. Wilson-Barnett and Carrigy concluded that those patients who have a highly emotional disposition probably respond to admission with negative emotions which will then persist for some time. Others may initially report feelings of anxiety and unhappiness but lose them after a day or two.

Privacy and territoriality

Privacy

One feature of day-to-day life which has to be compromised on admission to hospital is privacy. In addition to the discomfort caused by their illness, patients have to put up with exposing their bodies to strangers. Whilst this is accepted as a feature of being in hospital, it is not a normal feature of everyday life. Similarly, when people wish to have private conversations they are usually at liberty to do so, but in hospital it is not always easy to. In some instances patient privacy may be at odds with the nurse's need to effectively monitor their patients. Gadbois *et al.* (1992) analysed the spatial and temporal organisation of the work of nurses in medical and surgical units of a French hospital. The units were designed around a U-shaped configuration. An analysis of nurses' trips completing various aspects of their work indicated that this was not the best design as far as work load was concerned. Jaco (1979) found that the type of ward design most favoured by nurses for patient observation was a radial arrangement; however, this was the design least preferred by patients when privacy was considered. This illustrates an important point – that in many cases it will prove impossible for patients to have privacy when they are in hospital. The role of the nurse is to try to make them feel that they do have some control over their environment. If, despite the adverse circumstances, patients develop a feeling of control over their privacy, their levels of stress and anxiety will be reduced, leading to increased levels of health and well-being.

Placing screens and curtains around a patient's bed does afford some privacy, even though the barrier is acoustically imperfect. However, some patients are reluctant to ask for privacy, since they are scared of being labelled 'difficult'. Again, if it is not possible to give patients direct control over opening or closing curtains, blinds or screens, they must be made to feel that they can ask for assistance whenever they wish. Attention to what may be regarded as cosmetic, or even petty, details does have substantial psychological benefits which can be measured in both financial and medical terms. Cameron (1993) investigated what constituted comfort from a patient's perspective. The findings indicated that comfort was not viewed as a passive process, with patients waiting to receive help, but as a dynamic process, with each patient actively engaged in increasing comfort levels.

Territoriality

Territoriality is related to privacy in as much as it is also concerned with the use of personal and public space. People naturally feel more comfortable when they are on their home ground. Altman (1975) has classified territories into three types.

- *Primary territories:* places where people are able to exert complete control, such as their own homes.
- *Secondary territories:* these are semi-public areas affording limited access to strangers. Examples are the front path of a house or its doorway.
- *Public territories:* areas where access is provided to everybody, for example a park bench or a shopping mall.

Although these are defined territories, there can be a tendency in some cultures to try to change public territory into primary or secondary territories by placing items of clothing such as a coat or hat on a seat to discourage others from sitting there. Finding a spare seat on a bus or train is fine, but how much better it is when one finds a seat with three vacant ones surrounding it.

Schumaker and Reizenstein (1984) state that:

Hospitalised patients leave the comfort and security of their homes (primary territories) and enter an unfamiliar setting in which the classification of territory is ambiguous. Although they are assigned to their 'own rooms,' patients have no choice in the furnishings of the room and only limited control over who enters the room, or when a person enters it. In addition, patients are expected to perform behaviours in this environment that they have heretofore usually confined to their own primary territories (e.g. sleeping and resting, discussing personal issues with friends, and grooming).

They go on to suggest a number of 'benefits and barriers' to the personalisation of the hospital environment, including the following:

- Patients should have as much opportunity as possible to personalise their setting in the hospital, as this reduces the negative impact of the discontinuity between leaving the home environment and entering the hospital habitat.
- There should be consultation between patients, nurses and those involved with hospital design with regard to the personalisation of space.
- Although the specific details of personalisation may differ from one hospital to another, consideration should be given to such items as a bulletin board viewable from the patient's bed, a locker for clothes with shelves for grooming materials and a table within easy reach of the patient.

The following obstacles, or barriers, to the implementation of personalised patient space should be considered.

- Space in hospitals is a 'valued commodity', therefore consideration should be given to providing space for the patients and the space required for other needs.
- Often there is a requirement for technical equipment, which will compete with a patient's personalised space.
- Too much personalised space can disrupt the provision of appropriate nursing care.

Noise in the hospital environment

Noise is a psychological concept and is defined as sound that is unwanted by the listener because it is unpleasant, bothersome, interferes with important activities, or is believed to be physiologically harmful.

(Kryter, 1970).

Noise can inflict most irritation when people find themselves in a new environment. For example, people who go to live near a railway line, or on a busy road may have difficulty sleeping at first, but soon habituate to the noisy environment and after a while seem not to notice the noise at all. Indeed, when these same people are placed in a quiet environment, they often experience discomfort at the lack of noise.

In hospitals, while some of the sounds may not be loud, they may nevertheless still cause considerable irritation. The sounds which occur in intensive care units may cause significant stress, disturbance and sleep problems for patients, but at the the same time may be perceived as normal and necessary for patient care by the nursing staff (Topf, 1992).

Unfamiliar, unpredictable and uncontrollable sounds have been described as particularly stressful stimuli. With this in mind, it must be remembered that patients are often particularly sensitive to noise owing to the fact that they are ill and in many cases experiencing little, or no, stimulation. One has only to think of how we feel when we hear a strange sound in the middle of the night to appreciate what some patients may feel on their first night in hospital (Evans and Cohen, 1987).

The use of light in the hospital environment

Unfortunately, the needs of patients and hospital staff are often at odds where lighting is concerned. In many circumstances medical staff require high levels of illumination, whereas patients often prefer low levels. High levels of illumination produce greater productivity and increased accuracy and have also been evaluated as less stressful by staff (Barnaby, 1980). On the other hand, patients may need low levels of lighting to rest and sleep, and indeed, feelings of warmth, comfort and relaxation are usually associated with low levels of illumination. However, an experiment by Martynuik *et al.* (1973) illustrated that the different lighting needs of patients and staff *can* be accommodated in one unit. Groups of patients and staff were placed in a room with six different lighting systems and were asked to rate the lighting arrangements on perceptual clarity and spaciousness. The participants were also given pairs of words such as pleasant–unpleasant; satisfying–frustrating; relaxed–tense and asked to rate each lighting system on a scale within each pair of words. The most popular choice for all participants was a combination of overhead downlighting with peripheral and overhead diffuse lighting. The main implication of this and other studies is that appropriate hospital lighting arrangements *can* be produced if planners are prepared to consult nurses and patients on the type of lighting that reflects everyone's needs. In the same vein, expertise should be brought to bear on the design of windows, the type of glass used and the integration of natural and artificial lighting.

Pollution and smells

A polluted working environment can be at the least irritating and at the worst unbearable. It has been found that there are large individual differences in the sorts of odours that people find irritating, as people tend to habituate to odours. Some people who work all day in a 'smelly' environment become totally unaware of the odour and it can come as a shock when people unused to the smell reflect their distaste, either verbally or non-verbally. However, it should be recognised that some forms of pollution and some smells *can* be reduced. Many hospitals operate a 'no smoking' policy, where smoking is prohibited except in designated smoking rooms. This policy works well as long as the people who smoke do not feel victimised and help is provided for those wishing to give up smoking. Some hospital odours are unavoidable, and a good ventilation system is essential.

The hidden message

It may seem that to concentrate resources on developing 'user friendly' lighting systems or on reducing obnoxious smells is trivial in comparison with the 'real' needs for life-saving hospital equipment. This may be so, but consider the following points.

- All hospitals convey a 'hidden' meaning or message to patients. This message is communicated largely by the attention paid to the sorts of details mentioned. Often it is the 'little things' that have the most influence on a patient's first impression of the hospital.
- When designing new hospital environments, ideally patients and staff should be allowed to consult the designers and architects to produce a hospital that reflects the needs of the people who live and work there. This is not necessarily a matter of finance.
- The design and structure of the wards and rooms, the provision of plants and suitable furnishings, and attention to physical comfort and privacy can communicate warmth and personal control as well as professionalism and competence.
- The hidden message should be 'You are important!'

Sick role behaviour

When patients enter hospital they normally have some idea of what is expected and how they should behave. Lorber (1975) interviewed over 100 patients at the beginning of their stay in hospital. The patients were all over 40 years of age and had been admitted for surgery ranging from moderate to serious in terms of severity. The patients were asked to indicate whether they agreed or disagreed with the following series of statements.

The best thing to do in the hospital is to keep quiet and do what you are told.

I co-operate best as a patient when I know the reason for what I have to do.

When I am sick, I expect to be pampered and catered to.

On the basis of the patient's responses to these questions, they were allocated to either a 'passive' or an 'active' group. Thus, if a patient agreed with the first statement and disagreed with the second and the third, they would be assigned to the passive, conforming group.

At the end of each patient's stay in hospital Lorber interviewed them again. She found that the patients' sick role beliefs were an indicator of their reported hospital behaviour. Those patients who had been assigned to the passive group were less likely to argue and complain then those in the active group. Before the patients were discharged the medical staff were asked to rate the patients as 'good', 'average' or 'problem', and to provide descriptions of each patient's behaviour and their reaction to it. In most cases, the patients rated as 'good' were found to be co-operative, uncomplaining and stoical while those rated as 'problem' were unco-operative, complaining, over-emotional and dependent. Patients who were *too* passive could also cause the nurses problems. In one instance, a patient who was very ill did not want to bother the nurses, even when she really needed care. Consequently the nurses frequently had to check on her status, which disrupted routines.

The nurses in this study recognised that 'problem' behaviour could stem from a severe medical condition and distinguished between two types of patients:

- Those patients who are very ill and often have a poor prognosis. Because of the severity of their condition nurses accept their behaviour and realise that they need a lot of attention.
- Those patients who are perceived as taking up more nursing time than they actually need or is warranted by their condition. These patients, it is often felt, frequently complain, argue and fail to co-operate.

Problem patients

Why are some patients seen as 'a problem' in hospital? One answer to this question is that *reactance* has occurred. in Chapter 2 it was suggested that when people feel that their sense of autonomy is being denied they react against the source of the denial and the people associated with it. In the context of hospitalisation, some patients feel that their freedom and ability to think and act for themselves are being eroded. A patient may not be allowed to get out of bed because of their injuries, or to watch television late at night because it would disturb the other patients. The response to reactance is anger and a determination to be as unco-operative as possible. Taylor (1979) says that reactance can manifest itself in:

> petty acts of mutiny such as making passes at nurses, drinking in one's room, smoking against medical advice, and wandering up and down the halls. Such minor incidents tend to irritate nursing and custodial staff, but rarely do any damage. However, petty acts of mutiny can turn into self-sabotage, such as failing to take medications

which are essential to recovery, or engaging in acts which have potentially fatal consequences.

Although the ideal way of dealing with such patients is to respond in an assertive rather than an aggressive manner, giving reassurances and providing explanations, this does not always occur. There can often be a tendency to ignore or criticise a patient's problem behaviour and to respond less quickly to their calls for attention.

Another explanation for 'problem' patients is based on the notion that the main fault with studies such as Lorber's (1975) is that they cast the patient in the role of either good or bad. In their review of 'good' and 'bad' patients Kelly and May (1982) suggest that patients come to be defined as good or bad not because they have a particularly 'difficult' personality or possess behavioural quirks but as a consequence of the interactions that take place between nurses and patients. They say that nurses symbolically take on the role of the patient both to make, and to make sense of, their own role, and it is in doing so that the labelling of patients inevitably takes place. The good patient is one who confirms the role of the nurse while the bad patient denies that legitimation.

Essentially, Kelly and May are saying that sick role behaviour should be viewed not as a patient *characteristic* but as an *interaction* between medical staff, the hospital environment and the patients. This perspective suggests that nurses have a much more positive role to play in affecting the behaviour of patients, and by looking at their own actions they can analyse how they react to specific situations. Johnson and Webb (2004) support this view. In their study of 'popularity' in one medical ward they say, 'Our argument is that social evaluations are not, in any way, tied to traits or variables which patients do or do not possess. Rather, evaluations of people in the ward were socially constructed in relation to a complex web of powerful social influences.'

One of the main problems associated with hospitalisation is not the label 'good' or 'bad' patient but the label 'patient'. Effectively, the message associated with the patient role is one which ascribes powerlessness, helplessness and insignificance. A 'patient' sits or lies passively while all responsibility, decisions, procedures, basic care functions and planning are undertaken by the medical staff, often without the person involved being told what is happening. All this strips away personal status, dignity and control (Nichols, 2003). One factor that has been found to be instrumental in the development of feelings of lack of control on entering the hospital environment is *confusion*. Kornfield (1972) suggested that there were three sorts of confusion.

- *Geographical confusion.* What is 'patient territory' and what is not? Finding one's way around large hospitals can be very daunting, and signs can often be confusing and use unfamiliar terminology. Arriving for the first time at a hospital and not knowing where to go or how to get there causes a great deal of anxiety. If one works in the same environment for some time a 'cognitive map' develops, and what may have seemed a maze becomes commonplace to the extent that directions seem obvious.

However, this is not the case for the newcomer. What seem to be clear instructions to someone who has worked in a hospital for some time may not be so clear to someone who is new to the situation. The best way to help people find their way is to take them to their destination and say, 'I was just going there myself.' This may not always be possible, for a whole host of reasons, but one should try to give directions in a patient-centred fashion. It may seem trivial to give attention to helping patients find their way in the hospital environment, but their first impression is all-important. If on entering the hospital environs patients feel 'cared for', they will have developed a positive first impression which will often remain with them (see Chapter 2).

- *Subcultural confusion*: a state of wondering who does what and when. It refers to not knowing who people in the hospital are and what they are supposed to do or not do.
- *Role confusion*: where questions such as 'How am I supposed to behave in this situation?' or 'How are my needs going to be met?' and 'How am I meant to communicate with the nurses and doctors?' are asked.

Nichols (2003) says that one way to reduce confusion is for the nurse to adopt a teaching role. The nurse should try to determine which aspects of the hospital are confusing to the patient and which features of the environment cause particular difficulties. In an attempt to provide client-centred care in a renal unit, the unit psychologist and the nursing staff got together to produce the following aims.

- To attempt to produce an environment where patients perceive themselves as 'associates' of the health care team and as such are included whenever possible in decision making about their treatment.
- To require the patients to try to keep themselves informed, thus reducing the stress of 'not knowing'.
- To use the unit's educational facility to try to achieve self-efficacy in dialysis, diet and exercise.
- To take advantage of emotional care and support.

Although this regime puts pressure on patients to take an active role in their own care, Nichols suggests that the majority of patients do take up the invitation to work with the health care staff. Finally, he says that staff have needs too and a balanced, negotiated compromise is the situation most likely to succeed.

Children and hospitalisation

The process of hospitalisation can prove particularly upsetting for children. (See Chapter 2 for a discussion of the effects of hospitalisation on child development.) Super (1981) found that the distress associated with hospitalisation and short-term separations peaked at about 15 months of age in a wide variety of cultures. The experience can be made easier, however, if parents can be involved in preparing their children for a stay in hospital. Sarafino (1986) suggested that parents can:

- explain the reasons why the child has to visit the hospital;
- provide the child with opportunities to ask questions about what is going to happen to them and provide answers which are easily understood;
- if available, read through booklets on children's admission to hospital with their child;
- when taking the child to hospital, explain the procedures for going to the toilet and other such routines, and point out that they will be able to have breakfast in bed;
- tell the child when and how often they (the parents) will be able to be with them.
- preserve a calm and relaxed manner in order to convey a matter of fact approach to the changes in their child's circumstances.

Giving children information about their hospital stay

There is a certain amount of controversy concerning the amount of information children should be given prior to medical procedures. Melamed and Siegel (1975) investigated the use of a video entitled *Ethan has an operation* in preparing 4 to 12 year old children for hernias and tonsillectomies. The children were split into two groups and matched for age, gender, culture and the type of operation they were about to undergo. One group saw the operation video while the other group watched a video about a boy going on a trip to the countryside. The operation video portrayed the events that Ethan experienced from the time of his admission to hospital to the time of his discharge, and although he was visibly apprehensive at first, he gradually overcame his anxiety and completed the treatment without distress.

The experimenters used three methods to assess the emotional adjustment of the children to being hospitalised: *skin conductance*; *self-reports of anxiety*; and *observers' ratings of emotional behaviour*. The two groups were assessed the evening before the surgery and again three weeks after discharge. The results indicated that all three measures demonstrated that there was a significant difference between the two groups' anxiety levels. The group that watched the 'operation' video experienced less anxiety before and after the operation than those who saw the 'trip to the country' film.

Monitoring and blunting

Thus there seems to be evidence that children may benefit from exposure to materials such as videos which portray events in hospital. However, it must be recognised that some children employ a *blunting* strategy to deal with stress and anxiety. These children do not want to know what is about to happen to them, as they are attempting to deny the stressful elements of the procedure, and preparations of this type may make them more anxious. For instance, Buchanan and Niven (2003) found that whilst children tended to adopt blunting procedures when given information liable to produce anxiety, the adults providing the information were predominantly monitors

Dahlquist *et al.* (1986) suggested that timing, the child's age and previous medical experiences are other factors to consider when preparing children for hospitalisation. Children younger than 7 years of age seem to prefer being presented with information shortly before the medical procedure, whereas older children like to have the details some time before the event. Also, young children appear to be made *more* anxious by information if they have previously experienced uncomfortable medical experiences.

It can be difficult for nurses who are familiar with the hospital environment and the medical procedures that occur within it to appreciate what it is like from the patient's point of view. However, it is important to try to see things from the perspective of the patient who is unfamiliar with, and somewhat apprehensive about, what is going to happen to them. The more one is able to understand the needs and concerns of patients, the less daunting an experience hospitalisation will be for them.

The ecology of human development

Bronfenbrenner (1979) once criticised the number of psychology experiments conducted in the laboratory by saying that developmental psychology had become 'the science of the strange behaviour of children in strange situations with strange adults for the briefest possible periods of time'. Possibly the same could be said of studying health behaviour in a hospital environment – it is an attempt to study the strange behaviour of people in strange situations with strange adults for brief periods of time. Working in the community at least enables nurses to observe people in their familiar and usual environment. As mentioned before, people do not exist in a vacuum but interact with their environment in such a way as to influence and be influenced by their habitat. Therefore, in order to gain a more appropriate view of human behaviour one must study it in relation to the surroundings. Bronfenbrenner (1979) proposes that we view the development of individuals within their ecological environment, which he defines as a nested arrangement of concentric structures, each contained within the next. He refers to these structures as the *micro-, meso-, exo-* and *macrosystems* and defines them as follows.

- *The microsystem.* This is a pattern of activities that occur in a particular setting such as a school, day care centre or the home. It refers to the personal relations between people and the roles they play in these settings.
- *The mesosystem.* The mesosystem is in fact a group, or system, of microsystems. For a child these might be the relations between home, school and friends; for an adult, between family, work and social life.
- *The exosystem.* This refers to one or more settings not directly involving the individual, but having an indirect effect on their behaviour. The exosystem for a young child might be the parents' place of work or an older brother or sister's class at school.

● *The macrosystem.* This system is consonant with culture, subculture or ethnic group. The essential ingredients of settings such as schools, cafes and medical practices are the same in all countries, yet there are important differences which are determined by the diversity of cultural and ethnic groups.

Bronfenbrenner's framework allows us to view individual behaviour in a much broader perspective. It provides a template which nurses can use to represent individuals in their community context, thus facilitating the development of more effective care plans and health promotion programmes.

Social networks and support

We have seen in Chapters 9 and 10 that social support affects a person's physical and psychological well-being and that it is important to distinguish between different types of support (informational, practical, emotional) and different types of social network (large versus small; dense versus distributed). Community nurses are in an ideal position to aid the development of social networks and also to use established networks for the implementation of indirect care. (The area of social support and indirect care is discussed in greater detail in Milne, 1993: chapter 8.) However, a review by Gillis (1993) of the determinants of a health-promoting lifestyle point to social support being second only to self-efficacy as the best predictor of a health-promoting lifestyle.

The use of Bronfenbrenner's approach to describing the community enables nurses to locate individuals within a group of nested systems; however, it does not give an indication of the relationships between individuals within these systems. Constructing a person's social network gives the nurse information on who is in the network, the frequency of interactions, their duration, the nature of their content, and so on.

Exercise 11.1 *Support from social networks* © Glenys Parry,
from *Coping with Crises*, Blackwell Publishing, 1990

This exercise takes quite a time, but most people find the results interesting and, what is more, you will be able to use the technique with others if you have first practised it en yourself.

First, make a list of people in your social network in the spaces on the left of the grid in Table 11.2. (There is room for twenty people; if you want to include more, add more spaces.) How do you decide who to include and who to leave out? The following guidelines will lead to a workable network for understanding crisis support. Write down the names of:

- *Members of your family* whom you see regularly. (Exclude distant relations you never see or see only at formal family gatherings.)
- *Friends* you see regularly or with whom you keep in contact by letter and telephone.
- *Neighbours,* if you regularly go into each other's homes. (Exclude neighbours with whom you pass the time of day in the street.)
- *Colleagues,* if you have frequent contact and feel there is a personal relationship but exclude those with whom you have only formal, impersonal contact.
- *Include* anyone else who is emotionally significant to you although you may be temporarily estranged or separated.
- *Exclude* casual acquaintances, purely professional contacts (e.g. dentist, accountant) or people you know only through someone else.

After making the list, start with name 1 and go along the row: the numbers along the top refer to the other people on the list. Under each column ask, 'Do these two people have a relationship with each other?' If in doubt about defining 'relationship', use the same criteria as above. Place a tick in each box where a relationship definitely exists, and a question mark if there is only a weak relationship or if you are not sure. Repeat this procedure for name 2, name 3 and so on until the grid is complete

Next, for each person, tick (using the four right-hand columns) if you would turn to this person for support in a crisis The kind of support you would look to them for is as follows:

E emotional support.
P practical help.
C companionship.
A advice and information.

Then take a plain piece of paper and sketch out a diagram of your network, using circles to represent relatives, triangles for friends and squares for colleagues. Draw a solid line between two people who have a tick, and a dotted line for a question mark. You may need two or three sketches before you are happy with the best way of arranging the people and the lines between them.

Take four copies of the final diagram and take four different-colour pens to represent the four types of support. On each diagram separately, highlight your potential sources of support. (You can do this all on the one diagram, but it might become muddled and hard to see the different colours clearly.)

Table 11.2 Social network grid

Name	1	2	3	4	5	6	7	8	9	10	11	12	13	14	15	16	17	18	19	20	E	P	C	A
1	*																							
2	*	*																						
3	*	*	*																					
4	*	*	*	*																				
5	*	*	*	*	*																			
6	*	*	*	*	*	*																		
7	*	*	*	*	*	*	*																	
8	*	*	*	*	*	*	*	*																
9	*	*	*	*	*	*	*	*	*															
10	*	*	*	*	*	*	*	*	*	*														
11	*	*	*	*	*	*	*	*	*	*	*													
12	*	*	*	*	*	*	*	*	*	*	*	*												
13	*	*	*	*	*	*	*	*	*	*	*	*	*											
14	*	*	*	*	*	*	*	*	*	*	*	*	*	*										
15	*	*	*	*	*	*	*	*	*	*	*	*	*	*	*									
16	*	*	*	*	*	*	*	*	*	*	*	*	*	*	*	*								
17	*	*	*	*	*	*	*	*	*	*	*	*	*	*	*	*	*							
18	*	*	*	*	*	*	*	*	*	*	*	*	*	*	*	*	*	*						
19	*	*	*	*	*	*	*	*	*	*	*	*	*	*	*	*	*	*	*					
20	*	*	*	*	*	*	*	*	*	*	*	*	*	*	*	*	*	*	*	*				

Analysing the social network and support diagram
You now have a social network diagram which highlights the sources of four different types of help. The following questions will help you think about the results.

- How many people are there in your network? (An average size would be about twelve, but remember that quality is just as important as quantity.)
- Is your network high or low-density? That is, are there many lines between all the members or only a few?
- Are there sub-clusters of relatively dense groups linked only by ore or two solid or dotted lines?
- Is your network dominated by one group, whether relatives, friends or colleagues or does it contain people from all these domains?

Now look at the four types of social support Are you using the whole of your network for support or only a small proportion of it? Are the same few people being used for all four types of support or do you spread the load? Is there any one type of support which is dearly lacking in your network? Thinking about these questions will often reveal ways in which you are not mobilising help as effectively as you could.

Of course nurses do not have to construct formal networks for each individual but it is a good idea to have some knowledge of the main features of the network so that key members can be enlisted to give support. Dean (1986) describes a study where key members of a person's network were used to promote health. Women who were likely to give birth to premature and low birth weight babies were given information about smoking, drinking, labour, delivery and care of the baby. Throughout the project, members of the women's social network attended the sessions so that they got the same information as the prospective mothers, knew what to expect, and know what community services were available. Dean claims that the inclusion of network members in the process of health promotion led to a greater acceptance of information and greater use of community services. The study is also useful as it gives examples of the sort of questions to ask to obtain an idea of a person's social network. As suggested at the beginning of this section, nurses can also be influential in creating opportunities for social networks to develop, and this is a major feature of the community development approach to health promotion.

Community development

One of the main problems for nursing in the community is gaining access to those people who really need attention. Often the people who need help the most are those who are the most reluctant to have anything to do with health professionals. There seems to be a greater prevalence of ill health in the lower income groups (Whitehead, 1987). This has posed problems for nurses engaged in health promotion, since these groups of people do not seem to respond to the more traditional health promotion methods, such as mass media campaigns (Gatherer, 1980). The community development approach seeks to tackle such barriers to good health by:

- responding to the perceived and expressed needs of a particular community;
- not imposing predetermined ideas and prescriptive programmes upon the community;
- improving social skills, self-esteem, assertiveness and reducing feelings of powerlessness;
- developing and facilitating self-help groups.

By concentrating on trying to get people to gather information and learn for themselves, nurses can encourage people to become more empowered and self-reliant.

A community development health project: 'Health in the shop front'

In 1987 a project was set up to try to promote community health by providing individuals and local groups with appropriate information and support to make informed health decisions. The project was situated in the north-east of England and attempted to achieve its aim in two ways. These were: to provide a 'drop in' information and advice service on all aspects of health, its maintenance, and on health-related services (statutory and non-statutory); and to provide support for local self-help groups, offering a range of services to groups or to individuals wishing to set up local self-help groups.

The project was situated in a 'shop front' in the middle of a city centre so that people would notice and take advantage of the information centre. The centre was open four days a week for members of the public to drop in for free confidential information on all aspects of health. People did not need an appointment nor did they need to give any personal details, thus ensuring anonymity. As the site in the shopping centre of the city was non-medical in appearance, it tended to attract people who would not normally use medical-type services. The centre was staffed by a senior health education officer who was also an experienced nurse, and information was made accessible through face-to-face contact. The centre acted as a central information store and referral agent, not just for statutory services such as GPs and health visitors, but also for non-statutory services, such as voluntary and self-help organisations.

The centre also acted as a self-help support project. Many of the self-help groups in the area did not require any assistance, but for those that did, the centre was able to provide use of the centre for meetings; secretarial/duplicating facilities; help with publicity; mail and phone contact point; training; links between group and community; links between group and professionals; and act as a referral agency to groups.

During the twelve-month period (April 1988–March 1989) the project was evaluated (Niven and Milner, 1989). The main findings were as follows.

- *Enquiries*. During this twelve-month period there were 1,522 enquiries (395 males and 765 females). All age groups were represented except the under-20s, who tended not to make enquiries at the centre.
- *Information requested*. The three topics most requested were:
  1 Information about specific diseases, such as coronary heart disease, or arthritis.
  2 Nutrition.
  3 Women's health issues.
- *Referrals made*. These were mainly to:
  1 Self-help groups – local, regional and national.
  2 Other NHS professionals (not GPs), such as the Health Education Department, Health Visitors, screening services.
  3 Other organisations, such as the Community Health Council.

How did the people using the centre find out about it? The majority of clients using the centre did so because they were just 'passing by', although publicity material continued to play an important role in drawing attention to the centre. There was an increase in the number of clients using the centre as a result of 'word of mouth' recommendations of friends and relatives, and in those coming back to the centre having used it before. The self-help groups supported by the centre ranged from the Hyperactive Children's Support Group and the Parkinson's Disease Association to the Agoraphobics Support Group and the Menopause Support Group.

This example illustrates how health can be 'taken to' people in a community setting. Owing to the informal nature of the centre, people who were passing by, maybe doing their shopping, were encouraged to drop in and discuss health concerns. These discussions led in many cases to the client being referred to an appropriate self-help group or NHS agency. Of course, one is entitled to ask whether self-help groups succeed in their expressed aims. I feel that it is important to distinguish between different types of self-help group (Niven, 1990). The structure, aims and objectives of the group are related to factors such as decision-making skills and self-esteem. An important role of the centre was to provide training in the best ways to run self-help groups and to advise on issues as they occurred. In this way the project attempted to accommodate the principles of community development and to produce individuals who were able to determine their own health needs and obtain advice on how they could be achieved.

In their review of the strategies for the maintenance of health-promoting behaviours, Redland and Stuifbergen (1993) emphasise the removal of barriers, the creation of supportive environments and the development of a strong sense of self-efficacy as important aspects of the adoption and maintenance of health-promoting behaviours. They suggest that future attention should be directed toward promoting healthy lifestyles and the development of 'wellness' thinking.

Culture

People from different societies think in different ways, just as children think in different ways from adults. Herein lies the problem, for in order to understand what is going through a child's mind we must try to put ourselves in their position and attempt to view the world from their perspective. This can be very difficult, some would say impossible. Yet in order to communicate in an effective manner with children it is important to attempt the task (see Chapter 3). The same can be said about people from different cultures – they often view the world in a different way from ourselves. Therefore in order to communicate effectively with people from other cultures we must try to make the same 'quantum leap'. Of course, there are similarities of thought and behaviour across cultures, just as there are differences, but when working in a multicultural environment it is vital not to assume similarities on the basis of superficial evidence. Consider the following two extracts. The first is based on a study carried out in South America by Wellin (1955). The water supply in the town of Los Molinos in Peru was contaminated. Boiling water before drinking it could reduce the risks of typhoid and other waterborne diseases. A rural hygiene worker called Nelida was employed to visit the households in the town and tell them the reasons why they should boil their water. A few of the families already boiled water before Nelida arrived, but after two years of visiting the town's 200 households, only eleven had begun to boil their drinking water. Why were so few prepared to do this?

One of the women, Nelida, is a very thorough and meticulous woman, but has a household of seven to look after. She would like to boil their drinking water but does not do so. There seem to be a number of limiting conditions as to why she does not:

- The fuel for the stoves is limited so that fires can be lit only three times a day.
- Most hearths can accommodate only one pot at a time, so boiling water is ruled out during preparation of the meals.
- Any prepared food or boiled water left overnight is considered 'sleeping' food, and has to be cooked or boiled again the next day.
- Since most of the water is drunk during the midday heat, the only reasonable time to heat it is after breakfast. However, Nelida has to leave the house to perform essential chores after breakfast and cannot boil the water at this time. (Indeed, every 'housewife' in Los Molinos who does boil water does not leave the house or has someone to whom the task can be delegated.)

Thus the reasons for her not boiling the water seem fairly logical: there are a number of 'barriers' and her actions could be predicted by some of the models of health behaviour previously discussed. Therefore the job of Nelida is to try to remove or reduce these barriers but she isn't succeeding, maybe because women like Nelida just have to leave home. But what about those who *do* boil their water? Is it only because they are able to stay at home?

Mrs A boiled her water before the arrival of Nelida. She suffers from what she says her doctors have diagnosed as sinus trouble, and she is known in the town as a 'sickly person'. She thinks her sinusitis came about when 'cold' entered her respiratory passages. For all people in Los Molinos, 'cold' is associated with harm and must be avoided by the very young, the old, the pregnant and the sick. Wellin states that:

> At no point does the notion of bacteriological contamination of water enter the scheme. By tradition, boiling is aimed at eliminating not bacteria, but the innate 'cold' quality of unboiled water.

In fact the eight women who were already boiling their water when Nelida arrived were 'sickly'.

Can we apply the theories of health behaviour discussed in Chapter 6 to account for those who did and did not boil their water? Let us look at the following examples.

A nurse might say that it would be all very well if she were going to take up nursing in Papua New Guinea, but what application does it have to everyday life? What this nurse has overlooked is the fact that we live in a multicultural society. We do not have to move to Papua New Guinea to come into contact with people from different cultures. Therefore it *is* important for nurses to have some idea of how culture can affect behaviour.

Another example of the importance of considering cultural differences is given by Miner (1956) in the journal *American Anthropologist*. Although it is nearly fifty years old, his account of the magical beliefs and rituals of the Nacirema people bears some examination. He says whilst Linton (1936) brought their attention to anthropologists twenty years ago, the culture is still poorly understood. They are a 'North American group living in the territory between the Canadian Cree, the Yaqui and the Tarahumare of Mexico, and the Carib and Arawak of the Antilles'. He goes on to say that the

> Nacirema is characterized by a highly developed market economy which has evolved in a rich natural habitat. While much of the people's time is devoted to economic pursuits, a large part of the fruits of these labours and a considerable portion of the day are spent in ritual activity. The focus of this activity is the human body, the appearance and health of which loom as a dominant concern in the ethos of the people. While such a concern is certainly not unusual, its ceremonial aspects and associated philosophy are unique.

In fact each household has one or more shrines devoted to this activity and the most powerful in the society possess several such shrines.

> The focal point of the shrine is a box or chest which is built into the wall. In this chest are kept the many charms and magical potions without which no native believes he could live. These preparations are secured from a variety of specialized practitioners. The most powerful of these are the medicine men, whose assistance must be rewarded with substantial gifts. However, the medicine men do not provide the curative potions for their clients, but decide what the ingredients should be and then write them down in an ancient and secret language. This writing is understood by the medicine men and by the herbalists who, for another gift, provide the required charm.

When the members of the community become ill, there is another specific ritual to be observed. In every community of any size, the medicine men have an imposing temple or latipso, where the more elaborate ceremonies required to treat very sick people are performed. 'These ceremonies involve not only the thaumaturge but a permanent group of vestal maidens who move sedately about the temple chambers in distinctive costume and headdress.' Some of these latipso ceremonies can be quite harsh such that a fair proportion of the really sick natives who enter the temple never recover. Young children whose 'indoctrination' is incomplete resisted going to the temple saying 'that's where you go to die'.

The whole process is described by Miner (1956) thus:

> The supplicant first entering the temple is first stripped of his or her clothes. In every-day life the Nacirema avoids exposure of his body and its natural functions. Bathing and execratory acts are performed only in the secrecy of the household shrine, where they are ritualised as part of the body-rites. Psychological shock results from the fact that the body secrecy is suddenly lost upon entry into the latipso. A man, whose own wife has never seen him in an execratory act, suddenly finds himself naked and assisted by a vestal maiden while he performs his natural function into a sacred vessel. This sort of ceremonial treatment is necessitated by the fact that the excreta are used by a diviner to ascertain the course and nature of the client's sickness. Female clients on the other hand, find their naked bodies are subjected to the scrutiny, manipulation and prodding of the medicine man.

Although Miner (1956) describes this behaviour as an example of the 'extreme', maybe it is not too dissimilar to our own.

Another important principle of cultural research is never to assume that speaking the same language is equivalent to understanding. Cole and Scribner (1974) conducted an experiment with two members of the Kpelle tribe of West Africa which illustrates this point very well. The participants were asked to sit side by side at a table, separated from each other's view by a partition. In front of them on the table were a number of wooden sticks of different shapes and sizes. The experimenter, who could speak fluent Kpelle, instructed the subjects to pick out certain sticks from the piles, describing them as, for example, the long thin one or the short fat one. After they had done this, the partition was removed and the sticks were examined. In many instances the sticks that the two subjects had selected were different; exactly the same request had been given to each subject but had often resulted in a dissimilar outcome. Cole and Scribner explained their results by saying that what had seemed like a straightforward series of requests from the experimenter was confusing and somewhat alien to the participants because of the difference in the conceptual realities of the experimenter and participants. Since the Kpelle had never experienced anything like this before and were unsure what was going on, they had difficulty knowing exactly what was required of them.

Implications for nursing care

The implications for nursing in a multicultural context are that if the conceptual realities of the nurse and the patient are different, communication may be difficult; indeed, what the nurse thinks is a perfectly simple, straightforward task may seem incomprehensible to someone from a different culture.

It also signifies that models of health behaviour such as health belief, locus of control, and theory of reasoned action, etc., would have difficulty in predicting the reasons cultural differences in behaviour. A cultural perspective highlights the strengths and weaknesses of models of health behaviour. Sometimes health behaviour follows an ordered, logical route, and in these cases the models provide a useful framework for understanding the decisions made by individuals; however, sometimes behaviour is not so logical or predictable, and the only way to come to some sort of understanding of what is going on is to concentrate on the specific aspects of each individual case, be it a person or a culture.

Although the study of Nelida may seem somewhat dated, the principles it illustrates could not be more timely. We live in a multicultural society and this study illustrates the importance of taking a global perspective on human behaviour. Whilst I believe Wellin's example has implications for community nursing in Britain, it illustrates the importance of cross-cultural studies in examining the applicability of theories and models developed in the West to cultures elsewhere in the world.

Summary

Health and illness cannot be fully understood in isolation from the environment in which they occur. This chapter has taken a look at both hospital and community as health care environments in order to explore their impact on the behaviour of individuals.

People's experience of hospitalisation has been described in relation to the stress incurred by communication problems and uncertainty about procedures and information. Stress also occurs as a result of the environmental features of hospitals and as a result of role changes imposed on the individual.

Finally, the community has been described in relation both to specific environmental features and in terms of general structures. Nurses working in the community need to understand and take account of the wider environment in which people function and the cultural differences which exist between people in a multicultural society if they are to offer the most appropriate forms of care.

Conundrum revisited

We wonder if you agree with us that the truth of this assertion is highly questionable. Whilst the nurse might be expressing an aspiration (care should be seamless and standards should remain high wherever the patient is), the material in Chapter 11 makes it plain that patients' experiences in different health care environments change considerably and with that, we may venture, will come a change in their needs. Individuals are used to receiving several forms of care or support from their family or community and this is disrupted when they are admitted to hospital. That this sometimes causes misunderstanding is vividly illustrated when a 'traveller' is admitted to hospital. Travellers live in very close communities, on the road and within a culture that is cautious about conventional health care. When the traveller is admitted to hospital his family will try to sustain their own form of care by visiting in large numbers and in rotation so that a traveller presence is always maintained. The movement of the patient into an alien hospital is seen as threatening to his traditional way of life and to the family who wish to continue caring.

Treatment modalities also influence notions of stress and affect the patient's needs. Working on an oncology ward, I once asked a patient suffering from cancer how he felt about the fact that radical bowel surgery had been recommended, rather than less invasive radiotherapy. He observed that surgery was painful, disfiguring but preferable. 'With surgery you cut the tumour out . . . its like you get rid of it, away from your body.' The patient anticipated that this would necessitate intensive physical support for a few days but that longer term he would need less psychological support than with radiotherapy. 'I don't trust the idea of rays shrinking tumours you see . . . they might not have got rid of it like a surgeon.' In circumstances such as these the nurse needs to appreciate the patient's perceptions and to adjust care.

In many senses hospital are abnormal environments. Not only do they pose a psychological threat in terms of noise, light, risk of infection and disruption to the lifestyle of the patient, but they surround him with different definitions of what is 'normal'. Imagine a consultant surgeon ward round where the patient's laparotomy scar is revealed for inspection. The consultant beams to his entourage, 'There, look at that. When did you last see such a beautiful piece of suturing?' Onlookers nod appreciatively but the patient groans. To the patient the scar looks long, ugly and anything but 'beautiful'. Patient and professionals are working from completely different reference points of what is normal and the nurse needs to appreciate the patient's evaluation of this if care is to remain sensitive.

That some patients behave in a problematic way in hospital seems further indication that environment fundamentally changes the experience of illness or treatment and that it is necessary for nurses to ascertain exactly what the patient is thinking and feeling. To what extent is the problem inherent in the patient's behaviour and expectations and to what extent is the problem created through different assumptions held about the 'patient role'? Under these conditions nursing needs to be inquisitive rather than prescriptive, and the nurse becomes investigator and care adjustor, enabling the patient to manage the transition to a new environment.

In this chapter we have returned to the subject of social support networks. In the preceding chapter they were portrayed as a possible resource that enabled individuals to deal with change. Now though they may also be considered in terms of disruption caused when patients are admitted to hospital or (within the community) required to regularly attend clinic. Treatment protocols (irrespective of environment) can significantly affect social support networks. Consider the case of a patient who is diagnosed as suffering from visual and auditory hallucinations. These prompt him to feel persecuted and to feel suspicious of others' motives when talking with family or friends. For a short period of time the patient is treated in hospital and removed from his social support network. He commences anti-hallucinogenic medication and returns to the community, with the proviso that he attends a day hospital three times a week. At this juncture the patient's social support network are unsure what care they can deliver and how this should, could or ought to relate to that delivered by nurses. The nurse needs to understand the perceptions of patients and lay carers if care is to be sensitively fashioned.

? Questions for further consideration

1 How can the models of Bronfenbrenner or Moos be of use to community nurses?
2 Assess the importance of patients' perceived control during hospitalisation.
3 Are there such people as 'difficult patients'?
4 To what extent is it important to conduct cross-cultural studies of health behaviour?
5 Discuss the use of social networks in the provision of health care.

References

Altman, I. (1975). *The Environment and Social Behaviour: Privacy, personal space, territory, and crowding.* Monterey CA: Brooks Cole.

Anderson, E. A. (1987). Preoperative preparation for cardiac surgery facilitates recovery, reduces psychosocial distress, and reduces the incidence of postoperative hypertension. *Journal of Consulting and Clinical Psychology, 55,* 513–520.

Barnaby, J. F. (1980). Lighting for productivity gains. *Lighting Design and Application,* February, 2–28.

Baron, R. A. (1987). Effects of negative air ions on interpersonal attraction: evidence for intensification. *Journal of Personality and Social Psychology, 52,* 547–553.

Bronfenbrenner, U. (1979). *The Ecology of Human Development.* Cambridge MA: Harvard University Press.

Buchanan, H., and Niven, N. (2003). Self-report informational treatment techniques used by dentists to treat dentally anxious children A preliminary investigation. *International Journal of Paediatric Dentistry, 13; 9–12.*

Cameron, B. L. (1993). The nature of comfort to medical surgical patients. *Journal of Advanced Nursing, 18,* 424–436.

Carlsmith, J. M. and Anderson, C. A. (1979). Ambient temperature and the occurrence of collective violence: a new analysis. *Journal of Personality and Social Research, 37,* 337–344.

Cohen, S., Evans, G. W., Krantz, D. S. and Stokols, D. (1979). Physiological, motivational and cognitive effects of aircraft noise on children: moving from laboratory to field. *American Psychologist, 35,* 231–243.

Cohen, S., Evans, G. W., Stokols, D. and Krantz, D. (1986). *Behaviour, Health and Environmental Stress.* New York: Plenum.

Cole, M. and Scribner, S. (1974). *Culture and Thought.* Chichester: Wiley.

Corney, R., Everett, H., Howells, A. and Crowther, M. (1992). The care of patients undergoing surgery for gynaecological cancer: the need for information, emotional support and counselling. *Journal of Advanced Nursing, 17,* 667–671.

Dahlquist, L. M., Gil, K. M., Armstrong, F. D., DeLawyer, D. D., Greene, P. and Wuori, D. (1986). Preparing children for medical examinations: the importance of previous medical experience. *Health Psychology, 5,* 249–259.

Davitz, L. L. and Davitz, J. R. (1985). Culture and nurses' inferences of suffering. In Copp, L. A. (ed.) *Perspectives on Pain.* Edinburgh: Churchill Livingstone.

Dean, P. G. (1986). Expanding our sights to include social networks. *Nursing and Health Care,* December, 545–550.

Douglas, J. (1993). *Psychology and Nursing Children.* Leicester: BPS Books (British Psychological Society) and Macmillan.

Evans, G. and Cohen, S. (1987). Environmental stress. In Stokels, D. and Altman, I. (eds) *Handbook of Environmental Psychology* I. Chichester: Wiley.

Evans, G. W. and Jacobs, S. V. (1984). Air pollution and human behaviour. In Evans, G. W. (ed.) *Environmental Stress.* Cambridge: Cambridge University Press.

Fuller, T. D., Edwards, J. N., Vorakitphokatorn, S. and Sermsri, S. (1993). Household crowding and family relations in Bangkok. *Social Problems, 40,* 410–430.

Gadbois, C., Bourgeois, P., Goeh-Akue-Gad, M. M. and Guillaume, J. (1992). Hospital design and the temporal and spatial organisation of nursing activity. *Work and Stress, 6,* 277–291.

Galle, O., Gove, W. and McPherson, J. (1972). Population density and pathology: what are the relations for man? *Science, 176,* 23–30.

Gatherer, J. (1980). *Is Health Education Effective?* London: Health Education Council.

Gillis, A. J. (1993). Determinants of a health-promoting lifestyle: an integrative review. *Journal of Advanced Nursing, 18,* 345–353.

Guppy, A. and Gutteridge, T. (1991). Job satisfaction and occupational stress in UK general hospital nursing staff. *Work and Stress, 5,* 315–323.

Hollander, J. and Yeastros, S. (1963). The effects of simultaneous variations of humidity and barometric pressure on arthritis. *Bulletin of the American Meteorological Society, 44,* 489–494.

Jaco, E. G. (1979). Ecological aspects of patient care: an experimental study. In Jaco, E. G. (ed.) *Patients, Physicians and Illness: A sourcebook in behavioral science and health.* 3rd edn. New York: Free Press.

Johnson, M and Webb, C. (2004) Rediscovering unpopular patients: the concept of social judgement. In Robb, M., Barrett, S., Komaromy, C. and Rogers, A. (eds) *Communication, Relationships and Care.* London: Routledge.

Karlin, R. A., Rosen, L. and Epstein, Y. (1979). Three into two doesn't go: a follow-up of the effects of overcrowded dormitory rooms. *Personality and Social Psychology Bulletin, 5,* 391–395.

Kelly, M. P. and May, D. (1982). Good and bad patients: a review of the literature and a theoretical critique. *Journal of Advanced Nursing, 7,* 147–156.

Kenrick, D. T. and MacFarlane, S. W. (1986). Ambient temperature and horn honking: a field study of the heat/aggression relationship. *Environment and Behaviour, 18,* 179–191.

Kincey, J. (1989). Surgery. In Broome, A. K. (ed.) *Health Psychology: Processes and applications.* London: Chapman and Hall.

Kornfield, D. S. (1972). The hospital environment: its impact on the patient. *Advances in Psychosomatic Medicine, 8,* 252–270.

Kryter, K. D. (1970). *The Effects of Noise on Man.* London: Academic Press.

Kulik, J. A. and Mahler, H. I. M. (1989). Stress and affiliation in a hospital setting: preoperative roommate preferences. *Personality and Social Psychology Bulletin, 15,* 183–193.

Langner, E. J., Janis, I. L. and Wolfer, J. A. (1975). Reduction of psychological stress in surgical patients. *Journal of Experimental Social Psychology, 11,* 155–165.

Lewin, K. (1951). *Field Theory in Social Science.* New York: Harper.

Ley, P., Bradshaw, P. W., Kincey, J. A. and Atherton, S. T. (1976). Increasing patients' satisfaction with communication. *British Journal of Social and Clinical Psychology, 15,* 403–413.

Linton, R. (1936). *The Study of Man.* New York: Appleton-Century-Crofts.

Lorber, J. (1975). Good patients and problem patients: conformity and deviance in a general hospital. *Journal of Health and Social Behaviour, 16*, 213–225.

MacDonald, W. S. and Oden, C. N. V. (1973). Effects of extreme crowding on the performance of five married couples during twelve weeks' intensive training. *Proceedings of the eighty-first Annual Convention of the American Psychological Association, 8*, 209–210.

Marks, David F., Murray, Michael, Evans, Brian, Willig, Carla, Sykes, Marie Catherine and Woodall, Cailine (2005). *Health Psychology: Theory, Research and Practice*, London: Sage.

Martyniuk, O. P., Flynn, J. E., Spencer, T. J. and Kendrick, C. (1973). Effects of environmental lighting on impression and behaviour. In Kuller, R. (ed.) *Architectural Psychology*. Stroudsburg PA: Dowden Hutchinson Ross.

Maslach, C. (1982). Job burnout: how people cope. In: McConnell, E. A. (ed) *Burnout in the Nursing Profession*. St Louis: Mosby.

Maslach, S. and Jackson, S. E. (1982). Burnout in health professions: a social psychological analysis. In Sanders, G. S. and Suls, J. (eds) *The Social Psychology of Health and Illness*. Hillsdale NJ: Erlbaum.

McKinlay, J. B. (1975). Who is really ignorant – physician or patient? *Journal of Health and Social Behaviour, 16*, 3–11.

Melamed, B. G. and Siegel, L. J. (1975). Reduction of anxiety in children facing hospitalization and surgery by use of filmed modelling. *Journal of Consulting and Clinical Psychology, 43*, 511–521.

Milne, D. (1993). *Psychology and Mental Health Nursing*. Leicester: BPS Books (British Psychological Society) and Macmillan.

Miner, H. (1956). Body ritual among the Nacirema. *American Anthropologist, 58*, 503–507.

Moos, R. (1979). Social-ecological perspectives on health. In Stone, G. C., Cohen, S. and Adler, N. E. (eds) *Health Psychology*. New York: Jossey Bass.

Nichols, K. A. (1989). Institutional versus client-centred care in general hospitals. In Broome, A. K. (ed.) *Health Psychology: Processes and applications*. London: Chapman and Hall.

Nichols, K. A. (2003) *Psychological Care for Ill and Injured People*. Maidenhead: Open University Press.

Niven, N. (1990). Decision making, locus of control and self-esteem in self-help groups. Proceedings of the fourth European Conference in Health Psychology, Oxford, p. 45.

Niven, N. and Milner, S. (1989). Health Psychology in the Shop Front. Unpublished paper presented to the International Conference on Health Psychology, Cardiff.

Paulus, P. B., McCain, G. and Cox, V. C. (1978). Death rates, psychiatric commitments, blood pressure and perceived crowding as a function of institutional crowding. *Environmental Psychology and Nonverbal Behaviour, 3*, 107–116.

Redland, A. R. and Stuifbergen, A. K. (1993). Strategies for maintenance of health-promoting behaviours. *Nursing Clinics of North America, 28*, 427–442.

Sarafino, E. P. (1986). *The Fears of Childhood: A guide to recognizing and reducing fearful states in children.* New York: Human Sciences Press.

Schumaker, S. A. and Reizenstein, J. E. (1984). Inpatient stress in acute care hospitals. In Evans, G. W. (ed.) *Environmental Stress.* Cambridge: Cambridge University Press.

Simpson, M. and Perry, J. D. (1990). Crime and climate: a reconsideration. *Environment and Behaviour, 22,* 295–300.

Super, C. N. (1981). Cross-cultural research on infancy. In Triandis, H. C. and Heron, A. (eds) *Handbook of Cross-cultural Psychology* IV. Boston MA: Allyn and Bacon.

Taylor, S. E. (1979). Hospital patient behaviour: reactance, helplessness, or control? *Journal of Social Issues, 35,* 156–184.

Topf, M. (1992). Effects of personal control over hospital noise on sleep. *Research in Nursing and Health, 15,* 19–28.

Volicer, B. J., Isenberg, M. A. and Bums, M. W. (1977). Medical-surgical differences in hospital stress factors. *Journal of Human Stress, 3,* 3–13.

Wellin, E. (1955). Water boiling in a Peruvian town. In Paul, D. B. (ed.) *Health, Culture and Community.* New York: Russel Sage Foundation.

Westbrook, M. T., Legge, V. and Pennay, M. (1993). Attitudes towards disabilities in a multicultural society. *Social Science in Medicine, 36,* 615–623.

Whitehead, M. (1987). *The Health Divide: Inequalities in health in the 80s.* London: Health Education Council.

Wilson-Barnett, J. and Carrigy, A. (1978). Factors influencing patients' emotional reactions to hospitalisation. *Journal of Advanced Nursing, 3,* 221–229.

Further reading

Crossley, Michele (2000) *Rethinking Health Psychology.* Milton Keynes: Open University Press. She takes a critical view on health psychology – particularly the psychobiological approach. Perhaps it is better to look at Marks *et al.* first – but definitely a must-read book.

Marks, David, Murray, Michael, Evans, Brian and Willig, Carla, eds (2000) *Health Psychology: Theory, Research and Practice.* London: Sage. There are many books on health psychology but David Marks and Brian Evans have been teaching nurses health psychology for years. Hence, not only is this a particularly good book, it is relevant too. Also the reader accompanying this volume is a valuable addition.

Index